Career Choices for Veterinarians

Private Practice and Beyond

Other books by Dr. Carin Smith

Client Satisfaction Pays: Quality Service for Practice Success, AAHA Press, 1998, 2nd ed. 2009.

Career Choices for Veterinary Technicians: Opportunities for Animal Lovers, with Rebecca Rose, CVT, AAHA Press, 2009.

Team Satisfaction Pays: Organizational Development for Practice Success, Smith Veterinary Consulting, 2008.

FlexVet: How to Be One, How to Hire One. The Comprehensive Practice Guide for Relief & Part-time Veterinarians, Smith Veterinary Consulting, 2007.

House Call: The Housecall Veterinarian's Manual, Smith Veterinary Consulting, 1996, 2007.

The Relief Veterinary Technician's Manual, with Rebecca Rose CVT, Smith Veterinary Consulting, 2002.

Abridged Version of The Current and Future Market for Veterinarians and Veterinary Services in the United States, NCVEI, C. Smith, Editor; 2000.

The Relief Veterinarian's Manual and Survival Guide. Smith Veterinary Consulting, 1992, replaced by *FlexVet.*

Career Choices for Veterinarians

Private Practice and Beyond

Carin A. Smith, DVM

Contributing Author Nina Kieves, DVM

Smith Veterinary Consulting
Peshastin, Washington
USA

Smith Veterinary Consulting & Publishing
PO Box 698
Peshastin, WA 98847
(509) 548-2010
info@smithvet.com
www.smithvet.com

Career Choices for Veterinarians: Private Practice and Beyond
Second edition, 2011.
© 2011 Carin A. Smith, Smith Veterinary Consulting; Smith Veterinary Consulting &
Publishing

Cover design by Cathi Stevenson, Book Cover Express

ISBN 978-1-885780-17-1

Library of Congress Control Number 2010913438

BISAC Subject headings
MED089000   MEDICAL / Veterinary Medicine / General
MED081000   MEDICAL / Reference
BUS012000   BUSINESS & ECONOMICS / Careers / General

ACKNOWLEDGMENTS

This book includes insights from a large number of veterinarians who generously provided thoughts to help their colleagues. Their quotes throughout the book lend reality to many job descriptions, and their contributions are greatly appreciated. Each of them may serve as a role model for others to follow.

Many thanks also to those individuals who offered to review all or parts of the rough manuscript and provided insights to make the book even better.

Special thanks to contributing author Dr. Nina Kieves, who as a veterinary student volunteered to read and update key portions of the book.

PEOPLE QUOTED OR PROFILED IN THE BOOK

(See Appendix to decipher the acronyms)
Alwynelle Ahl, PhD, DVM; APHIS veterinarian, retired; www.aphis.usda.gov
John Albers, DVM; Albers Veterinary Strategies; www.albersveterinarystrategies.com
Janet E. Alsop, DVM, ABVP-SHM; Veterinarian, Disease Prevention-Swine; Ontario Ministry of Agriculture, Food and Rural Affairs, Canada; www.omafra.gov.on.ca
Elizabeth Bellavance, DVM, MBA, CMA; Canadian Veterinary Consulting Services, ON, Canada
Joe Bielitzki, DVM, MS; Former Chief Veterinary Officer, NASA; www.nasa.gov
Melissa Blauvelt, DVM, MS; Clinical pathologist, VCA Antech
Michael Briggs, DVM; African Predator Conservation Research Organization; www.apcro.org
Eric S. Dubbin, DVM; Organization Development Executive Coach, FDA Ctr for Veterinary Medicine; www.fda.hhs.gov
Catherine Filejski, DVM, MA, MEPA, PhD [ABD]; Ontario Ministry of Health and Long-Term Care, Canada; www.health.gov.on.ca/en
David D. Frame, DVM, DACPV; Associate Professor, Extension Poultry Specialist, Utah State University, Logan, UT; www.usu.edu
Douglas L. Fulnechek, DVM; USDA FSIS Supervisory Veterinary Medical Officer, Springdale, AR; www.fsis.usda.gov
Michael Gilsdorf, DVM; Executive Vice President, National Association of Federal Veterinarians; www.nafv.org
Danielle Graham, DVM; Ringling Brothers and Barnum & Bailey Circus; www.ringling.com
Dan Green, DVM; Industry veterinarian
Lesli Groshong, DVM; Chief Shelter Veterinarian, Humane Society of Boulder Valley, CO; www.boulderhumane.org
Karen L. Jacobsen, DVM; Farm Animal Resources and Management, Athens, GA; www.KarenJacobsen.net
Myron J. Kebus, DVM; Aquatic veterinarian, WI Dept of Agriculture; www.datcp.state.wi.us
Susan Kerr, DVM, PhD; Extension Educator, Klickitat County, WA; www.co.klickitat.wa.us
Cathy King, DVM; Feline Medical Clinic, Vancouver, WA; www.felinemedicalclinic.com
Justine Lee, DVM, DACVECC; Book author; Associate Director of Veterinary Services at Pet Poison Helpline; www.drjustinelee.com
Mira Leslie, DVM, MPH; Public Health Veterinarian, British Columbia Ministry of Agriculture and Lands, Canada
Marli Styskel Lintner, DVM; Avian Medical Clinic, Lake Oswego, OR; www.avianmedicalcenter.net
Kerri E. Marshall, DVM, MBA; Senior Director, Medical Informatics, Banfield, The Pet Hospital, Portland, OR; www.banfield.net
John Mattoon, DVM, DACVR; Professor of Radiology, Washington State University College of Veterinary Medicine; www.vetmed.wsu.edu.

PEOPLE QUOTED OR PROFILED IN THE BOOK (cont'd)

Melinda Merck, DVM; Senior Director, Veterinary Forensic Sciences, ASPCA; www.veterinaryforensics.com
Beth Miller, DVM; International consultant, educator; www.bethmiller.org
Michael Moyer, VMD; Rosenthal Director of Shelter Animal Medicine, University of PA; www.vet.upenn.edu
Nancy Murbach, DVM; Veterinary House Call Service, Scottsdale AZ
Deb Nickelson, DVM; Marketing Manager, Veterinary Products Laboratories, Phoenix AZ; www.vpl.com
Christy Novick, DVM; Associate veterinarian, Feline Medical Clinic, Vancouver, WA; www.felinemedicalclinic.com
Philip Pacchiana, DVM, MS, DACVS; Cutting Edge Veterinary Surgery, Danbury CT
Julia Ponder, DVM; Director, Raptor Center, University of Minnesota; www.cvm.umn.edu/raptor
Stacy Pritt, DVM, MS, MBA, CPIA; Director and General Manager, Biological Test Center, Irvine, CA
Stacy Pursell; President, TheVet Recruiter®; www.thevetrecruiter.com
Helen Roberts, DVM; Aquatic Veterinary Service of Western NY and 5 Corners Animal Hospital; www.nyfishdoc.com
Kim T Rock, DVM, MIH; USAID-Africa Bureau, Office of Sustainable Development, Washington, DC; www.avma.org/
　　advocacy/get_involved/fellowships.asp; www.usaid.gov
Max Rodibaugh, DVM; Swine Health Services, LC, Frankfort, IN
Patty Scharko, DVM, MPH, DACVPM; Field/Extension Veterinarian, Clemson University, Columbia, SC
Joni Scheftel, DVM, MPH, DACVPM; State Public Health Veterinarian, MN Dept of Health; www.nasphv.org
John Tait, DVM, MBA, CFP; Managing partner of the Ontario Veterinary Group, Toronto, Canada
Gregg Takashima, DVM; Parkway Veterinary Hospital, Lake Oswego OR
Jay Tischendorf, DVM; Director, American Ecological Research Institute, Great Falls, MT; www.easterncougar.org and
　　http://aerie--institute.org
Linda Tollefson, DVM, MPH; Director, FDA Europe Regional Office, Brussels
Aurora Villarroel, DVM, MPVM, PhD, ACVPM; Extension veterinarian, Epidemiologist, Assistant Professor, Oregon
　　State University, Corvallis OR; http://oregonstate.edu/vetmed or http://ans.oregonsate.edu
Carol Walton, DVM; CEO, Carol Walton Expeditions, LLC; www.carolwaltonexpeditions.com
Lisa Willis, DVM; Mid-Texas Veterinary Associates, Gustine, TX
Jennifer Gordon Wright, DVM, MPH, DACVPM; US Public Health Service, CDC; www.cdc.gov

REVIEWERS

The following people reviewed, edited, and/or critiqued portions or the entirety of the rough draft of the book.

Catherine Filejski, DVM, MA, MEPA, PhD [ABD]; Ontario Ministry of Health and Long-Term Care, Toronto, Canada
　　(Canadian government section)
Michael Gilsdorf, DVM; Executive Vice President, National Association of Federal Veterinarians, Sykesville, MD (federal
　　jobs section)
Sharon Curtis Granskog; Assistant Director, Media Relations, American Veterinary Medical Association (AVMA jobs)
Kent Fowler, DVM; Animal Health Branch Chief, CA Department of Food and Agriculture, Sacramento, CA (state jobs)
Kris Kruse-Elliott, DVM, PhD, DACVA; Redwood City, CA
Randy Lynn, DVM, MS, DACVCP; Summerfield, NC (industry section)
Beth Miller, DVM; Miller Consulting, Inc, Little Rock, AR
Kim Nicholas, DVM, MS, and Kathy Nicholas; Renton, WA
Deb Nickelson, DVM; Marketing Manager, Veterinary Products Laboratories, Phoenix, AZ
Janice L. Trumpeter, DVM; Deputy Executive Director; American Animal Hospital Association (AAHA jobs section);
　　www.aahanet.org
Aurora Villarroel, DVM, MPVM, PhD, ACVPM; Extension veterinarian, Epidemiologist, Assistant Professor, Oregon
　　State University, Corvallis OR; (rural veterinary practice section)
Sandy Willis, DVM, DACVIM; Seattle, WA
Rebecca Rose, CVT; Lakewood, CO

PREFACE

Writing this book included a combination of fun interviews with interesting veterinarians along with tedious hours of fact-checking. While the facts are essential for the reader, the stories bring the facts to life.

Stories are part of what mentors share with others to help them see new possibilities. The first edition of this book included a warm foreword by one of my mentors, Dr. Al Koltveit, who was the Editor in Chief of the *Journal of the AVMA* for many years. Sadly, Al passed away this year, making me aware of the transition in my life from being mentored to becoming a mentor for others. Since the first edition was published, it has been gratifying to hear the many stories of veterinarians' career journeys in which the book played a small part.

People enter the veterinary profession because they feel a connection with animals and the natural world. Then, upon graduation, they find themselves face-to-face with the reality of the working world—and that's where this book comes in.

A review of the first edition described the book as "brutally honest." This edition may elicit the same response, since it includes a mix of exciting opportunities and disheartening facts. However, I feel confident that each reader can find a career path that is rewarding both personally and professionally.

The year 2011 has been proposed as "World Veterinary Year." It is appropriate that veterinarians appreciate the opportunities available to them, and that the public comes to appreciate the many roles that veterinarians can fill.

Carin A. Smith, DVM

CONTENTS

TABLES

Note: Income and salary data will vary as the years pass; use these tables to consider comparisons among types of work.
  See the resources for citations to find current data.

INTRODUCTION TO THE SECOND EDITION

Veterinary medicine offers one of the most rewarding and diverse career choices available today. *US News* rated veterinary medicine as one of the 50 best careers of 2010, and *Money* magazine ranked veterinarians as number four for jobs with the greatest projected growth in 2009:

> Pet ownership has grown 17% in the past 10 years, and as more people embrace furry friends, more vets are needed to keep them healthy. The veterinary medicine field has echoed advances in human medicine, and veterinary specialists in fields like oncology and ophthalmology have found clients clamoring for services.

James Herriot's book, *All Creatures Great and Small,* created a fantasy for many veterinarians and students. They may dream of providing medical care to species of their choice, with grateful clients and, somewhere in the background, a magical staff. Most who have ever considered a career in veterinary medicine at some time imagined the world of a private practitioner working each day to benefit the lives of puppies and kittens, or helping a small farmer with dairy cows.

Choices today are much different. Veterinarians in general private practice have a more diverse workday than their physician counterparts. Veterinarians examine animals, perform anesthesia and surgery, evaluate radiographs, diagnose perplexing diseases, and work with multiple species.

Veterinarians have the opportunity to specialize, or to work in research, for industry, in public health, or for animal shelters. They are highly valued for their wealth of knowledge and are admired for their compassion in working with animals and people. The veterinary degree provides choice and versatility in daily work as well as in the long-term.

Economic and social challenges do exist in the veterinary profession, however. The last chapter of this book details those challenges and discusses opportunities for the future.

The 12 years since the first edition have brought many changes to veterinary medicine, yet many choices remain the same. In this edition, the information about private practice has been enhanced, including more information about specific interests and specialties within that segment. The section about government jobs reflects changes in government agencies, such as the addition of the Department of Homeland Security. The first edition of this book included a separate chapter on working with computers. Since computers are integrated into all jobs now, that chapter has been omitted; what was once only "writing" is now "information services." The final commentary about the current status and the future outlook of the profession has changed significantly since the first edition.

An important expansion in this edition of the book is the inclusion of web sites for almost every resource cited in the text, so the reader can easily investigate if further information is sought.

Who Should Read This Book?

- Veterinarians—not only those thinking of a career change, but also those interested in broadening their work or in volunteering.
- Veterinary students enrolled in a college of veterinary medicine.
- College students majoring in pre-veterinary medicine, health sciences, or other biological sciences.
- High school students who are seriously considering a career in health care or veterinary medicine.

Whether you're a seasoned veterinarian, a new graduate, or an aspiring veterinarian, you will find a wide array of career pathways available to you. After reading the review of the "traditional" practice, you'll get to the more unusual parts of this book—career choices beyond private practice. You will be amazed at the wide variety of options available within the veterinary profession.

Students

Some of you may have already decided on your area of interest in veterinary medicine, whereas others wonder about new choices not yet considered. Either way, you'll gain from taking a fresh look at your chosen career. Perhaps you will realize the advantages of obtaining a bachelor's degree in business to best prepare for veterinary school, or you may change your thoughts about the type of externships you want to take as a veterinary student. You may realize that it would be a good idea to take a summer job in a research lab or with a veterinary consultant to add "research experience" or "business" to your resume. Broadening your horizons will only enrich your opportunities.

Many young veterinarians are challenged by financial need. The average debt upon graduation is double the average starting salary today. Some recent graduates may have difficulty finding an ideal job in private practice, especially if they are limited geographically by family or other constraints. Yet private practice is not the only choice. The choice needn't be "either/or" when it comes to making a good living and having a job you enjoy. This book will help you explore new career options.

Veterinarians

Some of you may be new veterinary school graduates who are exploring all of your options before you select a job. Others may be associate veterinarians who are thinking of new choices. Some of you already own a practice but have not found the satisfaction you desire or, even after enjoying several years of practice, are ready for a change. After all, those who graduate from veterinary school at age 25 can potentially look forward to 40 or 50 more years of work. Why spend it all doing the same thing?

For many veterinarians, thoughts of a change to nontraditional practice start with dissatisfaction with their current jobs. However, to gain happiness in your new career path, you must be driven by more than the desire to get *away from* your old one. It's time to turn dissatisfaction into desire. This book can help you start or find a new career in veterinary medicine that you look forward to entering.

If you have been in private practice for some time, you may choose to skip over Chapter 3 on traditional practice, jumping right to other selections—yet you may return there to see whether there is a new practice niche that interests you.

This book includes information that is most pertinent to veterinarians in the US and Canada. However, parallel opportunities exist in nearly every country of the world. Licensing requirements may vary, of course, depending on the job niche. Veterinarians may apply the principles of networking and job searching that are outlined here to explore options anywhere they desire.

How to Approach Your Search and This Book

Most veterinarians received a short review of career choices in school. They know they could work in industry, government, or private practice, or could further their schooling and become specialists. But they have not heard, in an organized and detailed manner, about all of the opportunities that exist within those categories.

No matter what your situation, take this advice: *Dismiss all job stereotypes from your mind, and read the entire book before you start to narrow your choices.* Your own stereotypic views of "industry" and "government" jobs color your thinking. By reading this book, you will understand what choices really exist.

Seek out veterinarians who have nontraditional jobs and ask them about their work. Talk to people with jobs you think you won't like—you may be pleasantly surprised.

How the book is organized

Chapters are grouped in a somewhat logical order based on employer type. However a great deal of overlap exists among different areas of interest and among employer types. One example is the wildlife pathology business that is discussed under working with wildlife (Chapter 6), although it also fits under veterinary specialists (Chapter 4) or starting your own business (Chapter 7). Similarly, poultry medicine is described under food animal practice (Chapter 5), although it could also be classified as a job in industry (Chapter 11), government (Chapters 15-18), or even consulting (Chapter 9). Forensic medicine is discussed as part of humanitarian jobs because of its relationship with investigating animal abuse (Chapter 13), although its connection with pathology could tie in with that specialty (Chapter 4). Jobs in research are discussed in various parts of the book, so someone who is interested in these jobs would investigate academia (Chapter 14), industry (Chapter 11), and government (Chapters 15-18). Likewise, if a person is interested in a particular species, jobs with that species could be found in any of the categories or chapters in the book. Use the index and the cross references in the text to find your areas of interest.

Daily work, pros and cons, qualifications, and *how to apply* are described for each job, if that information was available; however, as you will see, that detail is brief or nonexistent for many job niches. Consider this book as a starting point, and find out more about different career paths using networking interviews as described in Chapter 1.

Accuracy and timeliness

Great effort was made to gather accurate information for this book during an exhaustive search. However, agencies and organizations continually change their internal structures or job descriptions. What's more, some positions do not have official job descriptions, and some inquiries went unanswered.

Various sections of this book include samples of job announcements to give you an idea of the type of work and qualifications required for various jobs. Obviously, these are not current announcements, but it is possible that similar openings are available. Contact the appropriate agency for current job announcements.

Likewise, pay ranges, if available, will not remain current for the lifetime of this book. This book, written in 2010, contains data from 2007 to 2009. The numbers herein may serve as guidelines when comparing one choice to another in future years. (Don't forget to factor in the large dollar value of benefits when comparing pay!)

Much of the information presented here was obtained from interviews with individuals who described their specific positions. It is possible that occasional inaccuracies exist in the text, and it is also likely that additional job opportunities exist that are not mentioned here. Contact the groups or hiring agencies listed in each resource list at the ends of the chapters for complete and timely information.

Before you dive in: Using resource lists

As you read, you will see references to books, articles, or online sources for further information. These references include groups affiliated with each job category; places to find job announcements; web sites that provide information, job applications, and links to related material; as well as books and articles.

The book is organized such that you see these references abbreviated within the text as the topic is discussed, with an alphabetical, detailed citation at the end of the chapter in which they appear. A final appendix lists all the resources in the book.

Every attempt has been made to include current information and relevant web sites. However, some groups use their president's address as their only contact point. To find the current address, look on the American Veterinary Medical Association (AVMA) web site (www.avma.org), or search for any group by its name on the Internet.

Finding veterinary meetings and conferences

In several sections it is recommended that you attend a major veterinary conference or meeting in order to attend specific educational offerings or to visit the exhibit hall and learn more from the people there. Conference web sites include www.aahanet.org; www.avma.org; www.navc.org; www.wvc.org; and www.thecvc.com. A calendar of veterinary events is posted at www.dvm360.com > events >calendar.

Accessing web sites

Much of the additional information you need can be found on the Internet. Whenever possible, we have avoided typing long URLs (web addresses), since these often change and are difficult to type correctly. Instead, you will see the domain name followed by arrows (>), which signify a menu item on that web page. For example, if you see "www.avma.org > jobs" then you would go to the AVMA web site and then find and click on the word "jobs." Much information is buried deep within web sites and thus requires clicking through several pages or menus. Patience is necessary!

If you enter a web site into your browser and find that it no longer exists, or if you get an error message, try reducing the web URL to its "trunk." For example, if "www.avma.org/jobs" did not work, you would delete the letters or words to the right of the last slash mark and try "www.avma.org." Finally, if the trunk name no longer works, use a search engine to enter the name of the group or item and find out if it has a new web address.

Don't let yourself get stalled by being unable to access information. Become a sophisticated Internet searcher. You will have better results from search engines if you learn to use their "advanced" features. For example, restricting your search to web sites that end in .org, .edu, and .gov will remove commercial sites from your search results. Putting a specific phrase in quotation marks will restrict your search results to sites with just that phrase, and not sites that simply contain those words individually at random. Also, try more than one search engine (Google, Yahoo, Bing, etc.).

Obtaining books

It is unlikely that you will find many of the books listed here just by looking on the shelves of your local library or bookstore. That isn't a big problem, though.

You can ask the librarian at your local public library to help you with a computer search on the topics of choice. Don't worry if your library doesn't have a particular book on its shelves or in its catalog. Just ask the librarian to order a copy through the interlibrary loan service. Some libraries may charge a small fee for this service. If you borrow a book of interest and you find it particularly helpful, you may decide to buy it later.

Any local bookstore can find and order specific titles on the computer. You can also use online searches to find what you need, and order books used or new through a variety of bookstores online. Read online bookstores' book reviews and readers' comments. This will lead you to many more choices than just the ones listed in this book.

Some books may be out of print, but may still be available from the library or from a used-book store. Being out of print has nothing to do with a book's quality—the nature of the publishing business is such that books go out of print quickly.

"Books" often include printed directories which are ceasing print publication and converting to online-only access. If you aren't able to find a printed resource as listed in this book, search online for an equivalent resource. For example, the AVMA recently discontinued the printed edition of its resource directory, transferring some but not all of the information to its web site.

Obtaining articles

You can get copies of articles in three ways: by ordering reprints directly from the magazine; by finding a copy online; or by ordering reprints from your library. Any of these may be free, or there may be a small charge.

Your library need not have a particular magazine or journal on its shelves to get you a copy of an article. Just ask the librarian to order the copy through the interlibrary loan service. If you know someone associated with a college or university, you may be able to gain access to journals through that person at no charge. Members of the AVMA can access articles from *JAVMA* on the AVMA web site (articles from *JAVMA News* are available to non-members as well).

You can sometimes find articles online simply by typing the entire article title into a search engine. Make use of free online databases, such as the National Library of Medicine, to look for specific articles within the veterinary literature. See www.ncbi.nlm.nih.gov > PubMed.

Terminology

All veterinarians will be familiar with the terms used in this book. For example, an "associate" veterinarian is a veterinarian working in private practice as an employee. This book uses "veterinarian" or "DVM" to refer to both associate and owner veterinarians, except when the distinction is important. (No disrespect is intended toward University of Pennsylvania graduates, whose degree is titled VMD.) Students may want to keep a pocket dictionary handy for looking up the occasional mysterious word.

The use of the term "career choices" in this book may differ from what you have used. You may be saying, "I thought veterinary medicine *was* a career!" A career, in this book, is a job pathway that a person takes over a long period. So a "career choice" in this book means a job or series of jobs that become a long-term occupation, still related to veterinary medicine. The words "career" and "job" are used interchangeably with "career field," "career pathway," or "practice field." Many jobs discussed here are temporary or short-term positions, such as fellowships, volunteer opportunities, or one-year positions. These jobs, in addition to the option of returning to school, can all be a part of your career.

The acronyms used in this book are defined at first mention in a chapter, unless they are common acronyms such as AAHA, AVMA, and DVM. In addition, all acronyms used in this book are defined in an appendix at the end of the book, which will be a useful reference for the reader.

Introduction Resources

Advanstar, Calendar of veterinary events, www.dvm360.com > events > calendar.
Herriot, J., *All Creatures Great and Small*, St. Martin's Griffin, 2004.
Money magazine, Best Jobs in America, 2009, http://money.cnn.com/magazines/moneymag/bestjobs > job growth.
US News online, America's Best Careers 2010: Healthcare; http://money.usnews.com > Money > Careers; Dec 28, 2009

1 GETTING STARTED

Although most readers of this book will be veterinarians and veterinary students, others will be high school or college students considering veterinary medicine as a career. Some readers may be graduates of veterinary schools outside the US. For information about pre-veterinary requirements, applying to veterinary school, and state and federal licensing requirements, see Appendix A.

Secrets of Success: How to Apply for Any Job

> "Social capital" consists of your contacts that help in you both obvious and subtle ways. Just like financial capital, the more you invest, the more you benefit! (Maybe more, since friends don't lose value.)— Beth Miller, DVM, Little Rock, AR.

There are two methods of applying for any job: the "official written description of how to apply" and the "unofficial tips about how to get the job." Each chapter of this book provides the "official" word on how to apply for a given job. New graduates and practicing veterinarians also have a good idea of how to find jobs in private practice. These openings are advertised in state veterinary newsletters and nationally distributed veterinary publications.

However, experienced veterinarians also know that many private practice jobs are filled by word of mouth or networking. This is also the best way to find jobs outside of private practice.

Networking and information interviews

Before you go out and apply for a job, take this different approach. Go on an information-gathering expedition. The purpose of this is twofold: first, to actually gather information; and second, to network—that is, to meet lots of people, and let them meet you. These contacts, over time, create a great resource for you.

Three excellent books on networking are:
- *Fine Art of Small Talk: How to Start a Conversation, Keep It Going, Build Networking Skills—and Leave a Positive Impression!* by D. Fine.
- *Never Eat Alone: And Other Secrets to Success One Relationship at a Time,* by K. Ferrazzi.
- *Talk to Me: Conversation Tips for the Small-Talk Challenged,* by C. Honeychurch.

How do you find people for networking? If you are an AVMA member, start with the AVMA web site (www.avma.org > AVMA member Directory); search by job category, city, and/or state to find people doing different types of work. Look in your state veterinary association directory (usually available online via their web site), perusing the listings for unusual job titles.

Call people who are doing the work in which you are interested, and ask them whether you can make an appointment to come in and talk about their job or their company (or invite them to lunch—you treat). Then do just that. Don't ask for a job, but simply find out as much as you can. Be honest in telling them that you are thinking of changing career pathways and are gathering information.

Another approach is participation in special interest groups. Throughout this book you will see listings of these groups, which vary from the National Association of Federal Veterinarians (NAFV, www.nafv.net) to the Society for Technical Communication (STC; www.stc.org). Find out when these groups meet and attend their conferences, no matter what topics are on the agenda. Be ready to introduce yourself and start a conversation. Asking people about themselves is a good start. You will then be able to meet a large number of people working in that field, and will get an in-depth look at the variety of opportunities that may be available.

Make a plan to tackle the exhibit area at a large veterinary meeting. Make your approach while lectures are in session, the exhibit hall is quiet, and exhibitors have the time and interest to talk to you. Prepare ahead of time by taking notes on the exhibits in which you are interested—whether that be companies devoted to computer software, pet food, pharmaceuticals, or equipment. (See the calendar of veterinary events at www. dvm360.com > events > calendar.)

No matter which approach or combination of approaches you take, be sure to give your business card to everyone you meet. If you are changing jobs or are a student, the card need only state your name, phone number, and mailing/email address. You needn't worry about having an official "job title" on the card. (*Note to students:* Use a stable street address, such as that of your parents, and an email address that will remain functional after you graduate.)

Once you have met a lot of people in different jobs, two things will happen: you'll have a much better idea of what's involved in specific jobs, and people will have met you and will remember you at a later date. Since you will be meeting a large number of people, make a habit of jotting short notes on their business cards to remind you of where you met and what you talked about. Then, organize the business cards you receive by date or type of job so you can access that information easily.

Now you have the contacts and the information you need to send in your job application. You know a lot about the job you want; you know to whom to address your letter and application; and you know what the company needs. When your application crosses the right desk, that person will remember you. If there is a job opening, you might be the first person who comes to mind.

Social networking online

Online networking can be useful. Many long-term, productive business relationships are forged through contacts made "virtually." The smartest way to view social networking web sites is as tools that are part of your tool box, and not ends in themselves. Use these tools along with personal contact through phone calls and in-person, real-time conversations, as appropriate.

The *Veterinary Information Network* (VIN), formed in 1991, includes several services, including discussion boards on diverse topics of interest (www.vin.com). There is a fee to join.

The *Network of Animal Health* (NOAH), through the AVMA, offers listservs (discussion groups) on a wide variety of topics (www.avma.org > My AVMA > NOAH). You must be an AVMA member to participate.

VetsU is a veterinary social network. If you have attended a university as a student, resident, alumni, or professional, you can connect with others in your field by selecting your university on their web site (www.vetsu.com) to create your account.

LinkedIn is a social networking site geared toward working people (www.linkedin.com). There is no fee to join. A large number of interest groups exist within the site, including many involving veterinarians and veterinary medicine. One advantage to using this site is that you are "findable" even if you change jobs or locations.

Facebook is a social networking site used for both personal and business interactions (www.facebook.com). It is much less formal than Linked In. If you use this or similar sites for personal interactions, never forget that business and work contacts could see the information you post.

No matter which sites you use, be professional. Don't annoy your potential future employers or coworkers with the "fun" quiz you just took ("What animal am I most like?"). Monitor the amount of posting you do, realizing that those who post numerous messages per day can be perceived as annoying.

Many other social networking sites exist or will be created. Balance the amount of time you devote to these with the amount of time you use making concrete and personal contacts. It is easy to spend hours of unproductive time online if you aren't careful.

Job Hunting and Applications

Online job announcements

While networking is the most important tool for job hunting, there are many good job-related web sites and association job listings that can also be helpful. Sometimes the hiring agency may not be aware of the veterinarian's training and thus the job announcement won't be one you'd obviously target. For instance, a job with the United Nations titled "agricultural scientist" revealed, on closer inspection, the requirement for a "veterinarian or PhD in animal science." That job was not found simply by searching for "veterinarian."

If you use your imagination, some "generic" job web sites could yield interesting possibilities. Job web sites include:

- Careers.com
- Careersniff.com
- Craigslist.org
- Monster.com
- Myveterinarycareer.com
- Advanstarvhc.com
- AnimalHealthJobs.com
- TheVetRecruiter.com
- USAjobs.opm.gov

- Cafevet.com
- Careerbuilder.com
- Naturejobs.com
- Newscientistjobs.com
- Sciencecareers.org
- Veterinarycareernetwork.com
- Vetmgrcentral.com
- Vetrelief.com
- Vin.com

The AAHA job bank

The American Animal Hospital Association provides a job bank for its members. AAHA provides free or low-cost access for students. Listed jobs are mostly those in private practice, including emergency, specialty, animal shelter, mixed animal, and small animal practices. Occasional large animal, government, industry and academic jobs are also posted. See www.aahanet.org > Career Center.

A recent search of the AAHA job bank revealed openings in these areas:
- Small animal practices
- Emergency clinic
- Exotics/avian internship
- Agricultural research service, USDA
- Shelter veterinarian
- Low-cost spay-neuter clinic
- Equine practice
- Beef cattle educator

The AVMA Veterinary Career Center

The AVMA's Veterinary Career Center (VCC) provides a job placement service and a Career Development Resource area for its members (see www.AVMA.org/vcc). AVMA staff members are available by e-mail (vetcareers@avma.org) or by visiting the AVMA membership booth at several large veterinary meetings throughout the year.

Opportunities are available in private practice, academia/research, government/ military, nonprofits, associations, and industry. There are usually a large number of private practice positions listed. The number of listings for non–private practice jobs is relatively small, but still useful. The job-seeker profile questions are extremely general, so don't worry about trying to focus on filling out the form in a way that targets a specific job. Leave your options open and you'll get a longer list of potential jobs. You can be notified when a new job has been posted that meets your chosen criteria.

A recent application submitted to the Career Center for a non-practice job revealed this variety of job openings, none of which required more than a veterinary degree:

- FDA position
- USDA-APHIS Veterinary Service position
- Veterinarian for US Army Corps
- Program director for veterinary technology program
- Veterinary technology teacher
- Shelter medical director
- Technical services representative for pharmaceutical or pet food company
- Lab animal veterinarian
- Primate facility veterinarian
- Clinical trials coordinator for pharmaceutical company
- Pet food sales representative
- Food animal clinical researcher for pharmaceutical company

Your resume or curriculum vitae

Job applications usually ask you to submit a resume. Most people in the business world use a resume to describe their job history and special talents. Veterinarians in academia are accustomed to using the curriculum vitae (CV) to describe their educational background.

The Latin words *curriculum vitae* mean "class life" or "life study course," and thus the CV is a list of academic accomplishments. It is a document of the course of your studies and everything relevant to them—including all the classes taken, papers or books published, and grants sought and awarded.

A resume is an abstract of the CV plus any job history, skills, and experience that are relevant to the employer. It may include special abilities, honors and awards, and groups or associations to which you belong. The resume is short—one or two pages at most. A resume offers the advantage of adjusting it to suit each situation, whereas the CV remains as is, adding only further studies or grants.

Many people use a combined resume and CV, where the resume summarizes the attached CV and includes the information that is relevant to the employer's needs and the CV shows only the academic information. The combined resume/CV is better suited to the working professional.

Many books have been written about how to write a successful resume; your local library or any bookstore will have at least one choice. Studying those will help you ensure that your resume is the best it can be. Have your resume edited or reviewed to clean up any grammar or spelling errors.

The interview

Imagine you are in an actual interview for a real job opening. To help you relax during the interview, think of it in reverse of the usual way: *You* interview *the employer* to find out whether you want to work for them. If you assume that you are qualified for the job (and you know this because you have done adequate research about the job opening, the company or governmental agency, and their needs), then your approach can only be "of course they will want to hire me," and your goals will be 1) to show them why they need you (i.e., what you can do for them); and 2) to find out whether you *want* to work for them. (Here's where the pre–job-hunting "information gathering" expedition helps, too.)

One big worry for an interview is how to dress appropriately. If you've been in that company's office before, or have met someone who works there, you had a chance to see how they dress, and you can match your style to theirs—always err on the dressed-up side.

A problem that may arise is that you find a job for which you're ideally qualified, but it is not advertised as a job specifically for a veterinarian. (For example, working with commercial fish raising, where health care has been performed by fish biologists.) You may face the hurdle of changing your interviewer's stereotype of what a veterinarian is before you will be seriously considered for the job. Unfortunately for veterinary medicine, some veterinarians have found that it is not in their favor to point out that they are veterinarians. Instead, that's just a "by the way" comment, with other qualifications being more important. This may be a necessary strategy for you to use to get a particular job, but if it works, then use your new position to re-educate your colleagues about the wide range of talents found in veterinarians.

The next chapter provides useful tools to help you evaluate your priorities, skills, and knowledge, and how those items fit with various career paths.

Your career and your budget

Individual priorities and interests vary, and of course money alone is not considered a "good reason" to choose, or not choose, a particular job or career. It is important to weigh both the return on investment (ROI) as well as non-financial priorities when making choices. However, among graduates with debt, the mean educational debt of veterinary graduates was double the mean starting salary in 2010. Students must plan, budget, and manage their debts. (See J. Wilson's Inviting the Elephant into the Room.)

John Tait, DVM, MBA, CFP, managing partner of the Ontario Veterinary Group, Toronto, Canada, points out that ROI is not the same as the entry level salary, but instead is based on the total return over your working life. ROI also includes non-financial return, such as lifestyle, having a job you love, and job stability, among other factors. Dr. Tait and economist John Livernois calculated the total return to be between 7.4 and 9 percent per year, assuming a 40–year career. They also calculated the difference between getting a bachelor's degree (in any field) and the DVM degree. Although some graduates with a bachelor's degree do start out with a higher salary, the DVM catches up and passes that for a total lifetime income. The initial debt is an investment that creates the opportunity for future wealth, particularly if one becomes a practice owner or pursues board certification.

When comparing job offers, calculate the value of benefits (e.g., health insurance) as well as the variable cost of living in different areas, using resources such as the salary comparison calculator at www.bankrate.com.

Financial information and resources

A variety of resources provide financial information. For example, the AVMA web sites provide information on veterinary resources for students (www.avma.org > Veterinary resources) as well as public resources (www.avma.org > Public resources). Reference reports include the *AVMA Report on Veterinary Compensation*, (www.avma.org > Scientific resources). See also the AVMA report, *Employment of Female and Male Graduates of US Veterinary Medical Schools and Colleges,* and *Employment, Starting Salaries, and Educational Indebtedness of Graduates of US Veterinary Medical Colleges*, both published periodically in the *Journal of the AVMA.*

AAHA also publishes two books on a regular basis: *Financial & Productivity Pulsepoints* and *The Veterinary Fee Reference.* The most current edition of either can be obtained through your local library's interlibrary loan service or through the AAHA bookstore (www.aahanet.org). The AAHA web site includes a student section with information about career planning, financial planning, and work-life balance (www.aahanet.org > Students).

The National Commission on Veterinary Economic Issues (NCVEI) resources include financial data from practices nationwide as well as a wide variety of articles that will help students and veterinarians with career planning (www.ncvei.org > Resource library).

VetPartners, an association whose membership includes veterinary practice management consultants, has published a No-Lo Practice™ guide for practice valuation. VetPartners also has a great deal of information for veterinary students about managing debt and budgeting (www.vetpartners.org > Resources).

Financial aid

Financial aid is aimed at veterinary students, although graduate veterinarians may be eligible for a few programs.

Student debt is not unique to the veterinary profession. A variety of scholarships, student loans, and work study programs are available to students, with information available through school counseling centers.

Some career choices may offer loan repayment assistance, although this is almost totally confined to those working in food animal medicine. See Chapters 5, 16, and 19.

The Veterinary Medicine Loan Repayment Program (VMLRP, www.nifa.usda.gov/vmlrp) offers assistance to veterinarians who work in underserved areas. The Veterinary Services Investment Act would provide grants to relocate or recruit veterinarians and veterinary technicians into shortage areas, and support veterinary students seeking training in food-supply veterinary medicine (www.avma.org >press releases).

The Food Animal Veterinarian Recruitment and Retention Program (FAVRRP, www.avmf.org/favrrp) is a pilot program designed to provide financial incentives in the form of current student loan debt grants for veterinarians who commit to four years of employment in food animal veterinary medicine. The program is a joint effort of the American Veterinary Medical Foundation (AVMF) and the AVMA, with funding by several industry partners.

Individual programs exist in many states. An example is the scholarship from the Wisconsin Farm Bureau Federation (www.wisconsinagconnection.com), which is awarded based on interest in practicing medicine with large, farm livestock, and on having a farm background.

Chapter 1 Resources

Groups and web sites

American Animal Hospital Association (AAHA) job bank, www.aahanet.org.

American Association of Veterinary State Boards, 4106 Central St., Kansas City, MO, 64111; www.aavsb.org; phone: 877-698-8482; fax: 816-931- 1604; e-mail: aavsb@aavsb.org.

Association of American Veterinary Medical Colleges (AAVMC), www.aavmc.org.

American Veterinary Medical Association
AVMA Veterinary Career Center, 1931 N. Meacham Rd., Schaumburg, IL 60173-4360; www.AVMA.org/vcc; phone: 800 248 2862; e-mail: vetcareers@avma.org.
AVMA Model Veterinary Practice Act, www.avma.org > Issues > Policy > Model Veterinary Practice Act.

Bankrate.com, Salary comparison calculator includes local cost of living.

Center for Veterinary Economics, see NCVEI

Educational Commission for Foreign Veterinary Graduates (ECFVG), www.avma.org/education/ecfvg.

Food Animal Veterinarian Recruitment and Retention Program www.avma.org > AVMA journals > *JAVMA News* > March 15, 2010, and www.avmf.org/FAVRRP.

National Board of Veterinary Medical Examiners (NBVME), www.nbvme.org.

National Commission for Veterinary Economic Issues (NCVEI), www.ncvei.org. (Note: The NCVEI may be forming a partnership with Kansas State University to form the Center for Veterinary Economics.)
NCVEI resources, www.ncvei.org > Resource library.

Veterinary Medicine Loan Repayment Program (VMLRP) www.gpoaccess.gov > Federal Register > April 19, 2010 75(74), pp.20239-20248. Web www.nifa.usda.gov/vmlrp; Email vmlrp@nifa.usda.gov.

Books and articles

AAHA, *Compensation and Benefits Review* (AAHA Press, published periodically), www.aahanet.org.

AAHA, *Financial and Productivity Pulsepoints: Vital Statistics for Your Veterinary Practice* (AAHA Press, published periodically).

AVMA, *Report on Veterinary Compensation*, www.avma.org > Scientific resources.

AVMA Communications Division, Shepherd A., Employment, Starting Salaries, and Educational Indebtedness of Year 2009 Graduates of US Veterinary Medical Colleges. *JAVMA*, September 1, 2009; 235(5): 523–526.

AVMA Communications Division, Shepherd A., Employment of Female & Male Graduates of US Veterinary Medical Colleges, 2009, *JAVMA*, October 1, 2009; 235(7): 830–832 (similar report published periodically).

AVMA Communications Division, Shepherd A., Employment, starting salaries, and educational indebtedness of year-2010 graduates of US veterinary medical colleges. *JAVMA*, October 1, 2010; 237(7): 795-798

Ferrazzi, K, and T Raz, *Never Eat Alone: And Other Secrets to Success One Relationship at a Time* (A Currency Book, Division of Random House, 2005).

Fine, D, *Fine Art of Small Talk: How To Start a Conversation, Keep It Going, Build Networking Skills——and Leave a Positive Impression!* (Hyperion, 2005).

Honeychurch, C., and A. Watrous, *Talk to Me: Conversation Tips for the Small-Talk Challenged* (New Harbinger, 2003).

Larkin M, Board Weighs In On Foreign Accreditation, *JAVMA News*, July 15, 2010: 130-133.

Rose, R and C Smith. *Career Choices for Veterinary Technicians: Opportunities for Animal Lovers*. (AAHA Press, 2009).

VetPartners, No-Lo Practice Valuation Worksheet, www.vetpartners.org.

Wilson, J, Inviting the Elephant into the Room: A Dialogue to Co-create a Financially Healthy Veterinary Profession. Presented at the North American Veterinary Conference 2008, www.vetpartners.org >Resources.

Wisconsin Ag Connection, WFBF Awards Scholarship to Future Veterinarian, June 4, 2010. www.wisconsinagconnection.com.

Wood, F., Is Purchasing Power Shrinking? *Veterinary Economics*, August 2007; 36.

2 PLAN AND PRIORITIZE

Reading this chapter will help you focus on the specific sections of the book that might best fit your needs. Practicing veterinarians as well as students may gain a different perspective of career choices by assessing your skills and knowledge, evaluating your priorities, and then making a plan. Whether you want to work in private practice or pursue laboratory research, your choices will be clearer if you plan and prioritize.

Review your choices for additional training, whether that be through formal university courses or self-structured learning. Prioritize your needs, taking a second look at career paths you may have previously dismissed. Budget your time and resources.

Assess Your Skills and Knowledge

The sample job announcements scattered throughout the book give a sample of the skills and knowledge required for various jobs. Notably, many such announcements include far more than veterinary medical skills. Use your answers to the following questions to help beef up your resume.

If you are a practicing veterinarian, the hardest part about broadening your career search is thinking of yourself in a new way. Rather than just being a "dog doctor" (or "horse doctor"), you have a compilation of skills and knowledge that is much broader than you think.

- What did you study as an undergraduate? Even if you have never officially "used" this knowledge or your Bachelor's degree, it is still a marketable attribute.
- What kind of volunteer work do you do? With what groups are you involved? (This means not just veterinary groups, but social groups, sports teams, Toastmasters, Rotary, and parents' groups, for example.) Have you ever been elected as an officer of any of those groups?
- Have you ever written a scientific paper, a case study for a veterinary journal, a pet column for your local paper, or a newsletter for your clinic?
- Have you ever spoken to your local Kiwanis or Rotary group, or been interviewed by local radio or television?
- Have you taught 4-H classes or community classes for adults?
- What specific things have you done as a veterinarian? List your skills and areas of knowledge: radiology, anesthesia, surgery, pharmacology, toxicology, disease processes, or medical terminology. Don't forget your ability to read and understand complex scientific reports.
- What about administrative and managerial skills? How many employees have you supervised? What duties have you held in managing a veterinary clinic? Be

specific (e.g., "wrote budget, handled employee payroll, hired and fired employees, handled inventory").

- What were your jobs before you became a veterinarian? Did you help out in a research lab in college? Did you begin work on a master's degree or PhD—even if you never finished? The skills you learned while doing that work should be listed on your resume. Many jobs in government and industry ask for knowledge of how to set up a research study or how to do research.

Once you've broken down your experience into specific topics, you might be surprised by the diverse knowledge and skills you have accumulated. Then you can start to see how your abilities can be applied to a wider variety of jobs than you'd ever dreamed.

Basic skills to broaden your choices

Specific qualifications needed for each job (besides holding a veterinary degree) are listed in the discussion of the job itself. However, no matter what the job, whether in government or industry, at the AVMA or in technical writing, you must possess some basic skills and knowledge, which needn't be obtained via a college degree. What you need, in almost every case, are:

- Computer skills.
- Oral communication skills.
- Business knowledge.
- Written communication skills.
- Leadership and organizational ability.
- A flexible attitude and a broad, diverse background.

How are you going to get these skills? There are many ways to learn. Some cost money, yes—but think of this as "going back to school" in a whole new way. Consider how much less time and money this will consume than would getting another degree!

Computer skills

> The inability to drive a car in the old economy cut people off from a host of job opportunities. It's the same today with computers.—N. Beck, in *Shifting Gears: Thriving in the New Economy*

Beware of assuming that because you grew up with technology, you have the necessary skills to use it in the workplace setting. If you are older, it is never too late to become comfortable with technology. Take classes given by your local school, adult education night classes, or online courses. Subscribe to a computer magazine, and try out some of the suggestions. Read books about how to use specific software, then apply that new knowledge. Become familiar with the following:

- Mac and PC operating systems; Microsoft Office (MS Word, PowerPoint, Excel, and Outlook).
- Using basic internet search engines and performing advanced searches using programs such as PubMed (www.nlm.nih.gov > pubmed).
- Financial programs (Quicken/ Quickbooks) or design programs (InDesign, Photoshop), are not usually required, but may give your resume a boost.

- Using web-based services for business purposes (e.g. GoToMeeting.com; Yahoo and Google groups).
- UVIS, the Universal Veterinary Information System, which used in university settings. (Veterinarians working in industry or academia will usually be trained in the use of specific software after hiring, although prior familiarity doesn't hurt.)
- Practice management software for private practice. These programs vary with practices, but you can still become familiar with the main products with a visit to any convention exhibit hall.

Business knowledge

No matter what your career niche, when you understand the business end of your potential career field, you are better able to tell your interviewers how your skills can enhance their company's goals.

Working successfully in private practice requires an understanding of the business of health care in your country. This includes client relations, communication, record keeping, and the basics of small-business financial management. *Veterinary Economics* magazine is essential basic reading to understand the business and management issues of any veterinary practice (see www.advanstar.com or www.dvm360.com).

If you want to work in industry, you must understand their business. If you work for a non-profit group, you need to understand fundraising and budgeting. If you want to write, you must understand the business of publishing (i.e., before a magazine will pay you to write an article, they want to know whether it's useful for their readers and subscribers).

To learn more:
- *Study.* This can include reading, but also includes talking to people.
- *Go to veterinary meetings.* Attend the lectures about practice management. Visit the exhibit hall and chat with the people there about what they do and about their company's goals.
- *Look at AAHA's management course offerings.* (See www.aahanet.org.)
- *Attend meetings of business associations.* These include the Society for Human Resource Management (www.shrm.org), the American Management Association (www.amanet.org), and the Veterinary Hospital Managers Association (www.vhma.org). Students can join their school's chapter of the Veterinary Business Management Association, (VBMA; www.vbma.biz). This student-run group provides lectures and hands-on training to students in various business-related topics. Most chapters also welcome local veterinarians to attend lectures at no cost.

Oral communication skills

Offer to give talks to local breeder's clubs, at veterinary luncheons, or for your local service organization. Keep a list of your speaking engagements for your resume.

Join Toastmasters! This is highly recommended. Toastmasters is a nonprofit organization that teaches anyone how to speak more confidently in any setting. Toastmasters has programs for all kinds of people to learn what they need most in their jobs. View the web site for presentations, courses, and location of groups nearest you (www. toastmasters.org). Look in your local newspaper for meeting times. Clubs generally meet before or after work hours, once or twice a month.

Written communication skills

Take a class in technical writing, magazine article writing, or other nonfiction writing given by your local school or college or in online or correspondence courses.

Write articles for your local breeder's club or saddle club newsletter, or for a veterinary publication. You needn't jump into publishing in refereed journals right away. Try *Veterinary Forum* or *DVM Newsmagazine* to start. However, if you do want to publish in a peer-reviewed journal, simple case reports are a good way to start.

Leadership and organizational ability

Volunteer to be an officer in your local veterinary association or civic group. Or help to organize a veterinary meeting. Getting involved is easy if you start by offering to complete a specific small task and go from there.

Good time management is critical for any job, but even more so for those who are self-employed (housecall, relief, consulting, and writing jobs). If you have time-management challenges, you may need to hire a personal coach, take a course, or create your own techniques to improve.

Flexibility and a broad, diverse background

You can't buy these attributes, but they're desired by most employers. Will you be able to change as a job changes, or as your employer's needs change? A diverse background is a plus in many jobs that require you to know a little bit about a variety of species, and to be knowledgeable about medicine, business, writing, and speaking. Employers know they can train you to do specific tasks if you are flexible and a good learner.

Improve Your Skills and Knowledge

Training without more school

The vast majority of veterinarians do *not* hold a degree beyond their Doctor of Veterinary Medicine. Perhaps you don't have the desire, time, or resources to go back to school. You may not be sure enough of your potential new career choice that you are willing to commit to a few more years of school. But school isn't the only route to a new career. You have many more options for change than you may realize. In addition, you can get *started* in a new career without going back to school, to find out if you really like the change—then, later, you can always go back to school to further advance in your chosen new career (and sometimes, your employer will pay for it!).

Although this book includes many jobs that do not require more than a veterinary degree, that *doesn't* mean that all veterinarians will qualify for all the jobs, nor does it mean that some kind of further experience or training isn't required. However, you should look beyond the traditional "going back to school and getting another degree" mentality, and see that your past degree(s) (BS or MS), work experience, seminars, internships, and independent study are acceptable ways to gain experience and become qualified for specific jobs. Often, you just need to get your foot in the door and you can go from there. A previous externship or volunteering in your area of interest might be enough to do just that.

Don't immediately discount job ads that *appear* to ask for an advanced degree. During the research for this book, we encountered many people who said, "I didn't have the degree that's usually required for this job, but I got the job anyway because of my special knowledge [talents, experience]." Close inspection of job announcements often reveals statements such as "PhD *or equivalent research experience*," or "MBA *or equivalent business experience*." You might have just the specific experience they're seeking.

Three resources that address nontraditional education opportunities are:
- Nontechnical Competencies Underlying Career Success as a Veterinarian, *JAVMA*, By R. Lewis.
- *Bears Guide to Earning Degrees by Distance Learning*, by M. Bear.
- *Earn College Credit for What You Know*, by the Council for Adult & Experienced Learning.

Create your own learning

You can use your imagination and creative time-scheduling to fashion your own new learning situation. Consider the following:
- Courses on tape.
- Correspondence or online courses; webinars.
- College courses via cable/satellite TV.
- Offerings through your community school or college.
- Night or weekend classes.
- Intensive learning courses; many colleges offer short-term (weekends or one to two months) intensive courses in a variety of areas.
- Workshops and seminars offered by the many associations listed in this book.
- Meetings of groups involved in your potential new career (Federal veterinarians' meetings, extension agents' meetings, writers' seminars).
- Foreign language training (combined with travel).
- Magazines, journals, and books (audio or printed).
- Military training (enlist part-time or full-time in the military and get free training in a variety of fields).
- Test-drive a new career through a working vacation, such as those described on www.vocationvacations.com.
- Become certified in a niche area, such as becoming a Certified Professional Coach or a Certified Mediator, then apply those skills to veterinary medicine.

Volunteer

Volunteering is a great risk-free way to build your resume, gain new and valuable contacts, and explore new career paths. Seek out an area where you need experience (e.g., writing, speaking, computer skills). Do volunteer work for a nonprofit agency, or ask to spend a few weeks (or one day a week) working with someone, either for free or at low pay—in exchange, you get to learn on the job, meet people, and find out what is involved in a career you may want to pursue. You would be amazed at the insights you can gain simply by asking to "shadow" someone for a few days; very few people will turn you down.

Attend veterinary seminars

Throughout this book you will see advice to "attend classes and labs offered at national veterinary meetings," or "attend educational courses offered by associations." Just about every one of the special interest groups mentioned in this book offers some kind of continuing education for its members.

In addition, a large number of state, regional, and national veterinary meetings are held throughout the US, Canada, and the rest of the world. State meetings are advertised through state veterinary associations. See www.avma.org > My AVMA > Member Resource Directory > Associations & boards. National meetings are advertised through most veterinary publications (e.g., *Veterinary Economics*, the Journal of the AVMA, *DVM Newsmagazine*), and are also posted online (e.g., www.dvm360.com > events > calendar).

Participate in externships

Externships are typically shorter training periods undertaken by students while they are still in veterinary school. However, externships are not just for veterinary students! Externships exist in almost all career pathways and are mentioned in various chapters of this book. They may be taken in private practice, academic institutions, industry, and government. For example, see Chapter 13 for externships with international and non-profit groups.

Also, the Center for Public and Corporate Veterinary Medicine (CPCVM, www.vetmed.vt.edu/org/md/cpcvm) serves as a national and international resource to train veterinary students and graduate veterinarians for career opportunities in the public and corporate areas of the profession. The CPCVM partners with academic institutions, government agencies, industrial corporations, international organizations, and nonprofit institutions, including coordinating externships.

Externships are usually not paid, but some may offer a small stipend. They differ from other volunteering (ideally) in that they are structured for learning. Learning may include observing as well as supervised hands-on experiences.

Apply for fellowships

A variety of paid fellowships are available for those who want to study or gain experience in a specific area, including those offered by federal government agencies, universities, associations, and industry.

Details about some of these are provided in the appropriate chapters of this book. As you investigate your area of interest, you may find other fellowship opportunities. For example, a new fellowship was created as an incentive for veterinarians switching to research. It is a partnership between industry, nonprofit groups, and academia. (The Pfizer Animal Health / Morris Animal Foundation Veterinary Fellowship for Advanced Study; see www.morrisanimalfoundation.org > for grant seekers). (See also Chapter 14.)

AAAS Fellowships are an untapped resource

The American Association for the Advancement of Science (AAAS) offers a variety of fellowships for which veterinarians may be eligible. Veterinarians may be aware of the AVMA Congressional Fellowship (see Chapter 12), but they may be eligible for many additional positions; there were a total of 65 fellows in 2010 (see http://fellowships.aaas.org > Fellowship areas). In fact, an AAAS staffer said that veterinarians are considered "hot commodities" by many agencies that offer these fellowships.

Fellows work with a specific government agency in the capitol for one year (some fellowships can be renewed for a second year). Fellows are placed through a process of selection and choice based on their interests and the needs of various agencies. For example, a veterinarian worked at the Office of Ocean and Polar Affairs in the State Department, where he was known as the "polar bear guy" who ensured polar bears are safe from climate changes.

Fellows need to be flexible with slow moving government processes but also adaptable to various situations. To increase your chances of acceptance, you may send in an application for up to two fellowships in each of four program areas:

1. Congressional: Applications are made through about 30 sponsoring associations; the AVMA is but one of those.

2. Diplomacy, Security & Development: You may be placed with agencies such as the State Department, USAID, Department of Defense, or the Department of Homeland Security.

3. Energy, Environment & Agriculture: You may be placed with the Environmental Protection Agency, the Department of Energy, the Department of Agriculture, or the National Science Foundation.

4. Health, Education & Human Services: You may be placed with the National Institutes of Health, the Department of Health & Human Services, the Veterans Administration, or the National Science Foundation.

Former fellows read and score the applications. Factors considered include your scientific background, whether and what you have published or performed research on, and why you want to work on policy issues. Finalists come in for a "placement week" where they interview with different agencies that want a fellow; a mutual ranking and matching process determines your final placement.

Also see the information about USAID in Chapter 16.

Restart your career in mid life

For some veterinarians, the "change" they contemplate is simply changing from large animal to small animal practice. Others may have taken a "time out" from their veterinary career to pursue other activities. Either way, such veterinarians do not feel equipped to enter the workplace without reviewing their skills and knowledge.

To revive your lapsed skills, consider volunteering to get up to speed. Volunteer at a nearby practice to re-familiarize yourself with medicine and surgery. Volunteer to assist and to perform spay-neuter surgery for a nearby shelter. Volunteer at an emergency clinic so you feel comfortable with those situations. If there are specialists in your area, ask if you can volunteer and/or observe with them.

Practical continuing education is available from many sources. Attend hands-on "wet labs" that are offered at major national meetings. View special-interest associations for their CE offerings. Some veterinary teaching hospitals offer unique educational opportunities, such as the Low Fellowship at the University of California at Davis, which is a 20-day learning experience (www.vetmed.ucdavis.edu/ce/lowfellowship.html).

Find a mentor

One way to get help is through a mentor. Mentor relationships can develop informally or can be planned. Where can you find a mentor? It need not be the supervisor or practice owner where you work. In fact, some people would recommend that a good mentor is someone who does not work in the same place—that way, you can discuss workplace challenges that otherwise might be uncomfortable to address. Some workplaces have mentor programs in place; many associations also arrange such relationships. Mentors can work with you in person or remotely, via the internet, e-mail and telephone.

The most important aspect of the mentor/mentee relationship is an open discussion of expectations, roles, and responsibilities. Be realistic about what you are able to do. Don't over-promise. Set aside specific days and times when you will meet. For more details about how to create a mentor-mentee relationship, see the AAHA mentor guidelines, which can apply to any mentoring relationship, not just those in private practice (www.aahanet.org).

Beyond the DVM: Going back to school

Additional training: What's useful?

Follow your dreams and your interests, of course! And also, be aware of the impact on your budget and the potential for finding a job. Although income is not the only driving factor for one's career selection, it will impact your expectations. Similarly, while following your interests is always advisable, you can also match interests to training that might yield the greatest chances of finding work.

Internships

An internship is a one-year position taken by some veterinarians to achieve additional training. Internships are normally taken immediately after graduation from veterinary school, but can be done later. Internships can be taken in many fields of interest. Specific positions are mentioned in various chapters of this book. For example, international and government internships are described in Chapters 13 and 16, respectively.

An internship is usually required before one can proceed into a three-year residency program; residencies are designed to train veterinarians for board certification (see Chapter 4).

An interesting development in the past decade has been the increasing number of students entering internships; the percentage rose from 19 percent in 1998 to somewhere between 26 percent and 43 percent by 2010 (depending on which studies you read). The reasons cited most are to increase the quality of care and to pursue a residency. However, in one study, while the vast majority said they planned to continue with a residency, fewer than half actually did so. See the AVMA data in *JAVMA* and the *Trends* article by E. Choca.

Veterinarians should carefully analyze their expectations before deciding to undertake an internship. While cost is only one factor that influences the decision, it is important to be aware of the cost and return on investment. The AVMA reported the mean salary for all graduates entering advanced education programs in 2010 to be around $29,000, which is drastically less than the $67,000 mean starting salary for associates in private practice. Another study reported that while those who completed an internship were paid more than their peers upon entering the job market, the amount was not enough to make up for the lost income of their internship year. It is unlikely that the lost income from that first year will ever be recouped. (See Table 2.1, and Choca.)

In addition, private practice employers may not be willing to pay more for someone who has done an internship over a new grad who has not done so. Many employers state that they want to hire veterinarians with good client-communication skills, and internships often emphasize medicine or surgery, not client communication. Others point out that the skills gained in an internship can be obtained in any private practice job with a good mentor. Finally, private practice veterinarians are often paid based on their production, not on their expertise. It is not clear that higher expertise results in a higher income, other than for those with board certification. Board certification does offer a good return on investment (see Table 2.1, and *JAVMA* article by M. Gordon et al.).

One practice owner offers this insight:

> When evaluating a potential associate, I would not necessarily offer a higher salary to someone who had completed an internship. The qualities we seek include excellent interpersonal communication skills, understanding and embracing our Core Values (honesty, compassion, competency, professionalism, teamwork), time management skills, and seeing this profession as a lifestyle, not just a job. I have not seen that interns are consistently more qualified than someone who has been in practice for a year.—Gregg Takashima, DVM, Parkside Veterinary Hospital, Lake Oswego, OR.

Nonetheless, other factors may make an internship worthwhile. Interns report increased confidence in their skills and knowledge. Those working with horses or in small animal emergency medicine report that many employers prefer applicants who have completed an internship. Finally, an internship is a prerequisite for entering a residency.

The Veterinary Internship and Residency Matching Program lists internships and residencies that are available using a match program (www.virmp.org). See Chapter 4 for details.

Additional degrees or board certification

One way to modify your career choices is to go back to school—train in a different field or specialize in a particular area of medicine or surgery. The AVMA membership database showed that at least 12 percent of veterinarians reported having at least one additional postgraduate degree in 2008. However, providing this information is voluntary, so the actual percentage is likely to be higher. Of the veterinarians who held at least one additional degree, the top five degrees (excluding associate's and bachelor's degrees) are shown in Table 2.2. (See *Complete Idiot's Guide to Going Back to College* by D. Mize for down-to-earth tips.)

About 11 percent of veterinarians are board-certified specialists (see Chapter 4). You can become a cardiologist, toxicologist, or laboratory animal specialist by going back to school. Although board-certified specialists appear to be in high demand, not all specialties are in *equal* demand. Employer type also impacts income. For example, the average income of someone with only a veterinary degree who works in industry is higher than the average income of a board-certified veterinarian working for the government.

Another path is to obtain an MBA or law degree and work in veterinary law or business (see Chapter 9). Some private practice owners have pursued an MBA, but it is not clear that this additional degree provides a significant advantage to them. Furthermore, the MBA/DVM must then decide whether to concentrate on using medical/surgical skills, or on managing the business. However, an MBA may be useful or required for some jobs. (See Chapters 9, Consulting; 11, Industry; and 19, Future Outlook.)

Veterinarians who go into research will need an additional degree—a Master's or PhD—to advance. With increasing emphasis on "One Health" (the overlap of human and veterinary medicine, see Chapter 19) comes the opportunity for more cooperative research. Veterinarians may work in research positions in industry, academia, or government (see Chapters 11, 14–18), and may focus on a wide variety of areas, from pathology to infectious disease.

Another possibility is the Master of Public Health (MPH) degree. Many state and government job openings, as well as international positions, are suitable for the DVM-MPH; advancement in these jobs often requires the MPH. Many MPH programs can be completed via distance learning and require little classroom time. However, with government budget cuts, this niche may carry less demand over the coming decade. Some recent grads who focused on epidemiology or public health have expressed dismay in the scarcity of jobs and low pay being offered. (Public Health Reality Check, *DVM Newsmagazine.*) See Chapters 15–19.

No matter which avenue interests you, do your homework so your expectations are in alignment with reality. Following your heart is essential, of course. In addition, one must be aware of economic realities. Although returning to school means a longer delay before you can earn a decent income, board certification or pursuing a PhD *will,* on average, result in higher lifetime earnings. What's more, many student loans may be deferred until further training is completed. (It is important to note that the same financial increase cannot be said of simply completing an internship. Board certification or further specialization is needed to realize these financial benefits, as well as to be able to focus on one area of interest.)

The increase in income that results from further training is also related to the employer and the type of work done. Advanced training yields far greater financial rewards for those who work in industry than for those who work at a university or for the government. See Chapter 3 on traditional private practice, Chapter 11 on industry, and Chapters 15–18 on government for more details.

Also, further training may open up new choices but also may narrow your choices, because sometimes there are fewer job openings in which to utilize your specific knowledge and skills.

Table 2.1 may serve as a gauge of the spread and differences among various categories, although absolute numbers will rise over the coming years. Table 2.3 presents the median incomes of various veterinarian specialties (see also Chapter 4).

Table 2.1: Median incomes of veterinarians with various postgraduate training

Employment and postgraduate degree		Median income
Private practice DVM, no additional training		$91,000
	Associate veterinarian (employee)	79,000
	Practice owner	121,000
Private practice DVM		
	With master's	97,000
	With internship	79,000
	With doctorate	127,000
	Board-certified	145,000
Academia (college or university) DVM		85,000
	With master's	103,000
	With internship	31,000
	With doctorate	115,000
	Board-certified	115,000
Federal government DVM		91,000
	With master's	103,000
	With internship	103,000
	With doctorate	109,000
	Board-certified	115,000
Industry DVM		139,000
	With master's	151,000
	With internship	97,000
	With doctorate	178,000
	Board-certified	181,000

AVMA Report on Veterinary Compensation, 2009 (published biennially; 2009 edition reflects 2007 and 2008 data).

Table 2.2: Top five postgraduate degrees held by veterinarians

Degree	Veterinarians with degree
MS/MSc, Master of Science	6,962
PhD, Doctor of Philosophy	2,927
MPH, Master of Public Health	693
MA, Master of Arts	595
MBA, Master of Business Administration	420
Totals	10,910 (about 12% of all DVMs)

AVMA data; www.avma.org/reference/marketstats/usvets.asp. Also see Table 19.1.

Table 2.3: Median incomes for various veterinary specialists

Specialty*	Median income
Lab animal	$169,000
Pathology	151,000
Surgery	127,000
Internal medicine	127,000
Emergency and critical care	121,000
Ophthalmology	121,000
Poultry	121,000
Radiology	121,000
Toxicology	97,000
Microbiology	61,000

* Insufficient data for many specialists due to their low numbers. Expect spread within specialist groups based on employer type. AVMA Report on Veterinary Compensation, 2009 (reflects 2008 data).

Making a Change

> Do you feel bad enough to change right now, or would you prefer to wait a little longer, until you feel much worse?—Shelle Rose Charvet, President, Success Strategies.

The discussion in this section is of particular value to practicing veterinarians who are thinking of changing their jobs, which usually means moving away from private practice. However, students should take note of this section, too—to get an idea of how veterinarians feel about changing their jobs. Anticipating that this could happen to you, might help you avoid feeling that your life is ruined if your first job choice doesn't turn out exactly as you'd hoped. It will also give you an idea of what opportunities are available, and allow you to potentially gain experience in nontraditional arenas prior to graduating.

Veterinarians most often start their careers in private practice. Reasons for a change vary widely. Midlife veterinarians may find they want new challenges. Injury, allergies, disability, disillusionment, or partial retirement all may influence one's choice of career.

Non-practice jobs

> People often trace their ultimate achievements back to a childhood dream. But that pattern is usually either the result of hindsight or a suggestion that their development was arrested by something early in their life journeys... the natural development pattern is not for people to keep the same dreams, but to relinquish old dreams and generate new ones throughout their lifetimes...The image for such a life is not an upward-trending diagonal of increasing achievement but a spiral of linked cycles—the completion of each leading to a new cycle of experience and activity based on a new dream.—W. Bridges, in *Transitions: Making Sense of Life's Changes*.

"Aren't I wasting my veterinary schooling if I'm not in practice?" you may ask. One of the biggest stumbling blocks to avoid is the negative perception you may have about non-practice jobs. Others may say to you (or you may say to yourself), "Gee, won't you feel like you wasted your time in veterinary school if you're not working in traditional practice?" Dr. Smith even heard someone introduce her as: "This is Carin Smith; she used to be a veterinarian." She had to explain that she still *is* a veterinarian—she just makes a living in a different way than their dog doctor.

Consider this: You spent four years in veterinary school, with, at most, half of that in clinics—and half of the clinics involved working with species you probably don't see in your current job. Is it worth staying in a job where you're unhappy, just to prove that you "used" those years of your schooling? Have you ever thought to ask this of a small animal veterinarian, "Don't you feel like you wasted your schooling? After all, you never use the bovine medicine, the herd health, the basic virology, or the histology that you learned!"

Unfortunately, most people have a specific, romantic idea of what "being a veterinarian" is all about. You will encounter disappointment from people who feel you aren't fulfilling your (their) dream. It's also hard to have a job that people can't immediately visualize in a positive way. When you say you're a veterinarian, they immediately visualize a specific picture of a dog, cat, or horse doctor. When you say you're the director of technical services for a pharmaceutical company, or that you do medical writing, or that you work for the government, it's harder for others to imagine what you do. This may be the case even if they themselves are veterinarians.

Get ready for people to ask, "So, when are you going to go back to practice?" or "Don't you miss working on puppies?" Prepare your animated, happy reply to "What do you do?" in a few sentences that include a brief description of what you actually do for a living (e.g., "I'm a veterinarian, but like many veterinarians, I don't have a typical practice. Instead, my job involves. . . I really love my work!" or, "I work on projects and products that benefit millions of animals!")

Another perspective on the "Aren't you wasting your schooling" thought: Aren't you wasting your time continuing to practice if it's not what you enjoy? What do you prove by staying in a job just because it's what you thought sometime in the past that you wanted to do? How will you feel five years from now if you make a change . . . or if you don't? Veterinarians are increasingly aware of finding a work-life balance. The first step is to find a job in a career that you truly enjoy doing day in, and day out.

Explore your limits

Self-Assessment Questionnaire

Before you zero in on a particular type of job, ask yourself some basic questions about your needs and your situation. The answers will narrow down your potential choices. For many people, the primary restriction to life choices is geographical because their families are living in one area, or their spouses have jobs that can't be given up. Others feel a need to continue to work with animals or to help people. Let's go through the list of "I-have-tos" and see what comes up. Look for specific information about these choices in the chapters that follow.

1. Am I (and is my family) able to move (to a different town in my state; to any other state; to another part of the world)? Do I want to travel as part of my work?
   • Yes: Any career is open to you. If you enjoy travel, consider industry, military, or international assistance jobs. Private practice, particularly practice ownership, may limit your ability to travel or to move.
   • No: Eliminate most industry, government and corporate practice jobs, or be ready to take a job that might not be your first choice, simply because its location is right for you. Consider private practice, relief work, housecall practice, teaching, writing, or consulting (involves travel, but you can live where you want).
   • Look to the AVMA's data to find out which jobs are most abundant in your state. See AVMA's veterinary demographic reports, containing demographic and employment trend data, updated periodically (e.g., *US Pet Ownership & Demographics Sourcebook*, available at www.avma.org > references > market statistics).
   • Of veterinarians who are employed in veterinary industry, the numbers are highest in New Jersey, Pennsylvania, Michigan, Kansas, and California.
   • Of veterinarians who work for state or local governments, the greatest number are employed in Wisconsin, North Carolina, Florida, Texas, and California. However, every state employs a few veterinarians.
   • Military jobs are concentrated in Maryland, Texas, and US Possessions (e.g., Puerto Rico, Guam).
   • Jobs with the AVMA are in Schaumburg, Illinois, and Washington, DC; jobs with AAHA are in Denver, Colorado (AAHA also employs consultants in other states).
   • Jobs you can create anywhere include housecall or relief practice; consulting; and technical writing. USDA-APHIS jobs are located all over the country, too.

- If you want to work in another country, consider relief work, volunteer/assistance work, nonprofit agency work, military jobs, or federal jobs.

2. Do I need a steady job with immediate good income and benefits (to support a family, get good health insurance, or pay off debt)?
- No: Any career is open to you.
- Yes: Consider a government job; look into the FSIS, which may offer loan repayment and recruitment bonuses. Students may investigate USDA's APHIS scholarships. Also consider industry jobs. If you are focused on private practice, look at corporate practices. Eliminate housecall practice, relief work, writing, volunteer or assistance jobs, or consulting.
- If you want to get further training paid for, consider the Commissioned Corps or other military position.

3. Do I like working with people?
- *No:* Consider writing, informatics, industry's research and development (R&D).
- Yes: Most jobs are open to you. Focus on traditional private practice, teaching, consulting, industry, or nonprofit work.
- If you want to work with or help people directly, consider working for a volunteer/assistance program; working for industry, in technical services; working for the government (APHIS veterinary services); international work; extension work; teaching; or working for the military. Also consider relief or housecall practice.

4. Do I like working as part of a team or in a large group?
- Yes: Consider private practice, industry or government jobs, working with organizations or associations, or a job with an international assistance group.
- No (I prefer working alone, unsupervised): Consider relief practice, housecall practice, writing, independent contractor work for corporations (e.g., sales). Some Animal Care jobs with APHIS are fairly independent positions.

5. Do I need action and movement, or is a desk job preferable or acceptable?
- Action: Consider traditional practice, relief or housecall practice; lower-level state jobs (advancement means moving to a desk job; lower levels involve the actual field work); APHIS Veterinary Service; FSIS (food inspector) jobs; sales jobs; or R&D for industry.
- Desk: Look at industry, consulting, federal or state non–field positions, writing.

6. Do I want regular hours, or am I able and willing to work odd hours or days? Would regular hours feel like a "rut"?
- Regular: Consider teaching, government, the military or urban companion animal or corporate private practice.
- Variety: Consider writing, consulting, and some industry jobs. Food inspection can also involve long hours. In private practice, consider rural, mixed, housecall, or relief practice.

7. Do I still want to work around or with animals?
- Not necessarily: Any job is open to you.
- Yes: Consider traditional practice, housecall or relief practice; shelter work; industry, in research and development; teaching; or government, in veterinary services, APHIS.
- If you want to work with small animals, consider working for APHIS in animal care; working for industry in R & D; or housecall or relief practice. Many government and industry jobs allow you to do relief work in private practice "on the side."
- If you want to work with horses, or horse owners, consider working for the APHIS in veterinary services; as an extension educator; or for industry, with companies that supply equine products or services.
- If you want to work with livestock, ranchers, or farmers, consider working in rural private practice; for a volunteer/assistance group in international positions; for the APHIS in Veterinary Services; as an extension educator; for the Agricultural Research Service (ARS); or for industry, with companies that supply livestock products or services.

8. Am I a new graduate, or do I have any private practice experience?
- No experience: Consider private practice, government FSIS, or if looking at industry, be ready to start in an area that may not be your primary interest, just to get your foot in the door. Do not consider consulting, housecall, or relief work until you have some experience.
- Experienced: Any job may be open to you.

9. Do I want to live in a city, or in a rural area?
- City: Most jobs are open to you.
- Rural: Consider rural private practice. Most state governments have veterinarians working in field offices. APHIS field service jobs may also be located in rural areas. Consulting or technical writing can also be done from a rural home. Some industry jobs allow you to live in at least a small city, where you could find a home in the semi-rural suburbs. Extension agents often live in rural areas.

10. Can I, or do I want to, work for someone else? If not, do I have what it takes to run my own business?
- Employee life is fine or preferred: Almost every career is open to you, except those listed next for self-employed.
- Self-employed is what I want: Consider private practice ownership, technical writing, consulting, housecall practice, or relief practice.

11. How do I feel about paperwork, policies, and regulations?
- That drives me nuts: Avoid working for associations, schools, the military, or government.

- I can live with that: Associations, schools, the military, or government jobs might suit you, as could corporate private practice.

Stuck? Take a Second Look

Are you placing so many limits on your job search that you have few choices left? If so, reconsider your "have-tos."

Why can't you move to a different location? Can you move to begin your career change, with the potential of moving back to your desired area later on? Can you work as an employee until you gain enough experience to start your own business? Can you enjoy your pets and spend time with animals, even if a new career doesn't involve hands-on animal work? (Get any job with regular hours and good pay, so you have time and energy to enjoy your own pets, train dogs, or ride your horse.) If you'd prefer an active job but can't find one, will the regular, predictable hours of a good-paying desk job allow you the time and energy to exercise (and money for club fees, ski vacations, and sports equipment)?

What are your priorities? What trade-offs are you willing to make? Is a job change really what you want? Make a list of the things you like and dislike about your current job. Which of these will be different in your new chosen field? Which may be the same? Will a career change really bring you the changes you desire, or will it simply postpone your troubles, eventually leaving you with the same problems you have now.

If you find that you've placed too many restrictions on your "requirements for a perfect job," then maybe there isn't one. Are you dissatisfied with your job, or is your dissatisfaction with other aspects of your life? That is, are you searching for an answer that cannot be found with a job change?

You may not be sure that you really want to change jobs. If that's the case, ask for a leave of absence and spend several weeks or months working with a volunteer or assistance group. Spend that time evaluating your life priorities. Or, look into short-term educational opportunities, externships, or short-term fellowships that allow you to explore a new field without making a long-term commitment. Test-drive a new career through a working vacation, such as those described on www.vocationvacations.com. Consult publications such as *What Color is Your Parachute?* by R. Bolles, and *Alternative Careers in Science: Leaving the Ivory Tower*, by C. Robbins-Roth.

Your search for the perfect job might result in the realization that you want to remain in your current niche in veterinary medicine. Great! Now you will feel less like complaining, and you will dwell less on your problems. Instead, you realize that your career path is the one you'd choose out of all the choices in this book. You can now get on with it, either finding a different position within that career path or making the best of your situation because you know you made a positive choice.

Another possibility is that you truly want to make a drastic change in your career. Perhaps you want to study art, accounting, or music. Such a dramatic change takes a lot of thought. A safe way to explore a new option is to study it part-time while continuing to work in the veterinary world (part-time or relief), thus keeping all your options open until you're sure enough to make the complete change. You will still find your veterinary experiences inform your future artistic or business experiences.

A final note about planning is necessary. There is emphasis in the management literature on planning and goal-setting as "the" route to success. Yet many successful people feel they "happened upon" an opportunity or a chance encounter which became a driving force in their career change. Let yourself be flexible enough to take advantage of unexpected opportunities and to change your goals as you learn and grow.

Chapter 2 Resources

Groups and web sites

American Association for the Advancement of Science (AAAS) fellowships, http://fellowships.aaas.org.

American Animal Hospital Association (AAHA), www.aahanet.org.

American Veterinary Medical Association (AVMA), 1931 N Meacham Road, Suite 100, Schaumburg, IL 60173; www.avma.org > public resources; www.avma.org > scientific resources; and www.avma.org > veterinary resources.

Center for Public and Corporate Veterinary Medicine (CPCVM), www.vetmed.vt.edu/org/md/cpcvm.

National Commission on Veterinary Economic Issues (NCVEI), www.ncvei.org > Resource library. (Note: The NCVEI may be forming a partnership with Kansas State University to form the Center for Veterinary Economics.)

PubMed, National Library of Medicine, www.nlm.nih.gov > pubmed.

Toastmasters, 23182 Arroyo Vista, Rancho Santa Margarita, CA 92688, www.toastmasters.org; phone: 949-858-8255; fax: 949-858-1207.

Veterinary Hospital Managers Association (VHMA), www.vhma.org; phone: 877-599-2707.

Veterinary Internship and Residency Matching Program, www.virmp.org.

VetPartners, www.vetpartners.org > Resources.

Vocation vacations, www.vocationvacations.com

Books and articles

American Veterinary Medical Association (AVMA)

AVMA, *2007 US Pet Ownership & Demographics Sourcebook,* www.avma.org > references > market statistics.

AVMA, *Report on Veterinary Compensation,* www.avma.org > Scientific resources.

AVMA, Center for Information Management, Demographic and Employment Trend Data (various years); www.AVMA.org > veterinary resources.

AVMA Communications Division, Shepherd A., Employment of Female and Male Graduates of US Veterinary Medical Schools and Colleges, 2009, *JAVMA,* October 1, 2009; 235(7): 830–832.

AVMA Communications Division, Shepherd A., Employment, starting salaries, and educational indebtedness of year-2009 graduates of US veterinary medical colleges, *JAVMA.* September 1, 2009, 235(5):523-526.

AVMA Communications Division, Shepherd A., Employment, starting salaries, and educational indebtedness of year-2010 graduates of US veterinary medical colleges. *JAVMA,* October 1, 2010; 237(7): 795-798

Bear, M., and T. Nixon, *Bears Guide to Earning Degrees by Distance Learning,* 16th edition (Ten Speed Press, 2006).

Beck, N, *Shifting Gears: Thriving in the New Economy,* (Harper Collins, 1992).

Bolles, R, *What Color is Your Parachute?* (Ten Speed Press, 2009).

Bridges, W, *Transitions: Making Sense of Life's Changes.* 2nd ed. (Da Capo Press, Cambridge MA 2004).

Choca, E. Confidence, Not Cash, Motivates Interns, *Trends magazine* Nov/Dec 2010.

Council for Adult & Experienced Learning, *Earn College Credit for What You Know,* 4th edition (Kendall/Hunt Publishing Company, 2006).

DVM Newsmagazine, www.dvm360.com.

Gordon, M., et al., Comparison of long-term financial implications for five veterinary career tracks, *JAVMA* Vol 237, No. 4, August 15, 2010: 369-375.

Lewis R, and J Klausner. Nontechnical Competencies Underlying Career Success as a Veterinarian. *JAVMA,* 2003; 222(12): 1690–1696.

Mize, D.A., *Complete Idiot's Guide to Going Back to College,* (Alpha, 2007).

National Research Council, Committee on Increasing Veterinary Involvement in Biomedical Research, National Need and Priorities for Veterinarians in Biomedical Research, (National Academies Press, 2004), www.nationalacademies.org/publications.

Public Health Reality Check. *DVM Newsmagazine* Opinion/letters, June 2009; 32.

Robbins-Roth, C, *Alternative Careers in Science: Leaving the Ivory Tower* (Academic Press 2005).

Veterinary Economics magazine, www.advanstar.com or www.dvm360.com.

Wilson, J, Inviting the Elephant into the Room: A Dialogue to Co-create a Financially Healthy Veterinary Profession. Presented at the North American Veterinary Conference 2008, www.vetpartners.org >Resources.

3 TRADITIONAL VETERINARY PRACTICE

A review of career choices in veterinary medicine begins with a discussion of traditional practice. This is the type of veterinary work most people envision when they say the word "veterinarian." Traditional practice refers to a hospital or clinic that runs as a small business and serves clients and their animals. Traditional *practice* may include both "Western" and "integrative" (alternative) *medicine,* as this chapter describes.

Data from the AVMA shows that of about 93,000 veterinarians in the US, at least 60,000 are working in private practice. Of those, 47,000 veterinarians are working in a practice that serves companion animals primarily or exclusively (2009).

Private Practice

Overview: Small to large animal practice

Traditional practice includes veterinarians who operate a small service business that provides health care for domestic animals. "Health care" includes preventive medicine, anesthesia, surgery, diagnosis and treatment of disease and injury, nutritional assessment, and emergency and intensive care.

The basic categories of private practice are first described, followed by details about each. The typical four-year veterinary program offered at US veterinary schools emphasizes small animal, large animal, and mixed animal practices. All veterinarians graduating from US veterinary schools will be prepared to enter private practice as described here, assuming they pass the appropriate testing and licensing requirements (see Appendix A).

The *small animal practice* (also called *companion animal practice*) typically is confined to dogs and cats. However, many small animal practitioners also work with birds, exotics, and pocket pets, which can include ferrets, guinea pigs, and reptiles. Companion animal practices may be located in urban or rural areas. Some veterinarians concentrate only on cats, exotics or birds, but such exclusivity requires the large population base of a city. Large cities are also the primary location of emergency clinics—veterinary hospitals that provide trauma management and critical care.

Traditional practice includes general private practice veterinarians as well as specialists. Specialists are described in Chapter 4. Traditional practice also includes housecall, mobile, and relief (temporary) veterinarians, which are discussed in Chapter 8.

A *mixed animal practice* provides services for a variety of domesticated animals—including dogs, cats, horses, sheep, cattle, pigs, poultry, and goats. Many mixed animal practitioners also work with exotics or pocket pets. The mixed animal practice is the typical practice across rural America. Since these veterinarians are often the only ones available to the public in remote areas, they must be willing to work on all animals that are presented to their clinics. Mixed animal practice is described in more detail in Chapter 5.

The *large animal practice* can be divided into equine and food /fiber animal practice. Food animals include sheep, pigs, poultry, and cattle, as well as ostriches and other exotic species. Some veterinarians work with all large animals, whereas others limit their practices to one or two species, or even to a specific type of animal within the species. For instance, within equine practice are veterinarians who may work only with race horses, show horses, or backyard "pleasure" horses; bovine practitioners may work only with dairy or beef cattle. Large animal practice is described in more detail in Chapter 5.

Daily work

Veterinarians examine, diagnose, and treat animals brought by their owners. Daily work is spent examining patients, doing medical procedures, performing anesthesia and surgery, and evaluating laboratory tests and radiographs. Minor procedures fill the day, from cleaning a cat abscess to removing stickers from between a dog's toes. Many practitioners view the "fun" side of practice as evaluating complex medical cases to find a diagnosis, or performing surgery.

One amusing fantasy is that of a conveyor belt, which would transport animals from their owners' arms to a room where the veterinarian performs necessary services and then places the animal back on the belt for its return trip to the owner. The reality, though, is that veterinarians spend a significant amount of time working with *people*, sometimes in difficult and emotional situations.

Daily work includes talking to clients and interacting with the veterinary team. That team, at a minimum, includes the practice owner (who may be *the* veterinarian), a receptionist, and an assistant (who may be a credentialed veterinary technician). Larger hospitals may have many other team members to add to this list, such as associate and owner veterinarians, administrator, practice manager, client services team members, technician team members (credentialed technicians plus assistants), and kennel assistants.

Pros and cons

> About half my time is devoted to business: Paying bills, ordering drugs,
> or calling the plumber.—Beth Miller, DVM, Little Rock, AR.

One concept is frequently overlooked: *veterinarians operate a small service business.* Veterinarians who are practice owners don't just practice medicine and surgery; they have to do all the work involved in running a small business—including supervising employees, marketing their business, and collecting payment from clients. Veterinarians share this dilemma with many other small business owners. Although they may be qualified to do their "service," owning a business requires doing well at their second job of small business management.

The amount of time the owner spends on management varies with whether and how much they utilize the services of practice managers or administrators. However, it is a myth that someone can simply hire a manager and totally ignore the business, since the owner is ultimately responsible for the business and "managing the manager."

Even associates (employee veterinarians) must have basic business knowledge. AAHA's *Associates Survival Guide* is great if you're just starting out. AAHA also offers multi-day management seminars (www.aahanet.org). See also books and magazines on veterinary practice management, such as

- *Client Satisfaction Pays: Quality Service for Practice Success*, by C. Smith.
- *Contracts, Benefits, and Practice Management*, by J. Wilson.
- *DVM Newsmagazine*.
- *Financial and Productivity Pulsepoints: Vital Statistics for Your Veterinary Practice*, by AAHA Press.
- *Practice Made Perfect, A Guide to Veterinary Practice Management*, by M.L. Heinke.
- *Team Satisfaction Pays: Organizational Development for Practice Success*, by C. Smith, includes tips on working with the people in any private practice.
- *Veterinary Economics magazine*.
- *Veterinary Fee Reference: Vital Statistics for Your Veterinary Practice*, by AAHA Press.

Veterinarians in private practice must come to terms with conflict of interest issues. Three conflicts of interest are inherent in their work: 1) the desire to hold down costs for the client versus the duty to act as strong health-care advocates using medical evidence for decisions; 2) the need to earn money for the business to survive versus the health-advocate role based on medical evidence; and 3) the divided loyalty between the interests of the pet and the interests of the client.

The tough reality in the US is that health care for animals is not free, yet love for animals causes veterinarians to feel torn between providing care and paying the bills. Veterinarians who are successful in mastering medical care, human psychology, and business skills are the ones who enjoy their jobs. They may also be the most financially successful private practitioners. Others may find themselves reaching for other choices, including housecall or relief practice (Chapter 8). Another alternative is to work in corporate practice, where others take care of much of the "business side."

With the increasing number of specialists in private practice, there is increasing pressure on general practitioners to avoid performing certain procedures and to instead refer those to a specialist. Disagreement exists between older practitioners, who became accustomed to performing many procedures, and younger veterinarians, who may have been taught to avoid some procedures and instead refer those to a specialist.

Most private practitioners belong to the AVMA, which publishes the *Journal of the American Veterinary Medical Association* (*JAVMA*) and the *American Journal of Veterinary Research*. The AVMA web site (www.avma.org) contains a large amount of information, including links to your state and local veterinary associations. The AVMA also publishes the *US Pet Ownership & Demographics Sourcebook* every other year.

Pay

Veterinarians in private practice may be paid a salary, paid based on production, or paid a combination thereof. With production-based pay, the doctor is paid a percentage of gross income, with "gross income" including or excluding certain categories of services or products. Practice owners are also paid those ways, but in addition they receive a portion of the profits of the hospital. Details about pay structure are discussed in other sources, such as *Contracts, Benefits, and Practice Management,* by J. Wilson; AAHA's *Compensation and Benefits Review,* and *Veterinary Economics* magazine.

According to the AVMA, the average starting salary for new graduates entering private practice in 2010 was $67,000, ranging from $38,000 for equine-only practices to $71,000 for small animal only practices (Table 3.1)

Table 3.2 lists median income by practice type. At the time of this publication, statistics by ownership status were not yet available for 2009, but the 2007 numbers show the dramatic difference that ownership makes. The median income for all private practitioners was $91,000, and the median income of all private practice owners was $121,000, compared with an associate median income of $79,000.

Table 3.1: Mean starting salary by practice type

Practice type	Associate median income
Companion animal	$71,000
Mixed animal	62,000
Food animal	69,000
Equine	38,000

Source: AVMA, 2010 (numbers rounded)

Table 3.2: Median income by practice type

Practice type	Associate median income	Owner median income
Companion animal	$85,000	$133,000
Mixed animal	67,000	103,000
Food animal	76,000	139,000
Equine	79,000	127,000

Source: AVMA, 2007 Report on Veterinary Compensation.

Companion Animal Practice

The typical small animal practice serves clients who own cats and dogs. However, many of these veterinarians also work with pocket pets, birds, and other "exotic" species. Companion animal veterinarians may become specialists in canine and feline medicine, through the American Board of Veterinary Practitioners (see Chapter 4).

The average companion animal practice includes two veterinarians, although larger practices are gradually becoming more common. The typical veterinarian works 40 to 50 hours per week, including some Saturdays. Shorter workdays and part-time work are possible in practices with more doctors. Veterinarians working in locations that have an emergency clinic will have more definite working hours than those who must care for their own clients' emergencies. Veterinarians working in more remote locations could potentially work on a broader range of conditions than those who work in cities with specialists readily available for referral. (See Chapter 5 for a discussion of rural practices.)

Two associations are of particular importance to companion animal practices. The American Animal Hospital Association (www.aahanet.org) offers a wide range of publications, courses, and resources; certifies practices that meet certain criteria; and publishes *AAHA Trends*, which deals with the news and business sides of the practice, and the *Journal of the American Animal Hospital Association*, which deals with the medical side (www.aahanet.org). Also of interest is the American Pet Products Association (APPA), which conducts a biennial survey of pet owners (www.americanpetproducts.org).

To apply

Companion animal practice jobs are advertised through the AVMA Career Center, the AAHA Job Bank, in veterinary state association newsletters, and on a wide variety of job-related web sites (see Chapter 1). It is highly recommended that you spend at least a day in any practice where you are considering accepting a job. Interviews alone cannot give you the same first-hand information. Explore the practice philosophy to be sure it matches with your own approach.

Corporate veterinary practice

Although any practice may be run as an incorporated business, the term "corporate practice" has been used to describe a situation in which several veterinary hospitals owned by one entity are run as a large business, often with practices in many cities and states.

The larger the practice, and the more locations it occupies, the more it must organize and manage. That can save money when compared with the typical geographic area that has, perhaps, 10 different practices, each with its own X-ray machine, surgical suite, and so on. The basic approach of a corporate practice is to reduce costs and streamline procedures such that veterinarians can concentrate on practicing medicine and surgery and spend less time running the business.

Comparing corporate practice to individual ownership

Although there are exceptions, veterinarians employed by corporate practices may get better benefits compared with that offered in typical private practices, which often don't provide any benefits at all. They also may be able to work more predictable hours.

Corporate practices may offer more or different opportunities for advancement, as is illustrated by the profile of Banfield's Director of Medical Informatics in Chapter 10.

Although all private practices do so, corporate practices may create more standards and policies, for many reasons. With more staff members comes an increasing involvement of professional management, and clearer adherence to federal and state employment laws, many of which do not apply to smaller practices. For example, the Family Medical Leave Act applies only to businesses with more than 50 employees.

Creation of medical and business standards reflects an effort to avoid inconsistencies among the various practice locations and among veterinarians' approaches. Whether that interferes with the individual veterinarian's ability to practice good medicine has been the subject of considerable debate. The reach of these policies varies tremendously among different corporate practices; some corporate practices are hands-off from veterinarians' daily medical choices, and still give doctors the autonomy to make decisions on a case-by-case basis, whereas other corporations have strict protocols for every diagnosis, and still others are somewhere between these extremes.

Lack of control over business decisions may create conflicts for some veterinarians (for example, in deciding which drugs and medications to keep on hand). Conversely, being less involved in business may be desirable for many other veterinarians.

Standards and protocols are not unique to corporate practice. Practices accredited by the American Animal Hospital Association must meet standards and criteria for that accreditation. Also, small practices create standards—it's just that the veterinarians may be "closer to the decision" in terms of being able to make changes. What's more, groups such as AAHA and the AAFP are increasingly creating medical "guidelines" for approaches to various medical conditions. These papers are intended to guide practitioners in decision-making; they do not dictate protocols for treatment, and are not intended to create a legal standard of care.

There are many shades of gray when you consider the types of practice that fall between the solo practitioner and the large corporate practice. Large urban practices may employ 5, 10, or 20 veterinarians at one hospital. They may provide additional services, such as grooming and boarding, and they may sell pet products. They may hire a business manager so the veterinarians can spend more time being doctors and less time with running the business. At the other end of the spectrum is one of the larger corporate practices, Banfield, which is owned by Mars (the candy company).

One difference is that small private practices are usually owned by one or more of the veterinarians who work there, whereas corporate practices have central ownership. However, the issue of veterinarian ownership is a separate one from the issue of corporate versus small practice. A non-veterinarian or a veterinarian may own or co-own a practice of any size or one that is organized in any way. Practice owners may or may not work directly in, or manage, a practice that they own. And finally, state laws may allow or disallow non-veterinarian practice ownership.

The difference between veterinarians working in corporate practice and in traditional practice is one of business management, and is not a difference in careers per se. The veterinarian in a small traditional practice will spend a significantly greater amount of time doing business management than will a veterinarian in a larger practice. Veterinarians interested in a career in traditional practice should examine their attitudes toward, and interest in, business when deciding where to look for jobs.

Two articles of interest regarding corporate veterinary practices are those by G. Glassman in *Veterinary Economics* and by H.B. Hayes in *Virginia Business News*.

Major corporate veterinary hospitals include the following:
- Banfield, the Pet Hospital (www.banfield.com)
- BrightHeart Veterinary Centers (www.brightheartvet.com)
- HealthyPet (www.healthypet.net)
- National Veterinary Associates (www.nvaonline.com)
- Veterinary Centers of America (www.vcapets.com)

Feline medicine

> My interest in cats and their challenging nature made me sure feline practice was what I wanted to do. They are so different from other species. I worked here during high school, returned here after vet school, and bought into the practice when given the opportunity. — Cathy King, DVM, co-owner, Feline Medical Clinic, Vancouver, WA.

> I was a little concerned, when starting a job at an exclusively feline clinic, that one species might become repetitive, but the variety of patients and clients keep life interesting every day.— Christy Novick, DVM, associate veterinarian, Feline Medical Clinic, Vancouver, WA.

Veterinarians who work with cats usually do so as part of a companion animal practice. However, there is a trend toward establishment of feline-only practices in many cities. Cats are not small dogs, but have unique personalities and disease processes.

With regard to feline-only practices, cat owners appreciate the quiet nature of the waiting room, the skillful handling of the feline patients, and the understanding of the feline species by the entire patient care team. From a practice management standpoint, a feline-only practice allows for more exclusive equipment, pharmacy, and pet food inventory. Hospital design is simplified, and team training and education can be concentrated on one species. Species-specific practice does, however, limit the potential pool of clients, and this may limit where such a practice can be established.

Qualifications

Learn more about feline medicine to be successful. Sources of information include the American Association of Feline Practitioners (AAFP; www.catvets.com), the CATalyst Council (www.catalystcouncil.org), the International Society of Feline Medicine (www.isfm.net) and the Feline Advisory Bureau (www.fabcats.org). Veterinarians may become specialists in feline medicine, through the American Board of Veterinary Practitioners (see Chapter 4).

Avian medicine

My greatest joy in avian medicine is to almost daily continue to "go where no one has gone before!" This is what makes it challenging and stimulating. I find avian medicine to be a special niche. The work is very difficult. Your patients often present in fragile condition. Most of my clients are Internet educated and frequently coming off a less than stellar experience at another vet clinic. Their bird may be a decades-old family member and the owners are extremely emotionally attached to them. These clients can stress even the most capable of staff.

While the medical information available has increased dramatically over the last 20 years, I daily see problems I have never dealt with before— even after 25 years of practice. I am so busy I can hardly see straight. There is a huge market out there for anyone who wishes to excel in avian medicine—Marli Styskel Lintner, DVM, Avian Medical Clinic, Lake Oswego, OR.

Veterinarians who work with pet birds usually do so as part of a companion animal practice. However, a few veterinarians have birds-only practices. According to the APPA, about five percent of US households owned a bird in 2008, which is about six million households. Bird-owning households had an average of 2.5 birds. Although the numbers are lower than households with cats or dogs, this is a market that is *greatly* underserved. A housecall practice can be useful for work with pet birds (see Chapter 8.)

Some avian veterinarians work with backyard poultry or with ostrich and emu farmers. Others work on larger poultry operations. These are described in Chapter 5 as part of "food animal" medicine.

Qualifications

Veterinarians should participate in lectures and "wet labs" (hands-on learning) to ensure they have the appropriate skills to handle pet birds. Such courses are offered at many large veterinary conferences. In addition, the annual meeting of the Association of Avian Veterinarians (AAV, www.aav.org) offers great courses on birds and the American Board of Veterinary Practitioners (ABVP, www.abvp.com) can help a veterinarian to become a specialist in avian medicine. There is a separate specialty group for poultry veterinarians (acpv.info; see Chapter 4, Specialists).

Exotic animal and pocket pet medicine

Exotic animal medicine is a growing area for companion animal veterinarians. Over the last decade, households have become smaller, and pets ranging from rabbits to hedgehogs are becoming more popular. Exotic pets also include snakes, rats, ferrets and fish.

The APPA's biennial survey of pet owners has categories including dog, cat, fish, reptile, equine, bird, and "small animal." (The general use of the term "small animal" in veterinary medicine refers to dogs, cats, and many other pets; however, the APPA survey defines that term as "chinchilla, ferret, gerbil, hamster, hermit crab, mouse, rat, pot-bellied pig, prairie dog and rabbit.") According to the APPA, households owning fish, reptiles, and those "small" animals presented the highest increases in the number of households owning a particular species in the last 10 years. They report that the number of US households that owned fish, reptiles, and small animals in 2009 were 14 million, 4.7 million, and 5.3 million, respectively.

There are very few "exotics-only" veterinarians. Large metropolitan areas may have enough of a case load to support a veterinarian who specializes in exotics, but most veterinarians will need to combine this with a more traditional small animal practice (i.e., cats and dogs) in order to make a living. A housecall practice is ideally situated to work with exotics that might be difficult to transport (See Chapter 8.) Any practice looking for ways to grow can benefit from seeing exotic pets, since so few veterinarians offer this service.

Qualifications

Exotic practice is not one you can just dabble in; seeing only a few cases isn't enough of a case load to sustain one's knowledge. Students can learn more by taking advantage of externships to work in practices that see many exotic species or by spending time at a veterinary college that has a specific exotics program, such as the University of Tennessee, University of California–Davis, Auburn University, and the University of Pennsylvania.

Post-graduate internships are also available. Veterinary colleges that may offer internships in exotic medicine include those in Texas, Pennsylvania, New York (Cornell), Georgia, Colorado, and Massachusetts (Tufts).

Additional information can be learned at veterinary conferences. For example, recent topics at the North American Veterinary Conference (www.navc.org) included "Incorporating non-traditional species into your practice," "Reptile training," "Common clinical presentations in geckos," and "Performing anesthesia on ferrets, rabbits, and rodents."

Associations such as the Association of Exotic Mammal Veterinarians (AEMV, www.aemv.org) hold annual CE meetings and programs geared specifically for practitioners working with exotics. AEMV members also get a subscription to the *Journal of Exotic Pet Medicine*. Also check out the Association of Reptilian and Amphibian Veterinarians (ARAV, www.arav.org).

Veterinarians may become board-certified specialists in exotic mammal medicine, avian medicine, and/or reptile and amphibian medicine (see Chapters 4 and 6).

Emergency practice

In rural settings, veterinarians answer their own emergency calls. Areas with more than a few practices may simply rotate among local practices for after-hours emergency calls. However, the trend in most cities is to have clinics specifically focused on emergency and critical care of companion animals. Sometimes a group of private practices may join together to create a cooperatively owned emergency clinic. Other emergency clinics are owned by the emergency veterinarians themselves or by corporate practices.

Emergency practices are always open at night and on weekends. In some larger cities, they are open 24 hours per day. Such 24-hour facilities may also include specialists board-certified in other areas such as internal medicine and surgery. Emergency practices may have more diagnostic tools available than do daytime practices because laboratory results are often needed in a hurry. They also include full surgical facilities with trained technicians. If you like working nights and don't mind weekends, the pay can be great for very few days worked per week.

Emergency work is always exciting because you never know what will come through the door. Work can include potentially high-stress situations with high-stress clients and their very ill pets. You will see more patient death than in general practice.

Organizations that can provide information on emergency veterinary practices include the Veterinary Emergency and Critical Care Society (http://veccs.org), the Veterinary Emergency and Specialty Practice Association (www.vespassociation.org), and the American College of Veterinary Emergency and Critical Care (http://acvecc. org). AAHA provides information through its Referral Guidelines (www.aahanet.org/ resources >guidelines.

Qualifications

Emergency veterinarians may hold only a veterinary degree, may have completed an internship in emergency and critical care, or may be board-certified in emergency and critical care medicine (see Chapter 4.) Emergency doctor pay is usually salary-based rather than production-based because case load can vary so greatly from one shift to the next.

Sample job announcement: Emergency veterinarian

> This 24–hour hospital is staffed with the area's best veterinarians and technicians. We are in a very upscale area and have an affluent and loyal clientele. Work 6 pm to 7 am, 1 week on then 1 week off, thus providing great flexibility. Generous base + 25% bonus. The ideal candidate will have a state DVM license, a strong interest in emergency/critical care, and ideally at least 1–2 yrs of clinical experience, preferably in an ER setting. Also needs to be team player with good communication skills, and teacher/mentor for techs and staff.

Special Interests

Private practitioners may focus on many different areas of interest, which include different species (discussed in following chapters) as well as different aspects of medicine and surgery.

The word "specialist" has a legal meaning and refers to board-certified specialists, which are described in Chapter 4. Controversy exists in the profession about which veterinarians may be qualified to perform certain procedures. For example, many private practitioners have an interest in dentistry, behavior, or surgery, yet are not board-certified in those areas. They must take care in the way they describe their services so the client understands the level of expertise provided.

Areas of interest include every aspect of medicine and surgery. Some veterinarians enjoy dermatology, while others prefer dentistry. Among those who prefer surgery are those who prefer orthopedics and those who like soft-tissue surgery. There are veterinarians who focus on canine reproduction and breeding, and others who work only with racing greyhounds.

To find a group of veterinarians who share your interest, just enter search words [veterinarian], [association], and the word describing the interest, into any search engine. For example, a search of [veterinarian greyhound association] revealed that there is a Society of Greyhound Veterinarians (www.greyhoundvets.co.uk), and a search using [dermatology] led to the World Congress of Veterinary Dermatology Association (www.wcvda.com). Practitioners may learn more about their area of interest through a variety of continuing education courses offered through those associations.

Behavior

Every pet owner has to learn to communicate with their pet and to manage its behavior. Basic training is easily taught through means such as puppy classes. The idea of cat and kitten socialization classes is only beginning to take root. While these classes do prevent some behavior problems, the veterinarian's expertise is needed when problem behavior persists or does not respond to basic training.

Many veterinarians provide consultation with pet owners regarding behavior issues. Housecall veterinarians are particularly well suited to this type of consultation, since behavior can then be observed as it occurs. Veterinarians may also become board-certified specialists in behavior (see Chapter 4).

For information, contact the American Veterinary Society of Animal Behavior (www.avsabonline.org) and the American College of Veterinary Behaviorists (www.dacbv.org).

The American Association of Feline Practitioners (www.catvets.com) has created "Feline Handling Guidelines," a paper which describes some of the actions veterinarians can take to improve interactions between humans and cats.

Dentistry

Dentistry has grown into a field of its own as awareness of its importance increases. Equine dentistry is described in Chapter 5, under equine practice. Other resources include:

- AAHA Dental Care Guidelines for Dogs and Cats, www.aahanet.org > resources > guidelines.
- Academy of Veterinary Dentistry, www.avdonline.org.
- American Veterinary Dental Society, www.avds-online.org.
- Veterinary Dental Forum, www.veterinarydentalforum.com.

Hospice and palliative care

Hospice and palliative care are becoming more important in veterinary medicine. Any practitioner may offer this service, but it is more commonly provided by a housecall veterinarian (Chapter 8) or oncologist (Chapter 4). Resources include:

- Animal Hospice Compassionate Crossings, www.animalhospice.org.
- *AVMA Guidelines for Veterinary Hospice Care,* www.avma.org > products.
- Colorado State University Animal Cancer Center, www.animalcancercenter.org.
- Delta Society, an international resource for the human-animal bond, www.deltasociety.org.
- International Association for Animal Hospice and Palliative Care, www.iaahpc.org
- More Veterinarians Offer Hospice Care for Pets, *JAVMA News* by A Rezendes.
- Nikki Hospice Foundation for Pets and the Annual Symposium on Veterinary Hospice Care, www.pethospice.org.
- Spirits in Transition, www.spiritsintransition.org.
- Veterinary Cancer Society, www.vetcancersociety.org

Table 3.3: Integrative medicine definitions

Holistic: Relating to or concerned with wholes or with complete systems.
Homeopathy: A system of medical practice that uses tiny doses of a remedy that would in healthy animals produce symptoms similar to those of the disease. Little if any evidence exists to support the effectiveness of homeopathy.
Hospice: A facility or program designed to provide a caring environment for meeting the physical and emotional needs of the terminally ill, with a focus on comfort and quality of life.
Massage: Manipulation of tissues (as by rubbing, stroking, kneading, or tapping) with the hand or an instrument especially for therapeutic purposes. Note: Some state regulators differentiate between "massage" and "massage therapy." The latter may be considered to be the practice of medicine, and thus must be done by or under the supervision of a veterinarian, depending on state law.
Palliative care: Medical or comfort care that reduces the severity of a disease or slows its progress rather than providing a cure.
Physical therapy: Therapy for the preservation, enhancement, or restoration of movement and physical function impaired or threatened by disability, injury, or disease that utilizes therapeutic exercise, physical modalities (as massage and electrotherapy), assistive devices, and patient education and training.
Rehabilitation therapy: The physical restoration by therapeutic measures. In veterinary medicine, includes the application of physical therapy techniques to animals.

Derived from Merriam Webster's Online Dictionary

Integrative medicine

Some veterinarians want to stay in private practice (traditional *career*) and practice *alternative medicine*. The definition of alternative medicine changes over time, as formerly "alternative" practices blend into "mainstream" medicine. However, the term generally refers to areas such as veterinary chiropractic medicine, homeopathy, and acupuncture. A new term, *integrative medicine*, more closely reflects the current approach to blending new and old approaches.

Many veterinarians integrate one or more of these modalities into their companion animal or equine practices. Others focus solely on one aspect of integrative medicine. For example, a few veterinarians work solely in rehabilitation medicine or acupuncture.

Many terms relating to these approaches are misunderstood and misused. Learn the correct definitions of all these terms so you are clear about each. For example, many doctors use solely "Western" medicine but still take a "holistic" approach, which means that they consider all factors that may influence the animal's health. See this Chapter's resource list for several pertinent books, and also see these resources:

- Alternative veterinary medicine, www.altvetmed.org.
- American Holistic Veterinary Medical Association, www.ahvma.org.
- AVMA, Guidelines for Complementary and Alternative Veterinary Medicine, www. AVMA.org >issues >policy.

Rehabilitation

The field of rehabilitation covers several areas of interest. Some veterinarians have additional training in orthopedic surgery, pain management, acupuncture, massage, chiropractic and/or rehabilitation that has led to specialization or certification in these fields. One of the leading university programs in veterinary rehabilitation is at the University of Tennessee, which offers a certificate program in canine and equine rehabilitation for veterinarians, veterinary technicians, and physical therapists. That university's Canine Rehabilitation Resource web site provides general information, job links, and a list of educational conferences (www.canineequinerehab.com).

Another certification program is offered through the Wellington Rehabilitation Institute in Florida (www.caninerhabinstitute.com). Colorado State University offers a veterinary medical massage course (www.colovma.org). The American Association of Rehabilitation Veterinarians held its first meeting in 2008 (www.rehabvets.evetsites.net).

A new specialty, the American College of Veterinary Sports Medicine and Rehabilitation (www.vsmr.org), was approved in 2010. Veterinarians may become specialists in canine or equine rehabilitation. See Chapter 4, Specialists. Additional information about rehabilitation can be found at the following web sites:

- American Massage Therapy Association, whose web site lists schools and courses in animal massage, www.amtamassage.org.
- Equissage, a training facility for massage continuing education, www.equissage.com.
- Federation of State Boards of Physical Therapy, Physical Therapy State Practice Acts, www.fsbpt.org.
- International Association of Veterinary Rehabilitation and Physical Therapy, www. iavrpt.org.
- National Board of Certification for Animal Acupressure and Massage, provides a Scope of Practice and Code of Ethics for animal massage and acupressure, committee listings, and other resources, http://nbcaam.net.
- National Certification Board for Therapeutic Massage and Bodywork, www.ncbtmb. org.

Also see the following publications:

- *Canine Massage: A Complete Reference Manual,* by J. Hourdebaight.
- *Canine Rehabilitation and Physical Therapy,* by D.L. Mills et al.
- *Essential Facts of Physiotherapy in Dogs and Cats,* by B. Bockstahler et al.

Acupuncture and chiropractic

Veterinary colleges in the US teach little, if any, acupuncture or chiropractic techniques. Exceptions include the acupuncture courses taught at a few veterinary schools (e.g., Pennsylvania, Florida, and Minnesota). One good reference is A. Schoen's book, *Veterinary Acupuncture.*

For those who are interested, several groups offer information and courses for graduate veterinarians to gain certification in the areas of acupuncture and chiropractic. Most programs are completed over a year's time and require travel to a location for a week at a time to complete modules (locations vary by session and occur throughout the US and Canada).

Certification programs are available for veterinary chiropractic through the Animal Chiropractic Certification Commission of the American Veterinary Chiropractic Association (www.animalchiropractic.org), which has over 600 members. The AVCA professional certification program is open to licensed doctors of chiropractic and of veterinary medicine. There were over 300 AVCA Certified Veterinarians in 2010.

The International Veterinary Acupuncture Society (www.ivas.org) offers post-doctoral education for certification in Veterinary Acupuncture and also in Veterinary Chinese Herbal Medicine. IVAS has about 1,800 active members and has certified approximately 5,000 veterinarians worldwide in the last 37 years.

Chapter 3 Resources

Groups and web sites

Academy of Veterinary Homeopathy, PO Box 9280, Wilmington, DE 19809; www.theavh.org phone: 866-652-1590.
AltVetMed, www.altvetmed.org.
American Animal Hospital Association (AAHA), www.aahanet.org; phone: 800-883-6301; *AAHA Guidelines (Referral guidelines; Dental care guidelines; Mentor guidelines)* www.aahanet.org >resources > guidelines; multi-day management seminars listed at www.aahanet.org > education.
American Association of Feline Practitioners (AAFP), www.catvets.com.
    AAFP Feline Handling Guidelines, in press 2011.
American Association of Rehabilitation Veterinarians, www.rehabvets.evetsites.net.
American Board of Veterinary Practitioners (ABVP), www.abvp.com.
American College of Veterinary Emergency and Critical Care, http://acvecc.org.
American Holistic Veterinary Medical Association (AHVMA), c/o Dr. Carvel G. Tiekert, 2214 Old Emmorton Rd., Bel Air, MD 21015; www.ahvma.org; phone: 410-569-0795; fax: 410-569-2346; e-mail: office@ahvma.org.
American Massage Therapy Association, www.amtamassage.org; phone: 877-905-2700.
American Pet Products Association (APPA), www.americanpetproducts.org.
American Veterinary Chiropractic Association, 442154 E. 140 Rd., Bluejacket, OK 74333; www.animalchiropractic.org; phone: 918-784-2231, fax: 918-784-2675; e-mail: avcainfo@junct.com.
American Veterinary Medical Association (AVMA), www.avma.org; phone: 800-677-3726.
American Veterinary Society of Animal Behavior. www.avsabonline.org.
Animal Hospice Compassionate Crossings, www.animalhospice.org.
Association of Avian Veterinarians, www.aav.org.
Association of Exotic Mammal Veterinarians, www.aemv.org.
Association of Reptilian and Amphibian Veterinarians, www.arav.org.
CATalyst Council, www.catalystcouncil.org.
Colorado State University (CSU) Veterinary Medical Massage course, www.colovma.org; phone: 303-318-0447.
    CSU Animal Cancer Center, 970-297-4195; www.animalcancercenter.org.
Delta Society, 425-679-5500; www.deltasociety.org.

Equissage, www.equissage.com; phone: 1-800-272-2044.

Federation of State Boards of Physical Therapy (FSBPT), Physical Therapy State Practice Acts, www.fsbpt.org; phone: 703-299-3100.

Feline Advisory Bureau, www.fabcats.org.

International Association for Hospice and Palliative Care (IAAHPC), www.iaahpc.org.

International Association of Veterinary Rehabilitation and Physical Therapy (IAVRPT), www.iavrpt.org.

International Veterinary Acupuncture Society (IVAS), P.O. Box 271395, Ft. Collins, CO, 80527-1395; www.ivas.org; phone: 970-266-0666; fax: 970-266-0777.

International Society of Feline Medicine, www.isfm.net.

National Board of Certification for Animal Acupressure and Massage (NBCAAM), http://nbcaam.net; e-mail: info@nbcaam.net.

National Certification Board for Therapeutic Massage and Bodywork (NCBTMB), www.ncbtmb.org; phone: 800-296-0664.

Nikki Hospice Foundation for Pets, 400 New Bedford Drive, Vallejo, CA 94591; www.pethospice.org; phone: 707-557-8595.

Society of Greyhound Veterinarians, www.greyhoundvets.co.uk.

Spirits in Transition, www.spiritsintransition.org.

University of Tennessee, Canine Rehabilitation Resource, www.canineequinerehab.com; phone: 800-272-2044

University of Tennessee, facilities offering physical therapy/rehabilitation, www.utc.edu/Faculty/David-Levine/Veterinary.HTM#Clinics; phone: 423-425-4111.

Veterinary Cancer Society, www.vetcancersociety.org; phone: 619-474-8929.

Veterinary Economics, 8033 Flint, Lenexa, KS 66214; www.advanstar.com or www.dvm360.com; phone: 800-255-6864.

Veterinary Emergency and Critical Care Society, 6335 Camp Bullis Road, Suite 12, San Antonio, TX, 78257; 210-698-5575, Fax 210-698-7138, http://veccs.org, email info@veccs.org.

Veterinary Emergency and Specialty Practice Association, www.vespassociation.org.

Veterinary Dermatology Association, www.wcvda.com.

Veterinary Hospital Managers Association (VHMA), www.vhma.org; phone: 877-599-2707.

Wellington Rehabilitation Institute, Wellington FL; www.caninerehabinstitute.com.

Books and articles

American Animal Hospital Association

Associates Survival Guide (AAHA Press, 2005).

Compensation and Benefits Review (AAHA Press, published periodically), www.aahanet.org > resources.

Dental Care Guidelines for Dogs and Cats, www.aahanet.org/resources/guidelines.aspx.

Financial and Productivity Pulsepoints: Vital Statistics for Your Veterinary Practice (AAHA Press, published periodically).

Referral Guidelines, www.aahanet.org/resources/guidelines.aspx.

Veterinary Fee Reference: Vital Statistics for Your Veterinary Practice (AAHA Press, published periodically), www.aahanet.org.

American Veterinary Medical Association (AVMA), www.avma.org.

AVMA Communications Division, Shepherd A., Employment of Female and Male Graduates of US Veterinary Medical Schools and Colleges, 2009, *JAVMA*, October 1, 2009; 235(7): 830–832 (similar report published periodically).

AVMA Communications Division, Shepherd A., Employment, Starting Salaries, and Educational Indebtedness of Year-2009 Graduates of US Veterinary Medical Colleges. *JAVMA*, September 1, 2009; 235(5): 523–526 (similar report published periodically).

Guidelines for Complementary and Alternative Veterinary Medicine, www.AVMA.org >issues> policy.

Guidelines for Veterinary Hospice Care, www.avma.org > products.

Report on Veterinary Compensation, 2009 (published biennially), www.avma.org > scientific resources.

US Pet Ownership & Demographics Sourcebook, www.avma.org > reference.

Bockstahler, B., et al., *Essential Facts of Physiotherapy in Dogs and Cats* (Lifelearn, 2005), www.lifelearn.com.

DVM Newsmagazine, www.dvm360.com.

Glassman, G., The New Era of Corporate Practice, (presents interesting facts regarding purchasing and statistics), *Veterinary Economics*, November 2007; www.dvm360.com.

Hayes, H.B., The Rise of the Corporate Veterinarian, Growing Presence of National Chains in Virginia Reflects Shifts in Industry, *Virginia Business News*, August 2006; www.virginiabusiness.com.

Heinke, M., and J.B. McCarthy, *Practice Made Perfect, A Guide to Veterinary Practice Management* (AAHA Press, 2001).

Hourdebaight, J., *Canine Massage: A Complete Reference Manual* (Dogwise Publishing, 2004).

Lloyd, J. W., Current Economic Trends Affecting the Veterinary Medical Profession, *Vet Clin Small Anim*, 2006; 36: 267–279.

Merriam Webster's Online Dictionary, www.merriam-webster.com.

Mills, D. L., et al., *Canine Rehabilitation and Physical Therapy*, (Elsevier. 2004).

Rezendes A, More Veterinarians Offer Hospice Care for Pets. *JAVMA News* August 15, 200Schoen, A. M., *Veterinary Acupuncture: Ancient Art to Modern Medicine* (Mosby, 2001).

Schwartz, C, *Four Paws, Five Directions: A Guide to Chinese Medicine for Cats and Dogs* (Celestial Arts, 2004).

Shojai, A, *New Choices in Natural Healing for Dogs and Cats* (St Martin's Press, 2001).

Smith, C.A., *Team Satisfaction Pays: Organizational Development for Practice Success*, (Smith Veterinary Consulting, 2008).

Smith, C.A., *Client Satisfaction Pays: Quality Service for Practice Success*, (AAHA press 2009).

Veterinarians www.avma.org > Animal Health > AVMA brochures > Veterinarians.

Veterinary Economics magazine, www.advanstar.com or www.dvm360.com.

Wilson, J., et al., *Contracts, Benefits, and Practice Management for the Veterinary Profession* (Priority Press, 2009).

Wynn, S. G., *Emerging Therapies: Using Herbs and Nutraceuticals for Small Animals* (AAHA Press, 1999).

Wynn, S. G., and S. Marsden, *Manual of Natural Veterinary Medicine: Science and Tradition* (Mosby, 2002).

.

4 VETERINARY SPECIALISTS

> The development of clinical specialties in veterinary medicine began with the recognition of the American College of Veterinary Radiology by the AVMA in 1962. From the 1960s until the mid-1980s, specialty practice was primarily confined to veterinary teaching hospitals. Since the mid-1980s, however, there has been an explosive increase in the number of private specialty practices, particularly practices that treat companion animals—John A. E. Hubbell et al., in *JAVMA*.

Veterinarians may choose to specialize in one area of interest. This chapter is fairly short since the actual jobs that specialists can fill are included in traditional practice, industry, academia, and government (Chapters 3, 11, 14-18). Veterinary students get a good idea of the range of specialties within veterinary medicine while they are in school because they are taught by many of these specialists. However, if you are not yet in veterinary school, you may not be aware of the potential areas in which veterinarians can specialize. It is also likely that if you graduated several years ago, there may have been new specialties recognized since you left your training.

The word "specialist" has a specific definition. All veterinarians receive basic training in all of the areas listed in this chapter. Veterinarians in private practice might perform work in one area (e.g., surgery, behavior problems), but they are not considered "specialists." A veterinarian cannot be described as a specialist unless further training, beyond the veterinary degree, has been obtained. This usually consists of a one-year internship followed by a three-year residency. The veterinarian must then take oral and written exams to become a diplomate of a specialty. Then the veterinarian can add official letters behind the DVM, such as DACVS (Diplomate, American College of Veterinary Surgeons; see Appendix, Acronyms).

Types of specialists

Table 4.1 lists AVMA-recognized veterinary specialty organizations and the number of diplomats in that specialty. Several specialty areas, such as internal medicine, have sub-disciplines in which candidates may become certified. (See www.avma.org > education > specialization.)

Most specialties are organized within areas of medicine, not by species. The exceptions are those specialties grouped under the American Board of Veterinary Practitioners (ABVP), a board certification geared toward veterinarians in general practice.

As of 2010 there were over 9,000 board-certified specialists in the US, or about 11 percent of all veterinarians (www.avma.org > market research statistics). The specialties with the largest number of board-certified veterinarians are internal medicine, pathology, surgery, lab animal medicine, and those under the ABVP umbrella. Several specialties have fewer than 100 board-certified diplomates: nutrition, toxicology, behavior, dentistry, pharmacology, and rehabilitation. Proposals have been made for specialties of shelter animal medicine (Chapter 13), animal welfare, and parasitology. The specialty of laboratory animal medicine is also discussed in Chapter 6.

The specialties of exotic mammal medicine, avian medicine, and/or reptile and amphibian medicine are included under the umbrella of the ABVP. The Exotic Companion Mammal Practice specialty focuses on small mammals commonly known as "pocket pets," including rabbits, ferrets, guinea pigs, mice, and other small mammals. A separate specialty of Reptile and Amphibian Practice includes snakes, lizards, crocodilians, chelonians, tuataras, anurans, caudates, and caecilians.

Veterinarians who pursue board certification in the American College of Zoological Medicine take a two-part examination. The first section covers 5 sub-disciplines: avian, herpetologic, aquatic, free-ranging wildlife, and zoo mammals. Once those are passed, each candidate selects one of those subjects for in-depth testing. However, there is no special notation on the ACZM certificate for individuals that pass the exam. This is different from internal medicine (ACVIM) where sub-specialties (e.g., neurology or cardiology) are listed on the certificate.

In Europe certification falls under the European Board of Veterinary Specialisation (www.ebvs.org); in Australia the certifying group is the Australian College of Veterinary Scientists (www.acvsc.org.au). Some some individual countries within Europe also have their own specialist recognition. Also see the AVMA Policy regarding veterinary specialty organizations (www.avma.org > Issues > Policy > Veterinary specialty organizations).

Daily work

> I love being a surgeon in private practice because of the people. I get to work closely with everyone in my hospital on a daily basis. We collaborate on all cases during rounds and throughout the day. Consults are easy to obtain, and it is never an issue to get another specialist's opinion. I also enjoy the variety of procedures I am able to perform in soft tissue, orthopedic, and neurosurgery.—Philip Pacchiana, DVM, MS, DACVS, Fifth Avenue Veterinary Specialists, New York, NY.

The possible career paths for a board-certified veterinarian include all those discussed in this book; specialists simply use different talents, they may be paid more, and they may achieve higher levels of promotion. The daily work of a specialist varies widely, depending on the area of expertise as well as the employer type. For example, a specialist in private practice would have daily work similar to that described in the section on companion animal or equine practice. A specialist working for industry or academia would have daily work described in those sections. And so on. Specialists simply have focused specific skills and knowledge that they apply in the many career paths described in this book.

Table 4.1: Recognized veterinary specialty organizations

Web site www.	Recognized Veterinary Specialty Organizations		Diplomates
abvp.com	American Board of Veterinary Practitioners (ABVP)		862
	Avian	134	
	Beef Cattle	12	
	Canine & Feline	460	
	Dairy	37	
	Equine	91	
	Exotic Companion Mammal Practice	11	
	Feline	78	
	Food Animal	22	
	Reptile & Amphibian	new	
	Swine Health Management	17	
abvt.org	American Board of Veterinary Toxicology (ABVT)		94
aclam.org	American College of Laboratory Animal Medicine (ACLAM)		718
acpv.info	American College of Poultry Veterinarians (ACPV)		270
theriogenology.org	American College of Theriogenologists (ACT)		342
acva.org	American College of Veterinary Anesthesiologists (ACVA)		170
dacvb.org	American College of Veterinary Behaviorists (ACVB)		45
acvcp.org	American College of Veterinary Clinical Pharmacology (ACVCP)		48
acvd.org	American College of Veterinary Dermatology (ACVD)		187
acvecc.org	American College of Veterinary Emergency and Critical Care (ACVECC)		263
acvim.org	American College of Veterinary Internal Medicine (ACVIM)		1,894
	Cardiology	164	
	Small Animal Internal Medicine	969	
	Large Animal Internal Medicine	449	
	Neurology	161	
	Oncology	224	
acvm.us	American College of Veterinary Microbiologists (ACVM)		163
	Bacteriology/Mycology, 35; Immunology, 46; Microbiology, 63; Virology, 59		
acvn.org	American College of Veterinary Nutrition (ACVN)		53
acvo.org	American College of Veterinary Ophthalmologists (ACVO)		319
acvp.org	American College of Veterinary Pathologists (ACVP)		1,524
	Anatomic Pathology, 1,275; Clinical Pathology, 284		
acvpm.org	American College of Veterinary Preventive Medicine (ACVPM) Epidemiology, 60		607
acvr.org	American College of Veterinary Radiology (ACVR) Radiation Oncology, 68		338
vsmr.org	American College of Veterinary Sports Medicine and Rehabilitation		26
acvs.org	American College of Veterinary Surgeons (ACVS)		1,228
	Small Animal	208	
	Large Animal	120	
aczm.org	American College of Zoological Medicine (ACZM)		112
avdc.org	American Veterinary Dental College (AVDC)		99

AVMA, 2008 data; ABVP, 2010 data. Subgroups may total more than the overall group due to multiple certificates held by some individuals.

Specialists in private practice such as surgeons and radiologists sometimes have "mobile" practices, traveling to different general practices in an area to provide their services. This allows them to have low overhead (i.e., no rent, no utilities, few or no employees); they have only the initial capital investment in the equipment that they require, such as surgical instruments or a portable ultrasound machine. Other specialists, even though affiliated with a clinic, also travel to provide their specialty services.

Some veterinarians form group practices with multiple specialists. Others work for themselves, offering care only in their specialty. Some build a "telemedicine" practice, offering services at a distance via computer. That approach works better for certain specialties, such as radiology.

Specialists in academia must perform research and teach in addition to their clinical work (see Chapter 14). Specialists in private practice can still participate in research if they choose to do so. Options may be better at large referral centers that see a larger case load. A large draw, however, to enter private practice is the lack of required research and the focus on primary case responsibility and patient care. This can be a big draw for many people who do not want to deal with academia's "publish or perish" requirements.

Pros and cons

When considering a specialty, think about whether you want to limit your practice to one particular area of veterinary medicine. Although some people love the idea of excelling in one area, others feel that the broad spectrum of being a general practitioner makes the job exciting.

Although it is generally true that there is a good return on investment with advanced study, in reality that is not true for some areas. The resale value of a specialty practice may actually be lower than that of a general practice since the pool of potential buyers is smaller and the practice depends more heavily on the individual specialists' abilities.

Specialties with little or no demand will provide lower incomes, in general, than those with higher demand (see budgeting in Chapter 2). Industry board-certified veterinarians may earn the highest incomes of all (Chapter 11).

The most popular specialties to enter are internal medicine (37 percent of all 2008 residency applicants), surgery (21 percent), and emergency and critical care (14 percent). However, the popularity of specialties, as measured by the number of veterinarians holding certification or by numbers entering the field, does not always correlate with the demand (and thus, pay or job opportunities) for those specialists. For example, the specialty of internal medicine includes many subspecialties with varying demand. There are very few job openings for large animal internal medicine specialists. A study by J. Hubbell (*JAVMA*) investigated the needs for veterinary specialists in academia:

> As an index of the degree that the need for new specialists was being met, the number of currently open positions in each specialty was subtracted from the number of trainees in that specialty divided by 3 (because most programs are three years in duration) to determine the projected surplus or deficit of specialists. Surpluses (in terms of academic opportunities) were identified in the specialties of theriogenology, behavior, emergency and critical care, small animal internal

medicine, large animal internal medicine, cardiology, small animal orthopedics, small animal general surgery, and large animal surgery. Deficits were identified in the specialties of anesthesiology, neurology, oncology, nutrition, ophthalmology, and radiology.—J. Hubbell et al.

One might assume that private practices are saturated in the same areas as is academia. A survey conducted by the American College of Veterinary Surgeons showed that salary and location were the biggest factors driving surgeons to select private practice over academia. (K. Burns, in *JAVMA*). As demand for private practice specialists increases, it is difficult for universities and teaching hospitals to keep faculty and recruit new staff when pay and hours are significantly better in private practice.

The demand for specialists from pet owners appears to be more sensitive to the economy than the demand for general veterinary services. During the economic decline of 2008–2010, veterinary medicine overall was not as highly impacted as were many other industries; however, there were anecdotal reports that specialists had a greater decline in client visits than veterinarians in general private practice. (K. Burns, *JAVMA*).

Qualifications / To apply
Veterinarians who want to specialize go through a postgraduate internship (usually one year) and then a residency (usually three years) in a particular area of interest. These are paid positions, but the pay is very low compared with that of the typical job in private practice. (Still, interns are being paid to learn as well as to work. See Chapter 2.) Internships and residencies involve long hours of work and study, plus being on call for emergencies, with little time for anything else.

The internship or residency can be done at a university or a large private practice. Apply through the Veterinary Internship and Residency Matching Program (VIRMP, www.virmp.org). VIRMP does not certify the programs on the match list, so applicants should do some research on the programs they are considering—all the internships and residencies listed are not equal.

Although the majority of programs use VIRMP, some (mostly equine) choose interns directly from applications submitted separately (see equine interest groups in Chapter 5). Some specialties such as nutrition or dentistry have only a few residency openings and take a new resident only every three years.

Board-certified veterinarians may find jobs at universities, in corporate practices, or in large cities in private veterinary practices that employ several different specialists. Others may be employed by the veterinary industry or the government, and still others may work as consultants. Jobs are as diverse as the Director of Veterinary Services at Pet Poison Helpline (Justine Lee, DVM, DACVECC) or MN State Public Health Veterinarian (Joni Scheftel, DVM, MPH, DACVPM).

Pay
According to the AVMA Report on Veterinary Compensation:

> Among all practice types, board-certified veterinarians earned substantially more than their non-certified counterparts. In 2007, median professional income for board-certified practitioners was $145,000,

compared to $91,000 for non-certified practitioners. . . . Food animal exclusive and companion animal predominant board-certified veterinarians earned the highest median professional income of $172,000, while mixed animal board-certified veterinarians earned the lowest median professional income of $103,000.

See Tables 2.1 and 2.3 in Chapter 2 for pay ranges for board-certified specialists. Pay is higher for specialists in demand. One area experiencing high demand is veterinary pathology. Veterinary diagnostic laboratories are major employers of veterinary pathologists (Chapter 11). A survey conducted by the American College of Veterinary Pathologists found 150 open positions for both anatomic and clinical pathologists, with half of those being in the industrial sector (private laboratories, not academic labs) (www.acvp.org > career opportunities > employer demographic survey). Although that was some years ago, this is a significant number of openings given the total number of board certified pathologists (see Table 4.1). The number of openings is rising due to a combination of increased demand and increased retirement of the current generation of pathologists.

The National Institutes of Health has "challenges recruiting veterinarians that specialize in laboratory animal medicine and veterinary pathology . . . both specialties are reporting significant shortages." In both academic and nonacademic settings, there is a high demand for specialists in lab animal medicine, with average starting salaries of $100,000 or more (see Chapters 6 and 16.)

Chapter 4 Resources

Groups and web sites

Association of American Veterinary Medical Colleges (AAVMC), www.aavmc.org.
Australian College of Veterinary Scientists, acvsc.org.au.
European Board of Veterinary Specialisation, ebvs.org.
Veterinary Emergency and Specialty Practice Association, www.vespassociation.org.
Veterinary Internship and Residency Matching Program, www.virmp.org.
Veterinary Specialists in Private Practice annual conference, www.vsipp.com.
See also the veterinary specialty organizations and their web sites in Table 4.1.

Books and articles

American Animal Hospital Association (AAHA)
    AAHA, *2005 Specialty & Referral Veterinary Practice Benchmark Study* (AAHA Press, 2006).
    AAHA Referral Guidelines, www.aahanet.org.
ACVP, Veterinary Pathologist Survey: Final Report, 2002, www.acvp.org/career/employsurv.pdf.
AVMA *Report on Veterinary Compensation*, 2009, (AVMA Press, published biennially).
Burns, K., Teaching Hospitals Short on Specialists, *JAVMA News*, August 1, 2006; 229(3): 337-346.
Burns, K., The Economic State Of Specialty Practice, *JAVMA News*, June 15, 2010:1278-1280.
Cockerell, G. L., and D. R. Patterson, Closing the Supply versus Demand Gap for Veterinary Pathologists. A Multifaceted Problem in Need of a Multifaceted Solution, *Can Vet J*, 2005; 46: 660–661.
Gordon, M., et al., Comparison of long-term financial implications for five veterinary career tracks, *JAVMA* Vol 237, No. 4, August 15, 2010: 369-375.
Hare, D., Challenges in Clinical Education, *Can Vet J.*, February 2007; 48(2): 121–123, www.AVMA.org/onlnews/JAVMA/oct03/031001i.asp.
Hubbell, J., et al, Workforce Needs for Clinical Specialists at Colleges and Schools of Veterinary Medicine in North America, *JAVMA*, November 15, 2006; 229(10): 1580–1583.

5 RURAL AND FARM PRACTICE

I am originally from a rural town where the ranch horses got vet care, but the beef cattle were mainly treated by the cowboys, so I did not realize that vets got to do that kind of work. I was attracted to food animal medicine through Auburn's awesome food animal department.

I worked with some progressive large animal veterinarians, then opened up my own large animal hospital. I do beef cattle herd work, bucking bull medicine and surgery, equine reproduction and performance medicine, and a lot of whitetail deer work. The whitetail deer are very similar to goats and sheep. I do daily care of animals; fix the fences the bucking bulls tore through; do paperwork, herd work, and performance evaluation of bucking bulls (radiographs, joint injections, blood work); collect semen from whitetail bucks or AI on the does; and general herd health for one dairy. Working with the bucking bulls requires a lot of patience and good facilities (I just purchased a $32,000 hydraulic chute and alley). I do a lot of "performance bull" medicine, as well as geriatric care of older valuable cattle. They are still "food animals," although the older famous bulls are likely to be buried on the ranch.

Consulting is the most fun and profitable part about my practice. I charge a good hourly fee ($150 -$200/hour) and sometimes a standard daily rate (comes out to about $1500/day for semen collection). Hopefully, I save the client money in the long run. I love my job and I am just so grateful to make a living doing what I do!—Lisa Willis, DVM, Mid-Texas Veterinary Associates, Gustine, TX.

Rural and farm practice are part of "traditional" veterinary practice as initially described in Chapter 3. A variety of terms have definitions that overlap and diverge:
- Equine practice: Horses only.
- Farm animal practice: Any farm animals, such as pigs, chickens, sheep, cattle, or horses. May include pets.
- Food and fiber animals: Food animals plus sheep, llamas, and alpacas.
- Food animal practice: Any animal raised for food, such as meat or dairy goats and cattle, chickens, or turkeys.

- Food-supply veterinary medicine: Includes private practice food animal veterinary services as well as government public health and food safety jobs.
- Large animal practice: Cattle and horses; may include food and fiber animals.
- Mixed animal practice: A variety of pets, livestock, and horses.
- Rural veterinary practice: Veterinary service located in a rural area.
- Production medicine: Food animal medicine that provides tools to improve animal productivity, such as nutrition, reproduction, and immunology.

Although these categories initially seem similar, there are important economic and demographic differences. The AVMA classifies veterinarians as "large animal exclusive," "large animal predominant," "mixed animal," "small animal predominant," "small animal exclusive," and "equine." However, the term "large animal" can refer to either or both livestock or horses. To make it even more confusing, the term "food animal veterinarian" has come to mean so many things: food supply veterinarian, food systems veterinarian, government food inspector, veterinarians in food animal production medicine, and veterinarians who provide individual cow care.

Some people mentioned in this chapter are extension veterinarians; this career path is also discussed in Chapter 15, since their employer is the government (in association with universities).

Daily work / Pros and cons

Most of these veterinarians go to farms and ranches, although some also have standing hospitals where people bring their animals. Farm animal work is frequently done outdoors in all seasons. Some veterinarians have a technician who rides with them on their rounds, but many others operate on their own, with the help of the animal owners or farm managers, who vary in their abilities.

Veterinarians who want to work with one particular species must be willing to live in an area where that species is raised. For example, dairies are abundant in Wisconsin and California; swine operations in North Carolina and Iowa; beef cattle in the Midwest and West; and poultry in Iowa, Georgia, or Minnesota. Areas with large numbers of horses aren't always the best locations for equine veterinarians, since it is the proportion of people to horses that creates sufficient volume to keep an equine veterinarian busy. As an example, Montana has a high number of horses but they are spread over wide areas with low (human) populations. Specific aspects of daily work are discussed under each type below.

Qualifications

The DVM degree qualifies anyone to work in rural, mixed, or large animal practice. In the past, most veterinarians who worked in rural and large animal practice came from rural, farm backgrounds. Today, many successful large animal veterinarians are people who made the transition from a city childhood to being comfortable with farm animals. To do so, they devoted a large amount of time to living among, working with, and studying the clients they serve and their animals. A person motivated to work in this area should not be discouraged by anyone who claims they don't have the "right" background. The veterinary literature abounds with discussion of a shortage of veterinarians in some of these areas. See Chapter 19 for a detailed discussion of supply and demand issues.

Veterinarians may become specialists in several different areas. The American Board of Veterinary Practitioners has subspecialty groups for beef cattle, swine and horses. The American College of Poultry Veterinarians certifies poultry specialists. See Chapter 4, Specialists.

Pay

Veterinarians who work in 100 percent food animal practice earn some of the highest incomes in the profession; those in mixed animal practice are in the lowest income group (see Chapter 3). A variety of state and federal programs are being created to provide financial assistance for veterinary students and veterinarians who agree to work in "underserved areas," which may include food animal medicine or working in rural areas (see Chapters 2 and 19).

Rural Veterinary Practice

Thanks to Dr. Aurora Villarroel, extension veterinarian at Oregon State University, and coauthors for contributing this section. Information and quotes are from respondents to a survey on retention of veterinarians in RVP in North America conducted in 2008. The survey was a joint project of 6 collaborators from Oregon, Ohio, Michigan, and Colorado State universities, and The Academy of Rural Veterinarians. (See resource list, Villarroel et al.)

> Do not rule out rural practice without giving it a real look. Living in, raising a family and becoming a real part of the community cannot be valued by money. It is a real pleasure to be walking down the street and knowing most of the people you meet. Many are clients, but many are not; the vet is a really influential person in the community.— Anonymous rural practice veterinarian

A rural community can be defined in several ways. Some of the more humorous include "two or less traffic lights" or "a community that will not support a McDonald's or a Starbucks." According to 1,339 veterinarians who completed an Internet survey, the definition of a rural veterinary practice (RVP) is a practice in an agricultural community that does not focus on any specific animal species. The population size of the community is of secondary importance to the culture and the individual understanding of "rural lifestyle." (A. Villarroel.)

Daily work / Pros and cons

> Choose a job you will enjoy. You have to enjoy the people (your clients) and the lifestyle. Your clients will become your friends and lifelong neighbors. You need to be professional, meaning you have to be true to your word. Be humble when you are right, and quick at admitting when you are wrong. Be prepared to learn from your clients. They have been around for a while and chances are they do know more than you do incertain aspects. They certainly do know their animals and places

better than you do. Listen and ask for ideas from them: two brains always can think better than one alone.—Anonymous rural practice veterinarian

A rural veterinary practice can be a fulfilling and rewarding career for veterinarians who enjoy a rural lifestyle. Potential practitioners should consider the qualities of the community as much as those of the practice that they are considering.

According to survey respondents, the most appealing aspects of rural practice are the lifestyle available to veterinarians and their families, the variety of cases, and the relationships with their clients. Rural communities are generally considered desirable places to raise a family. The cost of living in a rural community is often significantly less when compared to urban and suburban areas, and this should be considered as a monetary benefit. Veterinarians in rural practices are usually well respected and regularly become community leaders.

Species and case variety is another benefit of rural practice. Practitioners in RVPs can expect variety and some thought-provoking cases. The distance to referral practices may be prohibitive for some clients. Therefore, veterinarians in rural practices may perform some procedures that would usually be referred to local specialists by urban practices. In addition, practitioners in RVPs may have more opportunities to treat a variety of species. An RVP is traditionally regarded as multispecies; although some practitioners may deem this a disadvantage, many enjoy the variety. Much of a veterinarian's large animal work can be seasonal, and other species can provide a source of income during the slow times, enabling the practice to be economically sustainable. However, some rural veterinarians focus exclusively on a single species. Thus, the combination of community, challenge, and variety offered in a rural practice setting creates a lifestyle that has a strong appeal to some individuals.

Client relationships tend to be stronger in rural practice than in urban practice. Due to the low population density of rural areas, clients and veterinarians tend to have long-term relationships. This can be a disadvantage if a client asks for preferential treatment, but is usually an advantage due to the degree of trust and camaraderie developed with the clients.

The following summary of potential cons was extracted for this book from the RVP survey, from rural practitioners' advice to new graduates considering jobs in an RVP:

- *Income:* Although many rural practices generate income comparable to urban practices, gross income may be an issue in some areas, depending on the local economy. Monetary and nonmonetary factors need to be considered when deciding on employment.
- *Emergency duty:* Most commonly, emergencies are handled by the practice instead of referring them to an emergency clinic. Being a solo practitioner may feel like working 24/7. A multidoctor practice or an alliance with neighboring practices can reduce on-call time per doctor.
- *Time off:* The seasonal nature of some work related to rural practice can demand long hours. Compensatory time off in the off-season or some other type of benefit, such as extra pay or benefits can be negotiated.

- *Family concerns:* This can run the spectrum from the availability of jobs for the spouse, to quality of health care and educational facilities, to availability of cultural and recreational amenities, to time flexibility to attend family events.

Job openings in an RVP may not be readily apparent because many of these practices do not advertise positions in a conventional manner. It is important to note that many practices advertise by word of mouth. The Academy of Rural Veterinarians is good source to find RVP positions (www.ruralvets.com > Resources > Job Bank), as is direct communication with rural practices in areas of interest.

Mixed Animal Practice

Rural practice and mixed animal practice aren't necessarily the same. A few rural practices may not work with large animals, and a few mixed animal practices may not be located in rural areas. About 4,300 US veterinarians were working in mixed animal practice in 2008.

Daily work / Pros and cons

Mixed animal practitioners may work in rural or suburban areas, with small farmers or hobby farmers. They work with multiple species, including pets, horses, and small ruminants such as sheep, goats, and llamas. They do much of their work on farm calls (see Chapter 8), either as a solely mobile practice or more often as a service in addition to their work at a hospital.

Their clients generally fall into two different categories. Some clients may emphasize cost-effectiveness if they are running a farm business. Others are hobbyists who often view these animals as pets. There can even be a "special" animal such as a child's 4-H project, or a very valuable animal that is part of a herd of commercial animals on a business farm. The special animal category has created a gap between the veterinarian's assumptions about this client (as a livestock owner) and the clients' desires for health care. Savvy veterinarians are beginning to take a different approach to these clients— for example, by sending out reminders for health care in the same manner as do small animal veterinarians.

Mixed animal practitioners may work in an area that does not have sufficient clients to support a separate emergency clinic. Thus most mixed animal practitioners do have to be "on call" for emergencies after hours.

Equine Practice

Equine practitioners may operate out of a full-service equine hospital, a mobile unit alone, or both. In rural areas, horses kept as pets or used for recreation are often served by mixed animal veterinary hospitals.

About 3,600 veterinarians were working in equine practice in the US in 2008. That total has increased gradually each year for the past three years, but at the same time, the total number of horses in the US is decreasing. The existence of large established equine practices combined with flat growth in horse numbers make it difficult to open a new equine practice in some areas. However, those veterinarians who love horses and are willing to move to an area where they are needed will find rewarding work.

Daily work / Pros and cons

Those veterinarians who want to work with *only* horses will find that potential jobs are limited to certain areas of the country that have enough density of both horses and horse owners to be able to provide sufficient work.

In many areas, the amount of work available often precludes supporting more than a few veterinarians, leaving those who do such work on call much of the time. Hours may be long and unpredictable. Equine practices with enough veterinarians to share the load and provide reasonable working hours are limited in number. In larger practices this call is shared, but so far there are not "emergency only/after hours" services for horses as there are for companion animals.

In the past, some equine veterinarians and horse owners viewed horses as utility animals, and thus not worthy of receiving advanced medical or surgical care. Today, many horses are valuable investments or are dearly-loved companion animals for which many people are willing to provide top-quality care.

Focusing on one aspect of the equine business allows one to focus on a specific area of medicine. Some equine practitioners work for a racetrack or specialize in reproduction for larger horse farms. Racetracks keep specific hours and have calendars around which the veterinarian must work (e.g., training and racing schedules). Veterinarians who work in reproduction must work long days during breeding season and must be available at all hours during foaling season.

Another niche is equine sports medicine, focusing on horses used in athletic competition. These veterinarians may focus on horses used for three-day events, jumping, rodeo, dressage, calf roping, and many other activities.

Some equine practitioners are specialists in equine surgery or medicine. Because of the horse's large size, complex or advanced surgery requires the use of a facility with specialized equipment.

Other equine practitioners work with show horses or with horses kept as companions for pleasure riding. Working with pleasure horses usually includes all aspects of medicine and routine surgery.

Controversy in equine practice includes debate about the scope of practice, with specific attention to equine dentistry, chiropractic and massage. Long neglected by equine practitioners, these areas of interest were "taken over" by non-veterinarians, who arguably filled a void. State regulations vary widely with regard to who may perform these procedures. (Also see Chapter 3, integrative medicine, and commentary about technican roles in Chapter 19.)

One item of concern is the low average starting salary for equine practitioners, which was only $38,000 in 2010, down from $42,000 in 2009 (AVMA). While the overall median income is still close to that of other private practice, such a drop in starting salaries should be monitored by those considering this type of work. (See Tables 3.1. and 3.3.)

Qualifications

Successful equine veterinarians must be aware of their clients' needs. Like veterinarians who work with birds or cats, equine veterinarians must be skilled in the "language" of the species and the clients they serve. Working with horses does not require extraordinary physical strength, but it does require a working knowledge of equine behavior. Respecting and understanding horse owners' concerns is also essential. Having your own horse helps not only to learn how to manage horses but also puts you in touch with other horse owners in your area.

Good sources of information include the American Association of Equine Practitioners (AAEP; www.aaep.org > career center) and the International Association of Equine Dentistry (IAED; www.iaedonline.com). Also see the sections about rehabilitation and integrative medicine in Chapter 3, and Table 3.1 for income information.

Equine veterinarians may become board-certfied specialists through the American Board of Veterinary Practitioners or the American College of Veterinary Sports Medicine and Rehabilitation. The specialties of internal medicine and surgery also certify "large animal" specialists which includes those focusing on horses (see Table 4.1 in Chapter 4).

Food Animal Practice

Daily work / Pros and cons

Daily work for food animal veterinarians varies with the species focus and the size of the herds serviced. Work may be indoors or outdoors but is usually in barns or other facilities that house animals. While the work is physical, it does not require great strength; experienced food animal practitioners use tools, equipment, and their brains to work with large animals.

Food animal veterinarians work with small ruminants, poultry, swine, and cattle. They often focus on herd health rather than individual animals. Some areas of the country have enough small farms of one type that the veterinarian can concentrate on just one species while serving those small farms. For example, multidoctor, dairy-only, private practices may be found in parts of Wisconsin where many dairies are located.

Some food animal veterinarians do not necessarily practice veterinary medicine every day, but are hired because—in addition to their veterinary training—they possess a combination of animal husbandry skills and experience in data management, data analysis, and personnel training. As farm managers or production managers (as many of these veterinarians are called), they generally work for one larger farm or one complex.

The potential job market for these veterinarians is unclear. On the one hand, the incomes of this group are among the highest in veterinary medicine. On the other hand, only a small number of veterinarians actually work in this area—of about 75,000 veterinarians in the US for whom career information was available, only about 5,000 veterinarians work in a predominantly or exclusively food animal practice.

Current data suggest a decrease in demand for food animal veterinary services. For example, the numbers of cattle, hogs, breeding sheep, and turkeys in the US have all been declining. In 2008, US cattle feeders lost more money on average for each animal sold than at any other time in history. Low milk prices are contributing to a decrease in the number of dairies. Continued agribusiness consolidation and a focus on herd health rather than individual animal medicine means that fewer veterinarians may be needed to provide the same service to those larger farms.

Publications that address this situation in food animal veterinary include the *JAVMA* articles by G. Cima and J.B. Walker, and the Pew Commission's report, *Putting Meat on the Table: Industrial Farm Animal Production in America.*

It is also possible, however, that increasing fuel and transportation costs will cause somewhat of a return to local agribusiness. Veterinarians who can understand and help animal owners develop appropriate markets will have an advantage in this field.

Food animal practitioners may use veterinary technicians for some tasks, as described in a *JAVMA* article by D. Remsburg:

> [Technicians can be used] to administer injections, collect feed samples, assess animal body condition, monitor health program indices, and perform other technical duties. . . . Additional duties could include castration, dehorning, assistance with dystocia, repair of uterine or vaginal prolapse, venipuncture, hoof trimming, necropsy, collection of milk samples, and inputting and processing of data.

> [Technicians could] collect patient history and key objective patient data on the farm and then report to a veterinarian. . . . The veterinarian would make a diagnosis predicated on these data (as well as any additional information requested) and then prescribe treatment. When the treatment is within the purview of a veterinary technician, the technician would provide that treatment to the animal. When the treatment is beyond the skill level or legal right of a veterinary technician, the veterinarian would proceed to the farm and provide that treatment. In this model, the use of veterinary technicians to travel to the farm, assess a problem, and provide treatment would allow veterinarians to pursue duties more appropriate for their professional training.

Whether this model will become widespread (or whether it is currently legal under state regulations) is not certain but will probably be affected by agricultural and global economics.

Qualifications

> "City slicker gone country" is how *JAVMA* described my American Association of Bovine Practitioners presidency in 2003. You do not need to be from a farm to participate in food animal production medicine, but you do need to learn and understand livestock management in as much detail as possible. I am still learning! Take advantage of student externship programs to get more exposure to food animal veterinary medicine.

I became involved in food animals during my undergraduate years with Block and Bridle Club, then did an internship and residency in different areas of production medicine. The Residency and Master of Public Health in Epidemiology allowed me to apply for university positions.

Continuing education has and will always be a chance to hear how others deal with livestock diseases and issues.—Patty Scharko, DVM, MPH, DACVPM, Field/Extension Veterinarian, Clemson University, Columbia, SC.

In addition to being able to treat individual animals, veterinarians who are successful in food animal medicine help their clients save costs, and minimize negative environmental impacts. Environmental issues are especially important with regard to waste disposal in large facilities. Knowledge of herd health, risk management, and global economics improves veterinarians' usefulness to their clients. Animal welfare is a continuing focus; monitoring equipment may measure activity and eating behavior, which reflects well-being.

Food animal veterinarians have a wide variety of employers from which to choose; they may work in industry, government, or academia. Many food animal veterinarians work in private practice, serving farms of a variety of sizes. Veterinarians may be hired by large food producers, such as those who specialize in poultry, beef, or milk products.

Those interested in a career in food animal medicine should look to special interest groups and associations for educational opportunities. For example, the American Association of Bovine Practitioners offers workshops and lectures at its annual meeting, and its web site lists externships for students (www.aabp.org).

Chapter 19 addresses the future outlook for this career choice, as does K. Gwinner's article in *JAVMA* about attracting students. The American Association of Food Hygiene Veterinarians (www.avma.org/aafhv) and the American Association of Small Ruminant Practitioners (www.aasrp.org) can also provide information. AVMA's web site (www.avma.org/fsvm) discusses food animal careers and presents the Food Supply Veterinary Medicine Coalition Report.

Additional training in food animal medicine is offered at the University of Nebraska Great Plains Veterinary Educational Center (GPVEC; http://gpvec.unl.edu), which provides education to veterinary students and practitioners through a cooperative agreement with Iowa State University and the US Meat Animal Research Center. The teaching program is primarily in food animal health and production management of beef cattle. The Production Beef Cattle Production Management Series available at the GPVEC for veterinarians with two or more years of food animal practice experience provides in-depth interdisciplinary training in beef production and economics. Veterinary graduate students may complete a distance MS through this program.

Internships and residencies in food animal medicine are offered at many veterinary colleges. It is important to recognize the unique differences among residencies in food animal medicine, large animal medicine, and rural practice or field services. Large animal residencies focus on both food animals and equine patients, with a typical heavier emphasis on equine patients, followed by camelid patients. Rural practice or field service residencies typically focus on reproduction (theriogenology) and herd health, usually with cattle.

Food animal / livestock consultants

For at least 25 years, the talk about the future of large animal medicine has been that veterinarians will more often be in a consultant role. However, this has not become the reality for the majority of large animal practitioners today.

A few veterinarians do work in a consulting role. In this work, the veterinary consultant may give recommendations about:

- Animal management and health care.
- Preventive medicine (which vaccinations and dewormers are cost effective to use).
- Nutrition (balancing or analyzing rations, finding less costly feed ingredients, analyzing use of supplements).
- Genetic counseling and evaluation of breeding lines.
- Facilities and housing (size, number of animals per unit of space, cleaning procedures, sanitation, potential for disease transmission, ventilation).
- Data management requirements for profitable herd management, including available options.
- Interpretation of data analyses generated by a computer program.
- Defining a corporate mission, market segments, and market potential for a client.
- Evaluating pricing, promotion, distribution, and sales.
- Business and farm management.
- Staff training.
- Keeping up to date with new technical developments and global trends.

Livestock consultants usually start by working with individual clients, such as farmers or ranchers. Livestock consultants may depend on a small number of large clients, creating a risky business situation if one client is lost, or they may have multiple smaller clients.

Work for companies can be done as an employee or on a freelance basis. The consultant must be aware of and in contact with experts in related fields, such as nutritionists and geneticists, to make use of their expertise when appropriate. Sometimes several experts work together in one consulting firm to provide all necessary services to each client. Livestock consultants may sometimes find that their business advice is not solicited or followed due to economic constraints or because they are viewed as being experts in medicine only.

Livestock consultants also have an opportunity for international work, as described by Dr. Janet Alsop:

> From 1995–1997, I worked for a private company that implemented
> a bilateral (Chinese-Canadian) livestock development project for the
> Canadian International Development Agency (similar to USAID).

As the project veterinarian, I was responsible for the health of three project swine herds located in China. I lived at one site, where I was the site manager, and visited the others on a quarterly basis.

Certain aspects of the job were very challenging. For example, it was difficult to find some animal health supplies, such as biologicals and pharmaceuticals, and we had to create our own diagnostic support system for the farms. My daily work involved a lot of training and inter-action with my Chinese colleagues. This took the form of discussions and hands-on demonstrations, or, occasionally, more formal lectures. I also assisted with technical problems. I enjoyed problem-solving at the farms and seeing people use knowledge that they acquired as a result of the project.—Janet E. Alsop, DVM, ABVP-SHM, former project veterinarian, China-Canada Lean Swine Project, People's Republic of China.

Beef and dairy cattle veterinarians

Most dairy veterinarians today focus on reproductive work. My focus is different in that my practice is 100 percent consulting with a primary focus on dairy nutrition and farm profitability. I also provide advice on youngstock management programs, quality milk production, and mar-keting of farmstead products. In all of my herds, I encourage the dairy to work with a local veterinarian to do the pregnancy testing, surgeries, and sick cow work. I coordinate with that veterinarian to provide cow vaccination and treatment protocols, disease control programs, and consultation on reproductive programs and protocols.

It is exciting and rewarding work, but it is best suited to veterinarians with a lot of patience and with a skill with numbers. I formulate lots of rations, and these are different for every dairy. Each dairy is unique in that each has different forages and different feeding systems. I sell no product, and thus, am paid only for my knowledge and time. Because my clients know I don't sell minerals, feed additives, or even vaccines or medicine, they trust my opinions a good deal. The number of dairy clients you need to do this kind of work will vary with the size and type of dairies you serve.

What I like best about my work is that I have become a trusted part of the management team for family farms. I work hard to help keep the business profitable and I contribute to cow welfare by keeping cows healthy. For those considering a consulting practice with dairies, important skills will include a sound knowledge of bovine nutrition, a familiarity with the dairy industry and dairy farming in general, and strong people and communication skills. I believe that in the future, veterinarians will rely less on pharmaceutical sales for a large part of their income, and will need to gravitate more towards consultation. Veterinarians are ideally suited to be nutritional and management consultants because we are "value-added." Our training in cow health and physiology and in cow disease management gives us an advantage over others offering similar services.—Karen L. Jacobsen, DVM, Farm Animal Resources and Management, Athens, GA.

Veterinarians working with only cattle (rather than in a mixed practice) will typically work with either beef or dairy cattle. Some may work as ranch veterinarians, or as consultants (see Dr. Jacobsen's web site at www.karenjacobsen.net). Those focusing on dairy cattle may work as consultants to very large dairy operations, or may work full-time in private practices that serve a large number of smaller dairy farms. Academic positions focusing on cattle are available, although the work may include other ruminants as well.

The American Association of Bovine Practitioners includes both dairy and beef cattle veterinarians (www.aabp.org). The American Dairy Science Association (ADSA, www.adsa.org) publishes the *Journal of Dairy Science* and provides useful web site links. The National Cattlemen's Beef Association is the major group for beef cattle operators (www.beef.org).

Continuing education opportunities are provided by the Academy of Veterinary Consultants (www.avc-beef.org), which holds three meetings a year, often in conjunction with larger veterinary conferences. This group is involved in beef cattle medicine, herd health programs, and consultation. Also see Chapter 9, Consulting.

Small ruminant veterinarians

Animals used for food and fiber include a variety of ruminants which are usually lumped under the category of "small ruminants." These include sheep, goats, and camelids such as llamas and alpacas. All these animals are kept on small farms as well as on larger operations such as those raising sheep for their wool.

Llamas and alpacas are raised for their wool, used for pack animals, or simply kept as pets. The consumption of lamb, goat meat, and sheep and goat cheese is rising in popularity, along with interest in "buying local," and thus there is a need for veterinary services for those animals. Because there are few areas with sufficient small ruminants to keep a veterinarian busy full-time, these veterinarians usually operate out of a mixed-animal practice. Resources for veterinarians with this interest include the American Association of Small Ruminant Practitioners (AASRP, www.aasrp.org), the American Sheep and Goat Center (www.sheepandgoatsusa.org) and the British Veterinary Camelid Society (www.camelidvets.org).

Swine veterinarians

Veterinarians who work solely with swine could work for a large swine production company; they could have a private practice that works only with swine; or they could be individual doctors in large animal practices where others work with different animals.

The type of employment dictates the working hours and days. Herd-health, production veterinarians, and consultants see few, if any, emergency cases, whereas those working with smaller farms or show animals may have longer or less predictable hours. Some swine veterinarians expand their services to include management, which requires additional knowledge, as one veterinarian relates:

> As our practice evolved, we worked with fewer and larger farms. We used to make three or four farm calls a day and now it's one to three calls per day. Most of our work is not heavily hands-on; instead, it is consulting and discussion of production records, problem solving on a herd basis, conducting postmortem exams, and collection of blood or fecal samples. Our facility consists of an office, a lab, and a dispensing area for medications.

> Opportunities are good as long as you are willing to move to where the jobs are and are willing to look at all the different types of employers. Jobs are advertised in the swine literature, or through the AASV (American Association of Swine Veterinarians). I'd advise anyone interested in swine medicine to learn as much as they can about swine production, including using the more common record-keeping software—don't assume that you know practical use of technology just because you grew up with it. Learn diagnostic pathology, since you must help clients solve disease problems. Observation skills in the barn are critical—evaluate the environment, the feed, water, air, the pigs' health, everything. And of course you should like pigs and love being in the barn. My job is great because I get to work with pigs and people, and there is always the challenge of something new to learn.—Max Rodibaugh, DVM, Swine Health Services, LC, Frankfort, IN.

The University of Illinois has a multiple-weekend Executive Veterinary Program that offers a certificate in swine health management (www.evpillinois.org). Veterinarians with two years of experience are eligible for the program. Twelve learning modules are offered every other month for three days each over a two-year period. The training includes classes in consulting, leadership, economics, financial management, marketing, biostatistics, legal issues, nutrition, and epidemiology.

The American Association of Swine Veterinarians is the veterinary group for anyone interested in swine (www.aasv.org). The pork industry group is the Pork Board (www. pork.org). If you are interested in a global perspective, look up these organizations: Asociación Mexicana de Veterinarios Especialistas en Cerdos (www.amvec.org); Canadian Association of Swine Veterinarians (www.casv-acvp.ca); and International Pig Veterinary Society (www.ipvs.de).

Poultry veterinarians

> The fascinating aspect of working in poultry medicine is the challenge of using and becoming proficient in laboratory diagnostic work. Poultry medicine is population-based, and requires that one enjoy working with epidemiologic tools, such as disease control and preventive strategies, statistics, and animal health economics.—David D. Frame, DVM, Dipl. ACPV, Associate Professor, Extension Poultry Specialist, Utah State University, Logan, UT.

Most veterinarians working in the poultry industry will have either a PhD, Master's (Master of Preventive Veterinary Medicine, Master of Avian Medicine, or similar), and/or will be board certified in the American College of Poultry Veterinarians. Opportunities for residencies are available in only a few states and are extremely competitive. Salaries usually are high and national or international travel, with long periods away from home, are often required.

Poultry veterinarians may work with a genetics or feed/nutrition company. They can work for a production company such as Tyson or Perdue (broilers), Michael Foods or Sparboe (layers), Jennie O (turkeys), or ConAgra. They can work with primary breeders such as Hyline, Aviagen, or Hybrid Turkeys. Other employers of poultry veterinarians are pharmaceutical companies; the government, such as federal and state veterinary medical officers and field veterinarians; and universities involved in poultry research and extension courses (e.g., University of Minnesota, North Carolina State University, University of Arkansas, and University of Georgia). Some work as international consultants (see the discussion about DAI in Chapter 13).

A few veterinarians work with ostrich and emu farms, where these birds are raised for their meat. These veterinarians are sometimes avian veterinarians in private practice (Chapter 3), who see pet birds as well as these "exotic" bird species. (See the American Ostrich Association at www.ostriches.org and the American Emu Association at www.aea-emu.org)

The primary source for job opportunities in poultry veterinary medicine is the American Association of Avian Pathologists (AAAP; www.aaap.info). Also see www.poultrycareers.org > contacts and the poultry industry web site, www.thepoultrysite.com.

Global trends in agribusiness

The Harvard Business School offers an agribusiness seminar in January of each year. This is a leadership workshop designed to help the experienced manager anticipate, and take advantage of, new trends and opportunities in domestic and international agribusiness. The seminar has as its central theme a concept of a world food system and the implications of global trends for private and public policy makers. The course cost includes tuition, books, meals, and accommodations. For more information or to apply, contact the Harvard Business School Executive Education Office (www.exed.hbs.edu/programs/agb).

In addition, a national conference for agribusiness is held each fall on the Purdue University campus. Multimedia reports are available through Purdue University (www. agecon.purdue.edu).

Chapter 5 Resources

Groups and web sites

Academy of Rural Veterinarians, www.ruralvets.com.
Academy of Veterinary Consultants, www.avc-beef.org.
American Association of Avian Pathologists, www.aaap.info.
American Association of Bovine Practitioners (AABP), www.aabp.org.
American Association of Equine Practitioners (AAEP), www.aaep.org > career center.
American Association of Food Hygiene Veterinarians, www.avma.org/aafhv.
American Association of Small Ruminant Practitioners, www.aasrp.org.
American Association of Swine Veterinarians (AASV), www.aasv.org.
American Dairy Science Association, www.adsa.org.
American Ostrich Association, www.ostriches.org.
American Emu Association, www.aea-emu.org.
American Veterinary Medical Association (AVMA), food supply information, www.avma.org/fsvm.
Harvard Business School Executive Education Office, www.exed.hbs.edu/programs/agb; phone: 800-HBS-5577 (outside the US, dial 617-495-6555); fax: 617-495-6999, e-mail: executive_education@hbs.edu.
International Association of Equine Dentistry, www.iaedonline.com.
National Cattlemen's Beef Association, www.beef.org.
Pork Board, www.pork.org.
Poultry careers, www.poultrycareers.org > contacts.
Poultry industry, www.thepoultrysite.com.
Purdue University, National Conference for Agribusiness, 1145 Krannert Bldg., West Lafayette, IN 47907-1145; htpps:// www.agecon.purdue.edu/cab/programs; phone: 317-494-4325; fax: 317-494-4333; e-mail: wall@agecon.purdue.edu.
University of Illinois Executive Veterinary Program, UI College of Veterinary Medicine, CEPS/Extension, 2938 VMBSB, Urbana, IL 61801; www.evpillinois.org; phone: 217-333-2907, e-mail: ope@vetmed.illinois.edu.
University of Nebraska Great Plains Veterinary Educational Center (GPVEC), http://gpvec.unl.edu.
Veterinary Medicine Loan Repayment Program (VMLRP), www.nifa.usda.gov/vmlrp; Email: vmlrp@nifa.usda.gov.

Books and articles

AVMA, *Food Supply Veterinary Medicine Coalition Report,* available online at www.avma.org/fsvm.
Cima, G., Economists: Livestock and Poultry Producers Cutting Flock, Herd Sizes, *JAVMA News*, April 15, 2009; 234(8): 985–987.
Gwinner, K., et al., Attracting Students into Careers in Food Supply Veterinary Medicine, *JAVMA*, June 1, 2006, 228(11):1693–1704.
Pew Commission on Industrial Farm Production, *Putting Meat on the Table: Industrial Farm Animal Production in America*, final report www.ncifap.org/ www.pewtrusts.org or www.ncifap.org/_images/PCIFAPFin.pdf. Also see Letters to the Editor, *JAVMA*, October 15, 2008; 233(8): 1227–1228.
Remsburg, D., et al., A Proposed Novel Food Animal Health Care Delivery System, *JAVMA*, September 15, 2007; 231: 6.
Villarroel, A., McDonald, S., et al., A survey of reasons why veterinarians enter rural veterinary practice in the United States, *JAVMA*, April 15, 2010; 236(8): 849-857.
Villarroel, A., McDonald, S., et al., A survey of reasons why veterinarians leave rural veterinary practice in the United States, *JAVMA*, April 15, 2010; 236(8): 859-867.
Walker, J. B., Food Animal Medicine in Crisis, *JAVMA*, August 15, 2009; 235(4): 368–374.

6 SPECIES VARIETY: FISH TO ELEPHANTS

When one thinks of "species variety," jobs may land in one of several spheres. First, nontraditional pets such as hedgehogs and reptiles are often seen in private practice, as discussed in Chapter 3. Next, "production" animal medicine includes a variety of species used for meat, milk, and fiber; these were discussed in Chapter 5.

Many other species need veterinary care. Broad categories include:
- Aquatic animal
- Wildlife and zoo animal
- Environmental issues that affect wildlife and marine animals
- Laboratory animal

All veterinary colleges teach a bit about these species, but students and veterinarians seriously considering work with such species must make an extra effort to learn more. They may do so by spending extra time with the course instructor, by taking externships that involve that type of work, by enrolling in an internship program after graduation, or by independent study. Learning after graduation can be accomplished through a variety of formats, including seminars and longer workshops.

Where are the jobs? Veterinarians who learn about marine mammals or fish diseases may be hired by nonprofit groups, government agencies, commercial fish farms, or marine parks. Those who focus on exotic animals may work in zoos. Laboratory animal veterinarians work in research facilities, government agencies, or universities. Veterinarians in private practice may have clients that include smaller wildlife sanctuaries, aquarium hobbyists, or backyard koi owners.

Aquatic Veterinary Medicine and Aquaculture

Aquatic veterinarians can work with pet fish or food fish; in private practice, or as consultants; and in research, industry, for the government, or academia. Some of these positions will require a PhD or master's degree.

Aquaculture is the farming of freshwater and saltwater organisms and aquatic plants. The field is rapidly growing as demand for fish species grows and more and more people depend upon fish as a mainstay of their diet. It is estimated that production of farmed aquatic animals in the US more than doubled between 1985 and 1999, from approximately 400 million pounds to 987 million pounds; production was over one billion pounds by 2005. (National Aquatic Animal Health Task Force.)

The American Pet Products Association reports that about 12 percent of US households are fish owners, who each own more than 10 fish, on average. The vast majority of fish owners obtained health care information from pet stores, not veterinarians. This is likely because so few private practice veterinarians work on fish, although this number is increasing (see G. Cima's article in *JAVMA*).

Daily work / Pros and Cons

Private practice veterinarians may work with aquatic species as a part of traditional private practice or as a niche on its own. For example, Helen Roberts, DVM, runs the Aquatic Veterinary Services of Western New York, an ambulatory pet fish practice. She loves to see fish as a part of her practice at 5 Corners Animal Hospital in Orchard Park, NY, but she also works with cats, dogs, and exotics. Dr. Roberts is a founding member of the World Aquatic Veterinary Medical Association, has served as a member on the AVMA's Aquatic Veterinary Medicine Committee, and is the editor and a contributing author of *Fundamentals of Ornamental Fish Health*.

In contrast, aquaculture veterinarians focus more on production and herd health. Disease prevention is just as—if not more—important than disease treatment. Most fish farms have hundreds to thousands of fish, making cost a large concern for treatment. Environment plays a key role, so much time is spent assessing water quality.

Daily activities for aquaculture veterinarians vary by region and employer type. In the Midwest, most work is with private fish farms; in Maine, with large corporate salmon farms. Arkansas and Alabama have the country's largest catfish farms, which usually contract with universities for their aquaculture needs.

A few government positions are available. Veterinarians may work with agencies such as the National Marine Mammal Laboratory (Chapter 16), or state agencies (Chapter 15).

For example, Myron Kebus, MS, DVM, of the Wisconsin Department of Agriculture has been involved with fish veterinary medicine for nearly 20 years. For him, it is a full-time job; however, his position is unique. Few other state departments of agriculture have a veterinarian on staff working specifically with fish. He notes that in the Midwest most private practice veterinarians practicing aquaculture do so only about up to 40 percent of the time (most of this time is spent working for fish farms). The rest of the time is spent in other sectors of private practice, usually in large animal practice. Most work involves regulatory testing for diseases and writing health certificates for fish that are going to be brought across state borders.

Some veterinarians work for nonprofit rescue organizations such as The Marine Mammal Center in Sausalito, California, or the Mote Marine Whale and Dolphin Rehabilitation Center in Sarasota, Florida. Large public aquariums also have veterinarians on staff.

Qualifications / To apply

You do not need an advanced degree to get started in aquaculture, but you do need additional training beyond the basics provided in veterinary school. An aquaculture veterinarian must be familiar with basic fish anatomy, physiology, reproduction, and husbandry requirements for many different species and families of fish. Knowledge of disease types and transmission are important. One approach for students is to get experience through externships and/or internships working with fish.

Several training programs exist for graduate veterinarians, such as the online and in-person training program through the University of Wisconsin. The online course, which can be taken at any time, comprises five modules. The hands-on course is offered every May. To date, more than 200 veterinarians have taken the course. (University of Wisconsin Fish Health Medicine Certificate Program, http://vetmedce.vetmed.wisc.edu/fhm.)

Aquavet, a program in aquatic veterinary medicine presented jointly by the University of Pennsylvania and Cornell University, offers two- and four-week courses (www.aquavet.info). Other universities, such as the North Carolina State University College of Veterinary Medicine, have postgraduate programs in aquatic medicine (www.cvm.ncsu.edu > ecosystem health). The University of Florida also has a strong aquatic animal health program (www.vetmed.ufl.edu > extension > aquatic).

There are a few residency programs available; these are extremely competitive. The aquatic residency is run by the American College of Zoological Medicine (ACZM, www.aczm.org; see Chapter 4). The ACZM web site includes job openings, internship and externship listings, and CE offerings.

Other nonveterinary sources provide valuable information and continuing education, such as state aquaculture associations or professional organizations working with aquaculture and fisheries. Many universities offer classes for fisheries biologists or other scientists.

It is expected that national accreditation through USDA-APHIS will be offered in the field of aquaculture. This will eventually become a requirement for practicing regulatory medicine in the field. See www.aphis.usda.gov> Animal Health > Animal Diseases by Species > Aquaculture.

Because employer type varies so widely, it is tough to describe "typical pay." Networking is essential in this field since these jobs may not be considered typical for a veterinarian. The total number of job openings specifically set aside or labeled for veterinarians is small, although the number of jobs for which veterinarians may be qualified is larger. See these resources:

- Alliance of Veterinarians for the Environment, www.aveweb.org.
- American College of Zoological Medicine, www.aczm.org.
- American Fisheries Society, Fish Health Section, www.fisheries.org/fhs.
- American Goldfish Association, www.americangoldfish.org.
- Aquaculture Network Information Center, http://aquanic.org.
- Aquavet, www.aquavet.info.
- Associated Koi Clubs of America, www.akca.org.
- Association of Zoos and Aquariums, www.aza.org.
- Fish Health Medicine Certificate Program, www.vetmedce.vetmed.wisc.edu/fhm.
- International Association for Aquatic Animal Medicine, www.iaaam.org.
- Michigan State University aquatic links, http://cvmstudent.cvm.msu.edu/ac/aquarium.htm.

- National Oceanic and Atmospheric Administration Careers www.afsc.noaa.gov/nmml > education web > careers.
- Southern Regional Aquaculture Center Publications, http://srac.tamu.edu.
- University of Florida IFAS Extension, http://edis.ifas.ufl.edu.
- University of Wisconsin Fish Health Medicine Certificate Program, http://vetmedce.vetmed.wisc.edu/fhm.
- World Aquatic Veterinary Medical Association, www.wavma.org.

Working with Wildlife

Rehabilitation centers, zoos, circuses, and sanctuaries all employ veterinarians. Internationally, veterinarians may be part of an environmental project, such as protecting indigenous forest animals through managed forest programs. Some government jobs include working with wildlife. (See Chapter 16: USGS, FWS, NMML.) The World Organisation for Animal Health also has a wildlife working group (Chapter 13). Also see Chapter 14 descriptions of university research with wildlife.

Daily work / Pros and cons

Daily work at rehabilitation centers or zoos includes hands-on medicine and surgery. Wildlife management may involve herd health and epidemiology, which focus more on total populations, so there is more indoor desk work, and outdoor work is not with individual animals. The total number of job openings is small.

Qualifications / To apply

A working knowledge of birds and other wildlife is necessary. This topic does not receive a large focus in most veterinary teaching hospitals, so students must make an effort to seek out learning opportunities. Veterinarians who want to learn more should attend continuing education offered by the associations listed in this chapter. Also look for short term externship opportunities, where you can learn on the job (these are not just for students). If there is a wildlife rehabilitation center or a zoo near you, volunteering there is another way to gain experience.

Because jobs are few, it's beneficial to have specialized training in the field, such as an internship, residency, or a background or degree in epidemiology, toxicology, conservation medicine, or public health.

Salary ranges tend to be lower than average for veterinarians overall. Legislation proposed in 2010 would create new positions for wildlife and zoo veterinarians, limit their school debt, and provide incentives to study and practice wildlife and zoo medicine. (See http://alceehastings.house.gov > newsroom > 2010 press releases >January, and the 2009 *JAVMA* article by R. Nolen.)

The web sites of the following list of associations are excellent sources regarding wildlife medicine:
- American Association of Zoo Veterinarians, AAZV; www.aazv.org.
- AVMA, www.avma.org > meetings > environmental opportunities.
- American College of Zoological Medicine, www.aczm.org.
- Association of Avian Veterinarians, AAV; www.aav.org.
- Association of Exotic Mammal Veterinarians, AEMV; www.aemv.org.

- Association of Reptilian and Amphibian Veterinarians, ARAV; www.arav.org.
- Association of Zoos and Aquariums, AZA; www.aza.org.
- International Wildlife Rehabilitation Council, IWRC; www.iwrc-online.org.
- National Wildlife Rehabilitation Association, NWRA; www.nwrawildlife.org.
- University of Minnesota's Wildlife Information Directory, wildlife links and a list of rehabilitation centers, www.tc.umn.edu/~devo0028.

Sample job announcement: Internship position, primates

> We welcome applicants with a background and interest in animal husbandry, welfare and conservation, exotic veterinary medicine, biology, and related fields. The volunteer intern needs to be a mature team player with respect for others, a good communicator and coordinator (written and spoken English), and be able to make a long-term commitment to the primates and the staff.

Wildlife rehabilitation

Rehabilitation facilities provide care for birds and animals such as raccoons, opossums, songbirds, bats, and even reptiles. Wildlife rehabilitation centers are located in large cities and in key areas for wildlife, such as at Sanibel Island, Florida. The HSUS (Chapter 13) also operates animal care centers that handle wildlife rehabilitation.

Daily work

Many rehabilitation centers focus on species such as raptors that are of interest for wildlife conservation. One such place is The Raptor Center at the University of Minnesota.

After practicing companion animal medicine for 16 years, Julia Ponder, DVM, capitalized on the opportunity to pursue her lifelong passion for birds by volunteering at The Raptor Center, where the director and residents shared their knowledge. She was eventually hired as a staff veterinarian, and she now serves as its executive director.

The most difficult part of the job, according to Dr. Ponder, is having to make decisions based on resources available rather than what could be done in a best-case scenario, which is frequently the case in most wildlife veterinary positions. Dr. Ponder also comments on seeing the suffering that humans can inflict (unintentionally or intentionally) on animals.

A great way to get experience and see whether wildlife medicine is really something of interest to you is to volunteer your time, as Dr. Ponder did; this will also help you get your foot in the door! Dr. Ponder offers the following advice for those interested in the field:

> Create a strong network—meet people working in the field, benefit from their knowledge and experience and work closely with them. The learning curve is steep and much of the available information is not well published—much more information is still to be discovered!

There are very few full-time wildlife jobs for veterinarians; zoo jobs typically require a zoo and exotics residency. Be very sure you understand what your goals for your work with wildlife are. Depending on your goals, you can determine how to structure things: Is wildlife/rehab medicine something you do to give back to the community while pursuing private practice? Do you want to do fieldwork/research (which will demand education/experience beyond vet school)? Do you want to be in a zoo or one of the rare wildlife hospitals? If so, you will need skill, knowledge, experience and a bit of luck. Externships and internships are wonderful ways to develop a network, see the opportunities, and learn.

Daily duties as staff veterinarian at The Raptor Center include diagnosis, medical treatment, and surgical care for injured and sick raptors. Records kept for each individual bird must be filled out as legal documents, just as at a companion animal practice. Because The Raptor Center is associated with the University of Minnesota, there is also teaching of didactic classes and oversight of students on clinical rotations. Teaching extends to overseeing interns, residents, and externs, who come from all over the world to study at the center. Finally, there is general oversight of all cases under treatment (those assigned to other clinicians), and occasional work with clinical research studies.

Hours vary based upon the number of clinicians working and the financial status of the organization. Full-time work is typically more than 40 hours per week, and can be substantially more during the busy season. The senior veterinarian also backs up the interns, residents, and students on weekends.

Benefits at The Raptor Center are quite good, including health, dental, and life insurance, because it is part of the university system.

Qualifications / To apply

In smaller cities and rural areas, private practitioners may obtain a wildlife rehabilitation license and work in this area "on the side," often providing services at little or no charge. Small rehab centers may also utilize the services of local veterinarians.

Larger facilities employ a staff veterinarian. Knowledge of wildlife husbandry and health care is necessary. Because these positions are often linked with nonprofit organizations, knowledge of not-for-profit management and fundraising are helpful.

Before rehabilitators are given a license, they must pass oral and written exams. Their facilities must also pass inspection. In some cases, permits from the US Fish and Wildlife Service (FWS) are required. Each state's wildlife agency can advise on the permits, training, and facility that are required.

Resources include:
- American Association of Zoo Veterinarians (www.aazv.org), which coordinated volunteers for the oil spill disaster of 2010.
- International Wildlife Rehabilitation Council, which offers training, continuing education, and networking (www.iwrc-online.org).
- National Wildlife Rehabilitation Association; 24 percent of its members are either veterinarians, students, or veterinary technicians. Its web site (www.nwrawildlife.

org) offers job listings, educational opportunities, a list of registered veterinarians and licensed wildlife rehabilitators, and publications such as *Principles of Wildlife Rehabilitation.*

- Oiled Wildlife Care Network (www.owcn.org), which led the 2010 effort to care for oil-affected marine mammals and sea turtles in Louisiana, in partnership with NOAA-NMFS and the US-FWS. (See Chapters 13 and 16). The OWCN is the world's only oiled wildlife response organization. Its members include world-class aquaria, universities, scientific organizations and rehabilitation groups. Established as a result of the 1994 Exxon Valdez oil spill in Alaska, it is currently administered by the UC Davis Wildlife Health Center in the School of Veterinary Medicine.
- Also see Chapter 13 details about working with nonprofit and service groups.

Zoo veterinarian

Daily work

Veterinarians at zoos and wildlife parks work with a wide variety of birds, mammals, reptiles, and aquatic animals. Zoo work includes hands-on medicine and surgery, herd health, helping endangered species, and educating people about wild animals. Many zoos are run by nonprofit organizations, which means there is often a public relations component to the work.

Qualifications / To apply

Zoos exist in every major city, yet not all zoos employ their own veterinarian. Smaller zoos and wildlife parks often contract with a local veterinarian in private practice to perform necessary work. Larger zoos have sophisticated veterinary facilities with veterinarians, technicians, and students. Zoos may hire veterinarians for non-clinical positions such as "Education Director" or "Resource Development." For the zoo, having a veterinarian in this position increases their credibility.

The web sites of larger zoos usually have a page for jobs or careers (e.g., the San Diego Zoo, www.sandiegozoo.org/jobs, or the National Zoo, http://nationalzoo.si.edu > careers and internships; also see Chapter 16).

The Wildlife Conservation Society (WCS, www.wcs.org), founded in 1895 as the New York Zoological Society, is one of the first conservation organizations in the US. It includes the Bronx Zoo, Central Park Zoo in Manhattan, Queens Zoo, Prospect Park Zoo, and the New York Aquarium in Coney Island. The WCS helped to launch One World–One Health in 2004 to promote an international and interdisciplinary strategy for combating threats to the health of life on Earth (www.OneWorldOneHealth.org). The WCS offers a diverse array of jobs and internships suitable for veterinarians and veterinary students at their headquarters in New York City and offices worldwide. The WCS interns and volunteers based in New York City work within one of its zoos or the aquarium. Positions available in the WCS global offices range from field research to conservation diplomacy, financial administration, or program management. Many positions require technical and scientific expertise.

Resources include the American Association of Zoo Veterinarians (www.aazv.org) and the Association of Zoos and Aquariums (www.aza.org).

Sample job announcement: Zoo Veterinarian

> Graduation from an AVMA-accredited college of veterinary medicine. Two years of clinical veterinary experience, preferably with exotic animals in a zoo setting or in an approved internship or residency. Requires knowledge of: the zoo's mission and philosophy; zoo veterinary medicine including exotic animal care, housing and environmental requirements; nutrition; preventive medicine; diagnostic procedures; restraint; treatment; disease control; and epidemiological techniques. Knowledge of: occupational hazards and safe practices working with dangerous animals; government regulations pertaining to animal health and welfare; and personnel management. Skills: administrative skills, interpersonal skills including ability to get along with diverse groups with tact and maturity; analytical skills, reasoning abilities, prioritization, and time management; presentation and persuasive skills with ability to express oneself clearly and effectively in oral and written form. Ability to: establish and maintain effective working relationships with governmental agencies, donors and the general public; to prepare comprehensive reports and maintain complex records of a highly specialized, and confidential, nature; to interact courteously and respectfully with supervisors, fellow employees, volunteers, zoo visitor and general public.

Circus veterinarian

Yet another job that involves work with wildlife is that of a circus veterinarian, who works with wild cats, elephants, and monkeys, among other species.

Daily work

There are no daily routines in circus work. Three or more days each week are spent travelling. An important part of the job is making sure that each animal has a current health certificate and the correct paperwork; as circuses travel around the country, they must comply with all federal, state, and local regulations.

Circus animals are all entertainers or, in some respects, athletes who perform various routines. Part of the circus veterinarian's job is to ensure they are healthy and at peak condition. This involves speaking with the trainers and keepers about the animals, consulting with staff veterinary technicians, and performing veterinary health care. "Winter quarters" is where the circus is stationed for approximately six weeks to practice the new show that will go out on the road for that year (for Ringling Brothers Circus this is in Florida). During this very busy time, the veterinarian typically vaccinates all the animals and draws blood for any tests that might be needed. Research is also part of the job; this is one of the rare environments in which a veterinarian is able to study the medical and health needs of a wide variety of exotic animals in one place for the good of exotics all over the world.

Even though most circus veterinarian positions do not require an advanced degree, experience with exotics and zoo animals is necessary. Salary is competitive within the industry. Benefits include medical insurance, liability insurance, state licensing fees, association dues, and CE funds, as well as all travel costs.

Danielle Graham, DVM, has worked in the circus industry for many years. She started with the circus just two years out of veterinary school with no additional training. While working in a small animal private practice, she looked for the opportunity to join a zoo or similar facility that would allow her to both practice and advance her education. When she got a call that the Ringling Brothers and Barnum & Bailey Circus needed an associate veterinarian, and was offered an interview through a professor from vet school, she jumped at the chance and got the job. As Dr. Graham relates:

> Not only do I get to work with amazing animals, but I get to see the country while doing it! I also enjoy meeting new people and learning interesting things from our multi-cultural staff on the units. This job constantly keeps you on your toes. One minute you could be working with a dog, and the next minute an elephant. That is what I love about my job; it is never the same day twice, and you are constantly learning new things, and constantly being challenged.

Other wildlife projects

The groups discussed in this section are among the variety of small associations and groups that work with wildlife and conservation. Most of these groups are too small to hire additional veterinarians, but volunteer opportunities may be available. The groups outlined here illustrate the potential niches that veterinarians may fill.

One example of a unique niche in wildlife medicine is the Zoo/Exotic Pathology Service in Sacramento, California (www.zooexotic.com), which is owned by two veterinarians with backgrounds in wildlife and pathology. These individuals targeted their unique interests into a thriving business.

The Urban Wildlife Institute of the Lincoln Park Zoo in Chicago includes interdisciplinary teams that study ecosystem health in the urban setting (www.lpzoo.com/cs_centers_uwi.php).

Dr. Carol Walton used her veterinary degree and lifelong interest in wildlife and conservation to launch a full-time ecotourism company (http://carolwaltonexpeditions.com).

> I am the owner of a wildlife tour company, and I guide groups all over Africa, South America, Antarctica, the Arctic and other places, like Madagascar to see lemurs and Rwanda/Uganda for Gorilla trekking. I take people on nature tours and teach them about the wildlife and conservation issues in the area. I'm now organizing Veterinary CE

trips for the North American Veterinary Conferences under the name of "NAVC Expeditions." I've done trips for NAVC to Antarctica, the arctic to see polar bears, the rainforests of Peru and Ecuador and the Galapagos with plans for future expeditions to Africa, Panama, Fiji, Iceland and many other wild and exotic places! —Carol Walton, DVM, Carol Walton Expeditions.

Mountain Gorilla Veterinary Project

The Mountain Gorilla Veterinary Project (MGVP, gorilladoctors.org) was started nearly 20 years ago by one veterinarian. The MGVP tracks ailing gorillas, observing and treating them when needed in their native habitat, and providing them with life-saving veterinary care for human-caused or life-threatening illnesses and injuries. MGVP is also working with the Wildlife Health Center at the UC Davis School of Veterinary Medicine to form the Mountain Gorilla One Health Program.

The MGVP staff are of varying nationalities and have varying levels of training above and beyond veterinary degrees. Many have PhDs or have trained in zoo animal medicine. Veterinarians work in Central Africa (Rwanda, Uganda, and the Democratic Republic of Congo). In-country field veterinarians are stationed in these three separate locations, while regional veterinarians and project directors move about. The international headquarters is located in Maryland. You can read the profiles of some of the MGVP veterinarians at www.gorilladoctors.org > about us > doctors and staff.

African Predator Conservation Research Organization

Michael Briggs, DVM, is the co-founder and chief executive officer of the African Predator Conservation Research Organization (APCRO, www.apcro.org), as well as the principal investigator for several of its conservation projects. After graduating from veterinary school, Dr. Briggs spent 20 years at major US zoos as both staff and associate veterinarian. During this tenure, he obtained his master's degree in veterinary medicine with an emphasis on parasitology and theriogenology. Since the beginning of his career, he has worked in the field in Africa, including South Africa, Namibia, and Botswana, during which he gained field experience with game capture as well as myriad research projects, many of which have focused on carnivores. According to Dr. Briggs:

> The conservation of the wild carnivores is the most important direction I could take with my life and career. I intend to help improve the chances of these animals surviving long-term and to help any group with that common goal.

Volunteer opportunities are available with APCRO to work in Africa. Volunteers must be physically fit, commit to a minimum of two to three weeks in Africa, and be able to support all their own costs. Work is often in very remote areas without telephones, electricity, or e-mail. Due to the interest in this project, waiting time after acceptance may be one year or longer.

Eastern Cougar Foundation

Jay Tischendorf, DVM, is one of the original board members of the Eastern Cougar Foundation, a group whose mission is to facilitate the recovery of the cougar in suitable wild habitat in the central and eastern US (www.easterncougar.org). Dr. Tischendorf's story shows how there is always room to get involved with your passion; you can create your own opportunities. In his words:

> I feel incredibly fortunate to have done all the things I've done—working with some really amazing animals, both wild and domestic, and some really great people in some very special places (and truly to have survived some of these episodes, as well).

Jobs related to the environment

Environmental jobs usually involve working with wildlife in a broad sense. Veterinarians who are interested in helping others through environmental awareness may find a niche in international work (Chapter 13). Government jobs (e.g., with the EPA or FWS) might also be appropriate. Fellows for the US Agency for International Development (USAID) also can have a positive impact on the environmental awareness of people in other countries. (See Chapter 16.)

A group called the Alliance of Veterinarians for the Environment (AVE) encourages veterinarians to get involved with careers that have a positive impact on the environment, building upon the connections between animal health and well-being and environmental and ecosystem health (www.aveweb.org). AVE offers educational programs on the connections between environmental health and veterinary medicine, with a focus on greening veterinary practices and addressing the health impacts of climate change. They are working with Tufts University on a Green Veterinary Practice Handbook, and they will have a chapter on green zoo veterinary practice in the new 7th edition of the Zoo and Wildlife Animal Medicine book (in press, 2011).

The Envirovet Summer Institute is a collaborative program between the University of Illinois, the University of California Davis, the White Oak Conservation Center, Harbor Branch Oceanographic Institute, and other organizations that provide instructors (http://vetmed.illinois.edu/envirovet). Students spend the first part of a seven-week course at conservation and oceanographic institutes in the US, and then travel to developing countries for three weeks. Envirovet participants can be veterinarians or veterinary students.

The North Carolina State University College of Veterinary Medicine has a variety of programs addressing a range of ecological issues around the globe (www.cvm.ncsu.edu > ecosystem health).

Other organizations that offer jobs related to the environment are The Nature Conservancy (www.tnc.org) and the National Council for Science and the Environment (www.ncseonline.org). Many web sites focus on environmental job listings, such as www.eco.org and www.ecojobs.com (tip: search "biologist"). Two books related to environmental careers are *Careers in the Environment*, by M. Fasulo and P. Walker, and *Complete Guide to Environmental Careers in the 21st Century*, by the Environmental Care Organization.

Veterinarians may be involved with rehabilitation of animals after man-made disasters such as oil spills. See the earlier section on rehabilitation. Also see the information about global climate change research at CSU, in Chapter 14.

Laboratory Animal Medicine

Research

> The breadth and depth of today's biomedical research involving the development of new drugs and medical devices is mind boggling. By working in this field, I make contributions to furthering both human and animal health on a daily basis. This makes working in the field extremely satisfying. Laboratory animal veterinarians support biomedical research by contributing to the development of animal models and managing entire research programs. Boredom is not an option, as a multitude of species and the constant demand for new procedures is the norm.— Stacy Pritt, DVM, MS, MBA, CPIA, Director and General Manager, Biological Test Center, Irvine, CA.

Daily work / Pros and cons

Laboratory animals include mice and rats, but also larger animals up to the size of nonhuman primates. The primary function of the laboratory animal veterinarian is to provide for the health and well-being of research animals. Depending on the facility, the laboratory animal veterinarian may work with only one species, or with multiple species, such as dogs, cats, mice, rats, and primates.

Work includes the design and implementation of clinical and preventive veterinary medical programs, oversight of animal husbandry programs, and consulting with and training of biomedical researchers and technicians. These veterinarians also may perform independent research and serve as consultants and collaborators to research investigators. Their work can involve herd health, in caring for a group of animals, or individual animal care as necessary for any one project.

Laboratory animal veterinarians work in a variety of positions including academia (at both medical and veterinary colleges), in industry, and for the government. Their work has the pros and cons of all those career paths.

Laboratory animal veterinarians must be comfortable with the programs and policies of the institution for which they work. They must be aware of regulations regarding animal welfare, and of the ethical debates about use of animals in research.

Qualifications / To apply

Research laboratories do hire veterinarians without further training. However, additional knowledge will help to advance in this field. This may be through board certification (see Chapter 4) or other means. For example, the American Association of Laboratory Animal Science (AALAS) offers a Certified Manager, Animal Resources (CMAR) certification program.

In general, laboratory animal veterinarians are paid extremely well. Overall, the average income from primary employment for 2008 was $153,038, a rise of over 14 percent from the previous reporting period, with the highest salary reported being $438,000 for a senior director with more than 20 years of experience. Benefits usually include health insurance, dental insurance, and a retirement plan. Additional benefits vary by employer and can include life insurance, disability insurance, and stock options.

Articles related to laboratory animal veterinarian income include those in *JAVMA* by B.C. Gehrke and R.S. Nolen. Web sites related to laboratory animal medicine include:

- Academy of Surgical Research, www.surgicalresearch.org.
- American Society of Laboratory Animal Practitioners, has salary survey, www.aslap.org.
- American College of Laboratory Animal Medicine, www.aclam.org.
- American Association for Laboratory Animal Science, www.aalas.org.
- Association for Assessment and Accreditation of Laboratory Animal Care International, www.aaalac.org.
- Association of Primate Veterinarians, www.primatevets.org.
- Institutional Animal Care and Use Committee, www.iacuc.org.
- Wisconsin National Primate Research Center, www.primate.wisc.edu.

Also see Chapter 11, Industry (R & D); Chapter 14, Academia; and Chapters 16 and 18, jobs with the federal government, particularly NASA, Veteran's Affairs, and the Army.

Sample job announcements

Attending facility veterinarian

> Requires DVM. One or more years of relevant experience preferred. Must function independently in an animal facility. Provide veterinary medical diagnostic, surgical, and/or treatment services within the animal facilities; clinical care for laboratory animals (rats, mice, and rabbits); oversight for nonhuman primate studies. Should possess a broad knowledge of laboratory animal health/medicine, current use practices in laboratory animal medicine, study coordination, sentinel program, import/export, and SOP creation and revision.

University position: Director of laboratory animal facilities

> Oversee the daily operations of the university's Laboratory Animal Resources, including budgeting and staffing; develop and implement training programs in animal care; consult in the design and development of animal care facilities; provide clinical support for animal research projects; and assist in the review and approval of animal research protocols to ensure compliance with all state and federal regulations. DVM required.

Industry position: Laboratory animal veterinarian

> Works within a multifunctional team to provide scientific and clinical expertise as well as leadership in providing oversight for an accredited laboratory animal program. Requires DVM or VMD; knowledge and skills in laboratory animal medicine; excellent written and verbal skills; and a willingness to work in complex environments. ACLAM Board Certification is desired.

Chapter 6 Resources

Groups and web sites

African Predator Conservation Research Organization, www.apcro.org/id1.html.
Alliance of Veterinarians for the Environment, www.aveweb.org.
American Association for Laboratory Animal Science, www.aalas.org.
American Association of Zoo Veterinarians, www.aazv.org.
American College of Laboratory Animal Medicine, www.aclam.org.
American College of Zoological Medicine, www.aczm.org.
American Fisheries Society, Fish Health Section, www.fisheries.org/fhs.
American Pet Products Association (APPA), National Pet Owners Survey, www.americanpetproducts.org.
American Society of Laboratory Animal Practitioners, www.aslap.org.
Aquaculture Network Information Center, http://aquanic.org.
Aquatic Veterinary Medicine Links, http://cvmstudent.cvm.msu.edu/ac/aquarium.htm.
Aquavet, www.vet.cornell.edu/Public/FishDisease/AquaticProg/ceo.htm.
Association for Assessment and Accreditation of Laboratory Animal Care (AAALAC International), www.aaalac.org.
Association of Avian Veterinarians, www.aav.org.
Association of Exotic Mammal Veterinarians, www.aemv.org.
Association of Primate Veterinarians, www.primatevets.org.
Association of Reptilian and Amphibian Veterinarians, www.arav.org.
Association of Zoos and Aquariums, www.aza.org; phone: 1-301-562-0777.
Eastern Cougar Foundation, www.easterncougar.org.
Environmental Careers Organization, www.eco.org; phone: 810-960-5857.
Envirovet, http://vetmed.illinois.edu/envirovet.
Fish Health Medicine Certificate Program, www.vetmedce.vetmed.wisc.edu/fhm.
International Association for Aquatic Animal Medicine, www.iaaam.org.
International Wildlife Rehabilitation Council, www.iwrc-online.org; phone: 408-271-2685.
Mountain Gorilla Veterinary Project, www.gorilladoctors.org.
National Council for Science and the Environment, www.ncseonline.org.
National Wildlife Rehabilitation Association, www.nwrawildlife.org or nwrawildlife.org/pubs; phone: 320-230-9920.
The Nature Conservancy, www.tnc.org.
Oiled Wildlife Care Network, www.owcn.org.
One World–One Health, www.OneWorldOneHealth.org.
Southern Regional Aquaculture Center Publications, http://srac.tamu.edu.
University of Florida IFAS Extension, http://edis.ifas.ufl.edu.
University of Wisconsin Fish Health Medicine Certificate Program, http://vetmedce.vetmed.wisc.edu/fhm.
Wildlife Conservation Society, 2300 Southern Boulevard, Bronx, NY 10460; www.wcs.org; phone: 718-220-5100.
Wildlife Rehabilitation Information Directory, www.tc.umn.edu/~devo0028.
World Aquatic Veterinary Medical Association, www.wavma.org.

Books and articles

Cima, G., Finned animals increasingly seen as patients. *JAVMA News*, Aug 1, 2010:246-249.
Environmental Care Organization, *Complete Guide to Environmental Careers in the 21ˢᵗ Century* (Island Press, 1998).
Fasulo, M, and P Walker, *Careers in the Environment*, (McGraw Hill, 2007).
Gehrke, B. C., B. J. Weigler, and M. M. Slattum, Professional Income of Laboratory Animal Veterinarians Predicted by Multiple Regression Analysis, *JAVMA*, 2000; 216: 852–858.

Hastings, A. Hastings Introduces the Wildlife and Zoological Veterinary Medicine Enhancement Act January 21, 2010: http://alceehastings.house.gov or http://alceehastings.house.gov/images/stories/PDFs/Wildlife_and_Zoological_ Veterinary_Medicine_Enhancement_Act_of_2010.doc.pdf.

Huneke, R. B., Salary Survey of Laboratory Animal Veterinarians for the Year 2008, American College of Laboratory Animal Medicine & American Society of Laboratory Animal Practitioners, April 2009, www.aslap.org.

National Aquatic Animal Health Task Force, National Aquatic Animal Health Plan for the United States, August 2008, www.aphis.usda.gov > animal health > animal diseases by species > aquaculture.

National Wildlife Rehabilitation Association (NWRA), Principles of Wildlife Rehabilitation: Minimum Standards for Wildlife Rehabilitation, www.nwrawildlife.org.

Nolen, R.S., Congressman sees need for more zoo and wildlife veterinarians, *JAVMA News* March 1, 2009, 236(5):497.

Nolen R.S., Despite High Demand, Laboratory Animal Veterinarians in Short Supply: Economic Survey Shows Upward Trend in Specialists' Salaries. *JAVMA News*, October 1, 2003.

Roberts, H, *Fundamentals of Ornamental Fish Health* (Wiley Blackwell, 2009).

Wride, N, A Nose Job for a Sawfish: A Long Beach "Aquavet" Is among a New Breed of Specialists Bringing Human-Type Treatments to Ailing Marine Life. Fake Fish Eyes, Anyone? *Los Angeles Times*, November 10, 2006; A1.

7 STARTING YOUR OWN BUSINESS

Housecall practice, relief work, writing, and consulting, which are the topics of the next three chapters, have one thing in common: They often involve running your own business. Many of the jobs described in the next few chapters can be performed by a veterinarian acting as an employee, but they usually are businesses run by one person who is self-employed. In addition, veterinarians may breed, raise and sell their own animals; they may own and manage dairy farms, beef cattle ranches, dog breeding kennels, or commercial aviaries. Veterinarians have started cremation services, pet cemeteries, and grief counseling services. (See Chapter 3 for private practice ownership.)

Let's say you have come up with a great widget that every veterinarian should buy, and you want to start a business selling widgets. Or perhaps you have written a great software program for veterinarians. Whether you are selling widgets, software, or your housecall service, you must be proficient in two areas:

- You must know the technical aspects of your business (e.g., how to make a widget, or how to use computers).
- You must know how to run your own business.

The latter requirement is just as important as the former. The biggest mistake made by new business owners is thinking that their technical expertise will carry them through the process of starting their business. Nothing will lead to failure faster than that attitude.

Business management includes financial management, human resource management, marketing, and more. Your ability to market your services is one of the most important contributors to your success. You may have the greatest new invention, but if no one knows about it, your business isn't going anywhere. Once you get clients, your ability to manage your finances and manage your time are the factors that determine whether you make it in the long run. Organizational ability is essential. Many entrepreneurs are great at start-ups but fail because they have no interest or ability in the day-to-day detail work necessary to keep the business going. Others find they miss the camaraderie of the office or hospital environment; after all, running your own business, especially at the initial stages, can be lonely. If you have never been in charge of anything, it can be difficult to adjust to having the last word for everything; there is no safety net behind you—your decisions are your own.

Self-Assessment Questionnaire

- Before you start your business, be honest with yourself about your abilities. Answer the following questions:
- Are you interested in being your own boss, managing your time, disciplining yourself to work, selling your skills (or product), and tracking down new clients?
- Are you good at record keeping, or can you hire someone who is?
- Are you willing to study business management and make a business plan?
- What are your start-up costs? What equipment and supplies will you need? What ongoing costs can you project? What will you charge for your products or services?
- How will you target your market and analyze your competition?
- If your work involves travel, will you charge for travel time, travel costs, both, or neither?
- If you will have an office in your home, is your area zoned for home offices?
- Do you have a good attorney and accountant who can advise you in legal and tax matters?
- Are you proficient at desktop publishing so that you can create your own brochures, press releases, and other materials? (Your start-out budget often won't allow hiring someone for this! Local printing / copy shops are a great help, though.)
- Who are your potential customers, how will they pay for your product or services, and how will you handle late payments?
- Will you hire employees, and if so, to do what jobs? Do you have job descriptions for these positions? Have you had management training, or will you get it?
- Do you have unrealistic expectations of the personal benefits of being self-employed? You may expect that you'll have more personal time, but chances are that you'll work longer hours than ever.
- What kind of insurance will you need?
- How will you pay your bills during the three to 12 months it will take to get your business off the ground?
- Can you get a loan to cover your business start-up costs?
- Do you know how to write a business plan?
- Are you willing to give up some control to the people you hire?

Getting help / To start

One highly recommended reference is *Working from Home*, 5th edition, by Paul and Sarah Edwards. It is the classic book for any self-employed person with an office in the home—writers, housecall veterinarians, relief veterinarians, consultants, and the like. The books and periodicals listed in the chapter resources are also excellent references for any veterinary business.

The Small Business Administration (SBA) offers low-cost classes in starting a business, a wide variety of publications that deal with every imaginable question you may have, and a very informative web site (www.sba.gov). SBA loans are also available. The agency rarely loans money itself, but instead backs you with a loan guarantee at the bank. Also, a group called SCORE (Service Corp of Retired Executives) can help you with free advice. Find the nearest group by contacting the SBA or Chamber of Commerce.

The American Veterinary Medical Law Association (AVMLA, www.avmla.org) holds educational meetings and publishes a member newsletter that includes legal updates pertinent to veterinarians. You do not have to be a lawyer to join their group or attend their meetings.

The Edward Lowe Foundation (ELF, www.edwardlowe.org) provides information, research, and education experience that support small business. It provides access to information through online services, computer databases, and publications. The ELF web site contains a huge list of resources and links for all sorts of other business information providers.

The Small Business Resource Center (www.sbrcbaltimore.com) provides online links to articles on starting and operating a small business, including: How to Prepare an Effective Business Plan, How to Raise Money to Start Your Own Business, The Legalities and Tax Advantages of a Home Business, How to Start a Consulting Service, and Reorganize Your Time to Start a Home-Based Business.

The Society for Human Resource Management (SHRM) provides a wealth of information, articles, and continuing education pertaining to employee management, laws, and productivity (www.shrm.org).

The US Business Advisor gives information about government regulations, publications, and resources for small business (www.business.gov).

The Veterinary Business Management Association (VBMA, www.vbma.biz) is a student-run organization with information on general business knowledge in the veterinary field.

Don't forget your state government as a resource. Many states offer services or information for business owners. The names of these departments vary slightly from state to state. Typically, they are known by the department of taxation and revenue for state taxes, business registration, and licenses; the employment division for unemployment insurance or employment security; the department of labor for labor and industries or workers' compensation coverage; the veterinary board for licensing; and the licensing department for state business licenses and pharmacy or drug licenses.

IRS publications are all available online at www.irs.ustreas.gov (all documents are free). Start with #334, *Tax Guide for Small Businesses*. Also, most libraries carry copies of IRS publications, or you can write to the Superintendent of Documents, Government Printing Office, Washington DC 20402, or call 800-TAX-FORM (800-829-3676).

Chapter 7 Resources

Groups and web sites

American Veterinary Medical Law Association, www.avmla.org; phone: 312-233-2760.

Edward Lowe Foundation (ELF), 58220 Decatur Road, P.O. Box 8, Cassopolis, MI 49031-0008; www.edwardlowe.org; phone: 800-232-LOWE (5693); fax: 269-445-2648; e-mail: info@lowe.org.

Entrepreneur Media Inc., 2445 McCabe Way, Ste. 400, Irvine, CA 92614; www.entrepreneur.com; phone: 949-261-2325 (customer service) or 800-274-6229 (subscriptions).

BNet, tools for working professionals, www.bnet.com.

IRS Publications, Superintendent of Documents, Government Printing Office, Washington, DC 20402, www.irs.ustreas. gov; phone: 800-TAX-FORM (800-829-3676).

Service Corp of Retired Executives 9SCORE), www.score.orgt.

Small Business Administration (SBA), www.sba.gov; phone: 800-827-5722; e-mail answerdesk@sba.gov.

Small Business Resource Center, 1101 E. 33rd Street, Suite C307, Baltimore, MD 21218; www.sbrcbaltimore.com; phone: 443-451-7160; fax: 443-451-7169; e-mail: info@sbrcbaltimore.com.

Smart Business Supersite, www.smartbiz.com.

Society for Human Resource Management (SHRM), www.shrm.org; phone: 800-283-7476.

US Business Advisor, www.business.gov.

Veterinary Business Management Association, www.vbma.biz.

Veterinary Economics, 8033 Flint, Lenexa, KS 66214; www.dvm360.com; phone: 800-255-6864; fax: 913-871-3808.

Books and articles

Brabec, B., *Homemade Money: Bringing in the Bucks: A Business Management and Marketing Bible for Home-Business Owners, Self-Employed Individuals, and Web Entrepreneurs Working from Home Base* (Betterway Books, 2003).

Edwards, P., and S. Edwards, *Working from Home*, 5th edition (Tarcher/Putnam, 1999).

Hazelgren, B., *Your First Business Plan*, 5th edition (Sourcebooks, 2005).

Inc. magazine, www.inc.com.

Veterinary Economics magazine, www.dvm360.com.

Williams, B., *Complete Guide to Working for Yourself: Everything the Self-Employed Need to Know about Taxes, Recordkeeping and Other Laws*, with Companion CD-ROM (Atlantic Publishing Group, 2008).

8   HOUSECALL AND RELIEF PRACTICE

While housecall and relief work are different, they are included together here because many veterinarians consider both of these choices when they want to stay in private practice yet create more flexibility or control over their work. Both do offer flexibility in terms of time or hours worked, but they differ in the kind of flexibility that is possible.

With housecall work, you can set the hours or days that you work on a weekly basis. For example, you could decide to work weekday mornings only, offering your housecall services only during those hours.

With relief work, you can decide which days or weeks that you work—but the hours actually worked each day (on the days that you are working), are fixed. For example, if you take a relief job to fill in for Dr. Good next week, you will have to work in her place during the hours that she normally would work.

Either way, the previous chapter on starting your own business is "must" reading. Create a professional business so you will be viewed with respect by your clients and can sustain your success.

Housecall and Mobile Practice Veterinarians

In a housecall or mobile practice, the veterinarian goes to homes, farms, ranches or stables to perform requested veterinary services.

The typical small-animal housecall practitioner carries supplies in a vehicle, but performs work on pets in the clients' homes. Small-animal veterinarians sometimes perform work in a mobile clinic, which is usually a customized form of motor home converted into an exam room, laboratory, and surgical suite. The term "mobile veterinarian" is often used to differentiate these veterinarians from the typical housecall veterinarian.

When one is describing large-animal practitioners, the term "mobile veterinarian" is used for any practitioner who travels to farms or stables, regardless of the vehicle used. "Ambulatory practitioner" is another term used to describe these veterinarians. They usually drive a pickup truck or large vehicle with refrigerator, running water, supplies, and equipment in a self-contained unit.

Mobile veterinary units are made by companies including LaBoit (www.laboit.com), Dodgen (www.dodgenmobiletech.com/veterinary), Porta-Vet (www.portavet.net), and Lifeline Mobile (http://lifelinemobile.com). LaBoit's web site includes a great deal of information for housecall and mobile veterinarians.

Housecall and large animal (or ambulatory) practitioners often have a base somewhere to keep their inventory so they can restock their vehicle on a daily basis. Most housecall practitioners keep home offices, where they store client files, supplies, and equipment. Their base or home office may also include some basic laboratory equipment such as a microscope and centrifuge.

Some housecall veterinarians spend all their time on housecalls and refer any complicated cases to a full-service hospital; some may lease space in a clinic in which they perform in-hospital procedures (such as surgery) themselves; and others work out of a "base" clinic and conduct housecalls only part of the time.

Both housecall and mobile practitioners can work part-time or full-time. They can work as employees or they can be self-employed. See Chapter 3 on traditional practices and Chapter 7 on starting a business.

View the following resources for more information:
- American Association of Housecall Veterinarians (AAHV), www.housecallvets.org or www.homevets.org.
- American Association of Mobile Veterinary Practitioners, webinars and networking, www.aamvp.org.
- Veterinary Information Network (VIN), an online venue where housecall veterinarians may connect, www.vin.com.
- *House Call: The Housecall Veterinarian's Manual*, by C. Smith, a detailed workbook that will help you start your business, develop a marketing plan, and organize your time. Updated periodically, it includes setting up your home office, creating an agreement with a local veterinary hospital for in-hospital work, getting clients, setting fees, hiring employees, and more. See www.smithvet.com.

Daily work

> I learn so much more visiting a bird in the home than I ever could in an office setting. The location, size and furnishings of the cage, food provided, cage bottom covering—all are immediately available for viewing and this obviates the need for detailed questioning about these pieces of the bird's history. Demeanor is much more easily discerned in this setting as well. Very rarely will a bird show accurate signs of disease when presented to a veterinary clinic in a small travel cage, unless it is so desperately ill it can do nothing to hide the fact. The stress of putting many pet birds into a carrier and driving to a vet clinic, then being handled by strangers in a strange place, is immense.—Nancy Murbach, DVM, Veterinary House Call Service, Scottsdale, AZ.

During a typical day, the housecall veterinarian will see 10 clients and will spend quite a bit of time driving. The job requires self-sufficiency and self-confidence. Some housecall veterinarians work alone, while others work with a veterinary assistant or technician. These veterinarians become adept at drawing blood from a cat without restraint, helping clients deal with grief after euthanasia, and organizing their driving schedule to minimize time-consuming backtracking. Those who are able to work with birds and exotic animals as well as cats and dogs have an advantage because birds and exotics are difficult to transport to a veterinary clinic.

Housecall veterinarians see fewer clients per day than do hospital-based veterinarians, for two reasons: first, much of their time is spent driving; and second, they spend more time with each client. Housecall veterinarians may develop more personal relationships with their clients than do other veterinarians.

Housecall veterinarians with no mobile unit will focus on preventive medicine and minor procedures that don't require hospital equipment or staff. Those who do have a mobile unit will be able to perform a wider variety of procedures, but the lack of a standing facility limits cases to those that do not require hospitalization.

Pros and cons

Dr. Murbach found a unique niche with her focus on pet birds and on hospice care. Other housecall veterinarians also find that certain health issues are better dealt with in the home. Housecall veterinarians may focus on behavioral problems in pets; solving these problems is easier when the home environment can be evaluated. They may perform more euthanasias than the average veterinarian, because even people who ordinarily take their pets to a veterinary hospital will call upon housecall veterinarians for this service. Housecall veterinarians may also offer hospice and palliative care, which are becoming more popular and are a great service for pet owners (see Chapter 3).

Housecall practitioners can set their own schedules and hours, which also allows them to work around their clients' schedules more effectively. This career path is useful for veterinarians who are parents because they can create a schedule around their children's schedules. (However, it is not realistic for a housecall veterinarian to think she can take her children with her on housecalls—not only are there safety issues, but many clients won't assume the kids are as cute as she does.)

Professional benefits include working in a challenging environment that changes every day, working alone (often without responsibilities for employees), and owning a practice with low overhead costs. Housecall practitioners can also develop personal relationships with their clients, create more leisurely schedules, and enjoy the calmer behavior of animals not stressed by a car ride or clinic atmosphere. They may be able to assist clients who are unable to transport pets to a clinic or who cannot leave the home; evaluate the effect of a pet's environment on its health; and get more done at their own homes because they aren't sitting around at a workplace when there's no work to do.

Possible disadvantages to consider with this career path include:
- You may have difficulty separating your work and personal life.
- You are dependent on a vehicle that runs well.
- You may miss the camaraderie of working with other veterinarians.
- You can't perform much surgery.

- Clients who are friends may tend to assume you are always available or that you'll give them discounts.
- Your liability may be higher because pet owners often assist you (a main cause of lawsuits is injury to pet owners who restrain their own animals).
- You have daily driving and possible traffic headaches.
- You have less assistance than you would in a hospital.
- You see fewer clients per day due to the increased client interaction time plus the travel time.
- You aren't building up equity in something you can later sell, as you would with a normal clinic. It is difficult to sell goodwill and a client list; even if you are able to do so, the value is much less than the value of a standing practice. You must be careful to save sufficient retirement funds.
- You have all the administrative responsibilities of a business owner.

Qualifications

The housecall practitioner is the chief executive, the main employee, and in many cases, the bookkeeper, technician, receptionist, and veterinarian all rolled into one. Since housecall veterinarians have home offices, the local zoning code must allow for home-based businesses, and there must be space for an office in the home. Successful housecall veterinarians are comfortable working with people on a one-to-one, friendly basis, and are outgoing, personable, and self-assured. They have the self-discipline necessary to organize their working hours, manage their business, and schedule time away from work. They have enough veterinary experience to handle, by themselves, any situation that might arise. Housecall veterinarians know that if their abilities or the home environment are inadequate to perform a particular treatment, they will have to refer that patient, and they must give up performing certain procedures that are best done in a hospital.

Veterinarians who might not like housecall work include those who thrive on the exchange of ideas and information among veterinarians in a group practice. Veterinarians will be most successful with housecall practice if they have at least a year or more of practice experience. Those who are comfortable chatting with other veterinarians online via computer will minimize their professional isolation.

To start

Consult your state practice act and your city and state business licensing agencies to learn the regulations that apply to housecall and mobile veterinary services. Veterinarians may start a housecall practice by continuing at their current jobs and setting up the housecall practice as a separate business that they work on during their "off" time (with their present employer's agreement), and then leaving their regular job after a designated time period. Others work part-time at a veterinary clinic to keep some income, and start their housecall practice part-time. Some find that they can integrate housecalls into their current jobs, continuing as an employee or partner in the practice. Other choices are saving up money, getting a loan, or relying on a spouse's income while starting a full-time housecall practice right from the beginning.

Some people choose to work as relief veterinarians while they begin housecall practice. This, however, is difficult because most relief jobs last a week, and they aren't able to see any of their new clients during this time. If the "relief" job consists of working specific days of the week or specific hours each day, that is part-time employment—not being a relief veterinarian.

A fairly new and innovative approach to housecall practice is exemplified by VETdispatch (www.vetdispatch.com), a business which works with housecall veterinarians. VETdispatch sets up and manages all practice management functions such as advertising, answering the phones, scheduling, inventory management and medical record keeping. They also provide techs, supplies, equipment and a shared image (branding) to the housecall veterinarians. Under this model, all a veterinarian has to do is to practice medicine, with minimal housekeeping duties and fewer risks of starting and running a practice.

Pay

Housecall veterinarians can earn as much as most traditional practice veterinarians (see Chapter 3). Although it is not possible to see as many clients in a day as are seen in a typical clinic, that reduction in revenue is balanced by the lower overhead expenses and higher fee charged for each visit. However, the practice owner receives not only current income, but also (theoretically) a return on the investment in land, a building, and a client base; housecall veterinarians don't receive this.

Fees charged by housecall veterinarians may be similar to or higher than the fees charged by clinics in the area, with the addition of a "housecall fee" that is charged over and above the exam fee. Smart housecall veterinarians also make sure they have a "consultation fee," so they don't use a lot of unbillable time giving advice. That is particularly important for services such as behavioral counseling or educating clients about hospice care.

Relief Veterinarians

A relief veterinarian is someone who makes a living working a series of temporary jobs. The relief veterinarian offers services to other veterinarians for a short-term, temporary "relief" situation. Each job may last as short as a half day or as long as several weeks. The reliever can take enough jobs to work full-time or can work only part-time, as desired.

In *human* medicine, doctors and nurses who do relief work (also called locum tenens) get their jobs by going through an agency. These agencies provide several benefits, including insurance, transportation fees, housing arrangements, temporary state licenses, and set wages. In veterinary medicine, relievers are most often self employed, although some work through agencies.

Daily work

Typically, the relief veterinarian keeps a small home office from which jobs are scheduled and paperwork is completed. The relief veterinarian's abilities and interests dictate the types of jobs accepted. A typical month might include working a week at a nearby small animal clinic; working a weekend at an emergency clinic; and traveling to a nearby small town to work at a mixed practice, staying in a hotel or in the absent vet-erinarian's vacant home. These small-town jobs usually include taking emergency calls during the night. Relievers in larger cities might limit their work to daytime hours in small animal practices.

The amount of travel required depends on the type of work done and the size of the veterinarian's home city. Relief veterinarians who live in a large city may not need to travel at all. However, those who live in smaller towns may need to travel extensively to get enough work to keep busy full-time.

Relievers who have an unusual talent or niche may also travel more because hos-pitals that need those special services are less likely to find someone in their own geographic area. Thus relievers who are willing to work on large animals, exotics, or birds may find that their services are requested over a wide geographic area.

Relievers do not work regularly at any one clinic. If a veterinarian works every Monday for Dr. Jones, for example, then that veterinarian is a part-time employee, not a relief veterinarian. However, relievers can (and do) work more than once for any one hospital—for example, the reliever could cover for Dr. Jones during several veterinary meetings, holidays, and vacations scattered over a year's time.

Relief veterinarians respond to calls from interested veterinarians by first confirming they are available on the requested dates. Then the reliever states his or her fees, and the caller decides whether or not to hire the reliever. The reliever sends a contract or letter that confirms the verbal agreement.

Once on the job, the relievers see appointments, perform surgery, and care for animals in the hospital. Relievers are legally and medically responsible for any cases in the hospital where they are working, so it is important that they agree with the philoso-phy and medical standards of the hospital owner. Relievers walk the tight rope of trying to maintain the clinic's standard policies and procedures, but maintaining their own standards of practice at the same time.

Pros and cons

Many of the advantages of relief work are similar to those of a housecall practice. This career allows for great flexibility and control over personal time and income. The reliever who does a good job and is willing to travel (or who lives in a large city) will have no shortage of work. Relievers must work with new people all the time—some they may like, and some not. The reliever has little control over the clinic atmosphere and policies, and cannot easily follow up on cases.

Parents looking for a "flexible" job will not necessarily find an answer with relief work. The flexibility with this work is flexibility by day or week worked, and not by hours worked per day. For flexibility in hours worked each day, either part-time employ-ment or housecall practice are better choices. (Pros and cons of relief versus part-time work are detailed in the book *FlexVet*, by C. Smith)

Disadvantages include working on holidays and weekends. Relievers often have to go to less popular or out-of-area continuing education meetings, because they are likely to have relief jobs during local meetings. They plan their vacations at times when others typically don't take theirs, are ready to celebrate holidays on the day before or after the actual date, and plan their CE around other veterinarian's preferences. Relievers will get more work if they are willing to take emergency calls. However, doing so means working after hours, perhaps more than veterinarians employed in a traditional job.

Relief work is not always a good job for new graduates; the kinds of experiences gained when you are left alone are not necessarily good ones. You must be decisive and confident working on your own.

Qualifications

Consider the following questions when considering whether you would like relief work:

- Are you interested in operating your own business and being self-employed?
- Are you comfortable working with people with a variety of personalities? Are you outgoing, personable, and self-assured?
- Are you able to work alone, or are you accustomed to a qualified technician's assistance? Do you have enough experience to handle any situation that might arise when you are the only veterinarian?
- Are you comfortable with any and all anesthetic regimens? Are you able to use a variety of methods, medications, and equipment? Are you comfortable looking up information as needed?
- Are you able and willing to travel? Can you work on holidays and weekends? Are you flexible enough to work different hours each week?
- Are you meticulous with record keeping? Do you write every detail in the patient records?
- Can you write up charges at each clinic according to their policies, or are you accustomed to altering your fees as you see fit for each case?
- Are you comfortable referring a patient—even though you have the expertise to take care of the problem—if the facilities are inadequate to perform a particular treatment or surgery?
- Are you able to maintain your high standards of practice no matter what your surroundings?
- Are you ready to turn down jobs for clinics in which you are not comfortable, even though you need the work? If you take such jobs, are you ready to assume the liability for all cases handled there?
- Do you have enough savings to carry you through your initial slow time?

To start

Before beginning relief work, veterinarians must obtain sufficient experience in private practice to be comfortable in a wide variety of situations. New graduates should obtain regular work prior to embarking on a career as a relief veterinarian. Older veterinarians nearing retirement may also consider relief work as a segue to full retirement; their challenge is to learn about new approaches to medicine, since they may have worked in one place for some time, with little exposure to different approaches.

Relief veterinarians are self-employed (that is, they are independent contractors); they are not employees of the clinics where they work. Many people start doing relief work quite casually. However, to take the full tax advantages of being self-employed, they should go to the trouble of setting up a genuine business. They must estimate their expenses and establish fees and policies. They need to get a business license (not the same as the veterinary license) and write up a contract for every job, as well as have a plan for marketing their services.

A true relief veterinarian can take certain tax deductions that are allowed for self-employed people. In contrast, a part-time employee should receive benefits that are given to all employees. If the job is misclassified, the veterinarian and the person hiring him or her may be subject to penalties in the event of an audit.

Read Chapter 7, Starting Your Own Business, and the section on international relief work in Chapter 13. Some relief veterinarians are members of the Veterinary Information Network (VIN; www.vin.com), where they discuss business issues. Details about starting and running a relief veterinary business, including tax issues, are described in the book, *FlexVet: How to Be One, How to Hire One*, by C. Smith.

Pay

The fees charged by relief veterinarians vary according to the local economy and one's ability to create a realistic business plan. Fees may be charged by the hour or by the day. Most relievers charge a base hourly fee, with a minimum daily fee. In 2009, typical fees ranged from $200 to $800 per day, or $60 to $100 per hour (whichever is greater). Additional fees are charged for mileage to any clinic out of the area, for use of any of their own equipment, for hotels, and for taking emergency calls.

Over the long-term, relief work can provide a satisfying full-time or part-time career. Relief veterinarians sometimes work back-to-back shifts (e.g., day clinic or emergency clinic) in order to earn money quickly in the short-term.

Relief veterinarians must realize that because they do not own a practice, they aren't building up equity in something that will pay them back in retirement. Thus, the career relief veterinarian must take extra care to save adequately for retirement.

Using agencies

Although most relief veterinarians work on their own, a few veterinarians' relief agencies exist. Consider the advantages each agency would offer, and decide whether you could get the same results without an agency. Check out the agency's references. Ask other relief veterinarians who work for the agency how much work they have and whether any problems have occurred. What benefits does the agency offer? For instance, do they do the preliminary checking that you normally would, to gauge the practice quality?

Potential benefits to the reliever of using an agency include getting immediate work; getting consistent work; getting help matching your medical philosophy and style to the hospital; and reducing the headaches of marketing yourself, negotiating fees, and collecting payment. Agencies could help you get work in the geographic area you prefer at the times and days you want to work.

However, if you work through an agency you may be making less money than if you work independently (getting jobs on your own, without using the agency). With some agencies, you receive few or no benefits (e.g., insurance). If you change your mind about using the agency, the noncompete clause keeps you from working those same jobs again.

Chapter 8 Resources

Groups and web sites

American Animal Hospital Association (AAHA), www.aahanet.org.

American Association of Housecall Veterinarians, www.housecallvets.org and www.homevets.org.

American Association of Mobile Veterinary Practitioners, www.aamvp.org.

Animal Hospice Compassionate Crossings, www.animalhospice.org, 805-598-6496.

Dodgen, www.dodgenmobiletech.com/products.php.

International Association for Hospice and Palliative Care, www.iaahpc.org.

LaBoit, www.laboit.com.

Lifeline Mobile, http://lifelinemobile.com.

Nikki Hospice Foundation for Pets, 400 New Bedford Drive, Vallejo, CA 94591; www.pethospice.org; phone: 707-557-8595.

Porta-Vet, www.portavet.net.

VETDispatch, www.vetdispatch.com.

Veterinary Information Network (VIN), www.vin.com; phone: (800) 700-4636.

Books and articles

AVMA Guidelines for Veterinary Hospice Care, www.avma.org/products/hab/hospice.pdf; phone: 800-883-6301.

Berger, L., *Savvy Part-time Professional: How to Land, Create or Negotiate the Part-time Job of Your Dreams* (Capital Books, 2006).

Glassman, G., Tax Rules for Relief Veterinarians, *Veterinary Economics*, 2006.

Rezendes, A., More Veterinarians Offer Hospice Care for Pets. *JAVMA News*, August 15. 2006.

Smith, C. A., *Housecall: The Housecall Veterinarian's Manual*, (Smith Veterinary Publishing 2007) available through www.smithvet.com or www.vin.com.

Smith, C. A., Relief Veterinarian or Part-Time Employee? Washington State Veterinary Medical Association; WSVMA *Newsletter*, March 1992.

Smith, C.A., *The Relief Veterinarian's Manual*, out of print; see *FlexVet*.

Smith, C.A., Rose, R., *Relief Veterinary Technician's Manual* (Smith Veterinary Publishing, 2002).

Smith, C.A., *Client Satisfaction Pays: Quality Service for Practice Success* (AAHA Press. 2009).

Smith, C.A., *FlexVet: How to Be One, How to Hire One. The Comprehensive Practice Guide for Relief & Part time Veterinarians* (Smith Veterinary Publishing. 2007; this is a revision of the previous book, *The Relief Veterinarian's Manual*).

Tyson, E., Schell, J., *Small Business for Dummies*, 3rd edition (Wiley Publishing, 2008).

Williams, J., *Unbending Gender: Why Family and Work Conflict and What to Do About It* (Oxford University Press, 2000).

Wilson, J., et al., *Contracts, Benefits, and Practice Management for the Veterinary Profession* (Priority Press, 2009).

9 CONSULTING

A consultant is someone who charges a fee to share special knowledge and to give specific help or advice to a client. Consultants are hired for assistance in a specific problem area (e.g., business, medicine, computers, livestock, management, or just about anything else) for a specified length of time, which can range from weeks to years. A consultant is a combination of teacher, leader, and mentor who leaves each client with solutions and new ideas that can be put into practice long after the consultant has gone.

Veterinarians can work as consultants for businesses ranging from veterinary clinics to livestock feed companies. For example, a veterinarian with an extensive background in animal shelter work can be hired as a consultant by shelters to train their employees, or an international swine consultant can travel all over the world to gather and disseminate information about new breeds of pigs.

Several of the books listed in the resources at the end of this chapter address setting up and running a consultant business.

Daily work

> The primary reason I like this work is because I like veterinarians. They are generally trustworthy goodhearted intelligent people. The part I enjoy the most is when I come across a veterinarian who has worked their entire life in their practice and they are ready to take the next step into retirement. Hopefully they've come to me early enough so that I can make a difference. I like being able to give them good advice on how they can improve their practice value before they sell. It is reward-ing to know that I have influenced the value of the nest-egg available to them when they exit their business. Veterinarians deserve to be finan-cially rewarded for all their hard work during their career. On a more selfish note, I like the freedom that comes with operating my own busi-ness. I have other interests besides my consulting work and I am able to schedule my time to pursue these interests.—Elizabeth Bellavance, DVM, MBA, CMA, Canadian Veterinary Consulting Services, Ontario, Canada

Consultants can be self-employed or work for a company; they may work alone or as part of a team. They are most effective when they have seen and evaluated their clients' environments, so they usually travel frequently. Before an on-site visit, the consultant obtains as much information as possible about the client to maximize time efficiency during the visit. The consultant's office work may include studying demographics;

writing materials such as office manuals, contracts, and client educational materials; analyzing financial, medical, or nutritional data; writing articles and speeches; developing ideas for and planning seminars; and keeping up with reading in the consultant's area of expertise. Consultants may make on-site visits several times or only once before developing a final plan or recommendation for the client. Personal visits are often followed by telephone consultations.

Some consultants will work with clients on a "virtual" basis, never visiting in person at all. This works better for individual consulting, such as coaching someone through a specific project or action.

Veterinarian consultants may be hired by
- Other veterinarians.
- The food supply industry (e.g., livestock producers, livestock feed companies, or farm equipment companies).
- Veterinary medical equipment companies.
- Veterinary computer software companies.
- Pharmaceutical companies.
- Pet food companies.
- Attorneys.
- Nonprofit groups.
- Government agencies.
- International development agencies.
- Groups that operate strictly online (e.g., VIN, the Veterinary Information Network www.vin.com).
- Just about anyone!

The consultant working solo typically has a small office, which may be a home office. This work space requires a computer, telephone, and an answering system, at a minimum. Consultants frequently use computer programs to analyze data, to communicate with clients, and to keep their own records. Consultants have to market their own businesses, which is done via word of mouth, their web site, and paid advertising. They also attend trade shows and meetings that are likely to be attended by their potential clients, such as those for veterinarians, managers, producers, and equipment or feed companies.

Many consultants are regular speakers at veterinary and related industry meetings. Speaking is a way to educate as well as to let potential clients evaluate the consultant's expertise. Consultants may also create their own seminars or courses, which they offer independently from other veterinary meetings. Clients may attend these seminars as a way to pick up business tips, and then decide to hire the consultant for specific help.

Consultants also publish regularly in journals or magazines appropriate to their areas of expertise (e.g., business consultants may write for *Veterinary Economics* magazine, and livestock consultants may write for livestock publications, such as the *National Cattlemen's Beef Association newsletter*). Writing is done for the exposure—to disseminate word about their work, to establish their credentials, and to educate potential clients about the benefits or need for their services. See Chapter 10.

Pros and cons

Consultants are problem-solvers who make a living by helping people do things better, faster, cheaper, and easier. Consultants must travel frequently, be comfortable speaking, stay cheerful and positive with every client, be flexible, and enjoy working with and helping a wide variety of people. They spend a lot of time on the telephone. Consultants are team leaders. Consultants must continuously come up with new solutions for new problems, easily changing their approaches for different clients. Writing skills are necessary and are used often. For example, all verbal recommendations must be followed up in writing as a formal report. In addition, some consultants produce newsletters for their clients.

Consultants may work long hours and get little time off. They are often up against deadlines to finish reports for clients. Their businesses consist of blue sky (no product, just a service) based solely on their own work. Like other self-employed people, they must concentrate on creating a good retirement fund. It may be difficult to build up equity and create a saleable business—thus they may have nothing to show at retirement. Creating a team with several consultants is one way to create a longer-lasting business that might be sold.

The consultant often causes clients to be initially dissatisfied—by pointing out problems and by making changes, which no one likes—before they are satisfied. The consultant must differentiate between what their clients want and what they need. Consultants may carry a large accounts receivable, so collecting payment is a constant chore. (Asking for prepayment, deposits, and periodic payments are a way to reduce problems.) Soliciting new clients is an everyday need (via direct mail, attending meetings that potential clients might attend, speaking engagements). Some clients can be frustrating to work with. Some may be "management junkies," who revolve through a series of consultants without making any positive changes. Others may not take the advice given and thus won't see any benefit.

Qualifications

Consultants must have a great deal more (or different) experience and breadth of knowledge than do their clients. However, specific skills are required in addition to their technical knowledge. Many consultants have additional business training to aid in the business aspects of consulting (both to help them run their own business, and to apply that knowledge to help others). Consultants must also have analytic skills, and top-quality writing and speaking skills; they must be great communicators, able to interact with all kinds of personalities. They must be knowledgeable about human behavior, needs, and desires, and be effective at motivating people to work together as a team. They must understand the fear of change and how to help their clients overcome that fear with positive results. Computer skills are essential. At a minimum, consultants must be able to use a variety of software programs and online services. (Some consultants work to tailor specific software to clients' needs.) Consultants must be comfortable leading, working alone, selling their skills, and tracking down new clients.

Quite a few consultants to the veterinary industry are not veterinarians at all, but people with college degrees and expertise in marketing, management, communications, law, human resources, or finance. The veterinarian working as a consultant in any of these areas of interest must bring their skills and knowledge up to that of other experts in that field.

A consultant's expertise can be gained through work experience. However, experience in only one private practice is not sufficient. One way to gather more experience in the path to consulting work is to take a job with the government or in industry, getting paid and learning on the way. Consultants should take the opportunity to work in a variety of career paths to broaden their background and knowledge. See the chapters on industry (Chapter 11), service or nonprofit organizations (Chapter 13), associations (Chapter 12), and government (Chapters 15–18), for more details.

Learn essential skills in public speaking, impromptu speaking, persuasion, leadership and more through Toastmasters (www.toastmasters.org), a nonprofit group that helps people become better speakers in all situations. The National Speakers Association (www.nsaspeaker.org) also offers training workshops and professional certification.

Another route to expertise is to take classes or earn advanced degrees in business, finance, law, livestock management, economics, health care administration, or agribusiness. Attending management presentations at conferences and taking seminars are great ways to gain more experience in various areas. More and more universities are offering short-term intensive courses, correspondence or online courses, or branch programs targeted at working people. (These are often called "Executive level" courses.) These courses can be taken with or without the intention of getting a degree.

For example, AAHA and Purdue offer a Certificate in Veterinary Practice Administration that can be completed by attending Purdue's Krannert School of Management for four long weekends over the time span of one year. This course offers a broad history of business management theory and practice that can serve as a foundation for learning more about business. See www.krannert.purdue.edu > admissions > masters programs > nondegree programs > sponsored programs.

Consultants may become Certified Veterinary Practice Managers through the Veterinary Hospital Managers Association (www.vhma.org), whose members include veterinarians, managers, and administrators. Other consultants have qualifications such as Certified Professional Coach or Certified Mediator, which they apply to their consulting work. See the International Coach Federation at www.coachfederation.org and the Association for Conflict Resolution at www.acrnet.org.

Pay

Consultants need to be able to put a dollar benefit value on the advice they give. That is, they must be able to show with numbers that their fee will be recouped in higher profits for the client. Typically, consultants charge $100 per hour and up, a daily fee ($2000–$10,000+ per day, plus expenses), or an annual fee with monthly payments. Hourly fees may be broken down into increments (1 minute, 15 minutes), and variations of fee structure are common (e.g., fee per month, fee for basic job plus hourly fee on top). A retainer fee is often charged (this is a down payment made before work is done). An excellent resource that discusses value pricing is the book *Pricing on Purpose: Creating and Capturing Value* by R.J. Baker.

Management consultants may work for a client on a short-term basis (a few days, weeks, or months); they may be hired for a year at a time, to help with long-range projects; or they may be hired for repeated management services, such as helping with financial or human resource management.

Not all work time is billable time, however. Marketing, office record keeping, studying (when not for a specific client), preparing speeches, and some travel are done on the consultants' own time and at their own cost. Clients tend to prefer a basic fee with these "extras" built in, rather than to see a bill with all kinds of little charges added for phone, copying, etc.

Types of Consulting

Business consultant

Business consultants evaluate the internal operations of veterinary clinics or other businesses, then work with business owners or company managers to improve their performance, profitability, and goals. Consultant assistance may be offered in:

- Utilizing staff, assessing pay and benefits.
- Managing time effectively.
- Ensuring compliance with OSHA regulations.
- Developing teams.
- Communications training,
- Starting up and developing a practice.
- Improving paperwork (medical records, contracts, hospital manual).
- Targeting new clients.
- Monitoring income and expenses.
- Preparing a marketing plan.
- Managing tax issues.
- Initiating or updating computer and software use.
- Assisting with partnership negotiations or practice sales.
- Planning for the future.

VetPartners is an association of management consultants that includes people with a wide variety of expertise (www.vetpartners.org). Member businesses range in size from solo consultants to larger teams. VetPartners offers a searchable online directory and the *New Consultants Guide*, available to members.

Other groups of interest include the American Veterinary Health Information Management Association (AVHIMA, www.avhima.org), which works in the area of information management, promotes patient care through health information, and advocates for the profession on governmental, educational, social, and business issues that affect the management of veterinary health. The Veterinary Hospital Managers Association (VHMA, www.vhma.org) counts among its members both hospital managers and veterinarians with an interest in management. The American Management Association (AMA, www.amanet.org) is also useful, as is the American Society for Training and Development (ASTD, www.astd.org). For a view of practice management from Europe, you can subscribe to John Sheridan's Business Briefing, which is based out of the UK. See www.veterinarybusinessbriefing.com and www.veterinarybusinessvideo show.com.

Electronic medical records consulting

A new area of interest is that of diagnostic codes for medical records. Using consistent codes across the profession will help veterinarians share and pool data to learn more about disease incidence, treatment outcomes, and other health data. This is already implemented in human medicine and is becoming prevalent in veterinary medicine as more clinics begin using electronic medical records (EMRs). Creating diagnostic codes has been an endeavor of the American Animal Hospital Association:

> Following seven years of development by the American Animal Hospital Association (AAHA) Diagnostic Code Task Force and Review Board and working with the Veterinary Terminology Services Laboratory, the Association has finished mapping the AAHA Diagnostic Terms to the Systematized Nomenclature of Medicine-Clinical Terms (SNOMED-CT). The terms are now available under reciprocal open-source licenses, without fee or royalty. SNOMED CT is a systematically organized computerized collection of medical terminology. Most areas of clinical information such as diseases, findings, procedures, microorganisms and pharmaceuticals are covered within this system. It provides a consistent way to index, store, retrieve and aggregate clinical data across specialties and sites of care. It also helps organize the content of medical records, reducing the variability in the way data is captured, encoded and used for clinical care of patients and research.—AAHA.

AAHA hosted several "practice management software summit" meetings to discuss findings with the software leaders. View the AAHA Diagnostic Terms at www.aahanet. org > resources > guidelines.

SNOMED CT is a clinical terminology and is considered to be the most comprehensive, multilingual healthcare terminology in the world. More information about SNOMED may be viewed at www.nlm.nih.gov/research/umls/Snomed/snomed_faq. html. Also of interest is the International Health Terminology Standards Development Organization (www.ihtsdo.org), which develops and promotes use of SNOMED CT to support safe and effective health information exchange.

Veterinarians who wish to become involved on a technical level should contact various software vendors. One easy way to find them is to browse through the exhibit hall at a major national veterinary conference. Also see the description in Chapter 10 of a veterinarian working for a corporate veterinary practice with the title of Senior Director, Medical Informatics; and Chapter 11, Industry jobs. Additional resources include:

- International Health Terminology Standards Development Organization, www. ihtsdo.org.

- SNOMED, the Systematized Nomenclature of Medicine, www.nlm.nih.gov/
research/umls/Snomed/snomed_faq.html.
- Society for the Internet in Medicine, www.internet-in-medicine.org.

Legal consultant

A growing group of consultants includes attorneys who focus on animal law or veterinary business law. Some of these attorneys are also veterinarians. Veterinary business law is similar to law that applies to any small business in the health services sector. Animal law is taught in many, but not all, law schools in the US and Canada. To find out more, look into these resources:
- American Veterinary Medical Law Association (www.avmla.org). You do not have to be an attorney to be a member.
- Animal law section of your state bar association (for attorneys). Search the internet using the state name, "bar association," and "animal law" to find these.
- International Institute for Animal Law, www.animallawintl.org.
- National Association for Biomedical Research, Animal Law Section, www.nabranimallaw.org
- Northwestern School of Law at Lewis & Clark College, publishes the Animal Law Journal, www.lclark.edu/law > animal law.

Industry consultant

Industry consultants are likely to find work from small companies that cannot utilize someone on staff full-time to fill their intermittent needs. Industry consultants also work for larger companies when specific expertise is temporarily needed in areas that those companies don't usually handle. An industry consultant assists companies by:
- Tracing the source of poor product performance in the field.
- Evaluating the reason for equipment failure.
- Evaluating and reducing costs of doing business.
- Speaking about technical subjects to the company's clients or staff.
- Providing technical assistance to attorneys working for clients involved in a lawsuit.

Livestock consultant

A livestock consultant may focus on herd health, production management, and/or other aspects of managing the facility, from business to environmental concerns. The consultant may evaluate all aspects of a livestock production facility to increase profitability. Although many producers take care of their own vaccinations and treatments for common diseases, that approach may actually increase their need for a consultant—the veterinarian can advise the producer about which vaccines are most cost-effective and which antibiotics are appropriate for particular situations. Nutritional advice is a growing area of livestock consulting. See the food animal practice section of Chapter 5 for details.

Chapter 9 Resources

Groups and web sites

Academy of Veterinary Consultants, www.avc-beef.org.

American Animal Hospital Association (AAHA).

AAHA Diagnostic Terms, www.aahanet.org > resources > guidelines.

AAHA practice management software summit meetings, www.aahanet.org > Media > Press releases > 03/26/2009.

American Veterinary Health Information Management Association, www.avhima.org; phone: 662-325-1166.

American Veterinary Medical Law Association, www.avmla.org.

Animal law section of your state bar association (for attorneys). Search the internet using the state name, "bar association," and "animal law."

Association for Conflict Resolution, www.acrnet.org.

International Coach Federation, www.coachfederation.org

International Institute for Animal Law, www.animallawintl.org.

National Association for Biomedical Research, Animal Law Section, www.nabranimallaw.org.

National Speakers Association, 1500 S Priest Drive, Tempe, AZ 85281; www.nsaspeaker.org; phone: 602-968-2552 fax: 602-968-0911.

Northwestern School of Law at Lewis & Clark College, publishes the Animal Law Journal, www.lclark.edu/law > animal law.

Purdue University, Veterinary Management Institute, Krannert School of Management www.krannert.purdue.edu/programs/masters/NonDegree_Programs/vmi.

Society for Human Resource Management (SHRM), www.shrm.org; phone: 800-283-7476.

Stanford University, Medical Informatics Short Course, www.smi.stanford.edu/community; phone: 650-723-6979.

Toastmasters, www.toastmasters.org.

University of Missouri, health informatics master's degree program, www.hmi.missouri.edu; phone: 800-877-4764.

Veterinary Hospital Managers Association (VHMA), www.vhma.org.

VetPartners, www.vetpartners.org.

Books and articles

AAHA Releases Diagnostic Terms, Diabetes Guidelines, *AAHA NewsStat* 8(10), 5/12/2010, www.aahanet.org.

Animal Law Journal, www.lclark.edu/law > animal law.

Altman, R, *Why Most PowerPoint Presentations Suck* (Harvest Books, 2007).

Baker, R. L, *Pricing on Purpose: Creating and Capturing Value* (Wiley 2006).

Bellman, G., *The Consultant's Calling: Bringing Who You Are to What You Do*, revised edition (Jossey-Bass, 2001).

Blech, E., *Business of Consulting*, 2nd edition (John Wiley and Sons, 2007).

Block, P., *Flawless Consulting: A Guide to Getting Your Expertise Used* (Jossey-Bass/Pfeiffer, 2000).

Levinson, J. C., and M. W. McLaughlin, *Guerrilla Marketing for Consultants: Breakthrough Tactics for Winning Profitable Clients* (John Wiley & Sons, 2004).

Maister, D., et al, *Trusted Advisor* (Touchstone, 2000).

Weiss, A., *Value-Based Fees: How to Charge and Get What You're Worth*, The Ultimate Consultant Series (Pfeiffer, 2002).

10 INFORMATION SERVICES

"Information services" includes gathering, sorting, and disseminating information via a wide variety of media. The work includes writing, editing and publishing materials in print or online; working with information and data management; and multimedia work (speaking, recording, and broadcasting via radio, television, or the internet). Much of this work is an integral part of any career path, but can be a part-time or full-time job on its own.

The Society for Veterinary Medicine and Literature promotes the reading and discussion of literary works to explore important issues in veterinary medicine (www.vetmedandlit.org). It also promotes the exchange of ideas between writers and veterinarians, animal scientists, animal behaviorists, and others interested in animal life, and among the different areas of veterinary medicine. Membership is free.

When it comes to writing for work, veterinarians may think in terms of articles in professional journals such as the *Journal of the American Veterinary Medical Association*. In these cases, the writer is not paid to write; instead, the writer must publish in order to report research findings and to maintain his or her job in academia. Many academic positions require writing case reports and publication of research data.

In contrast, other veterinarians are paid to write or even write for a living. They may work as self-employed freelancers or may be employed by government or industry. Some veterinarians work full-time as technical writers.

Freelance Writing

"Freelance" refers to self-employed people who write and sell articles. For many veterinarians, freelance writing is something they do "on the side," with their main income coming from other work. Having writing published can earn a veterinarian the respect of colleagues, spread the word about other products or services offered, or provide a creative outlet. Others take a more dedicated approach. Whether writing full-time or "on the side," the veterinarian writer must understand the business of writing.

Writing articles

Veterinarians may write articles for a variety of magazines, journals, or newspapers, which may appear in print, online, or both. They may write animal health care articles for magazines such as *Bird Talk, Western Horseman*, or *Cat Fancy*. Although these articles may seem "simple" in subject matter, writing them is not as simple as it first appears.

Freelance writers begin by coming up with an article idea. The writer should contact magazines and ask for their "writer's guidelines," which outline the style and format in which articles must be submitted. The article's length, subject, and style are considered when deciding which magazine to approach. The writer sends a "query letter" to the magazine's editor, outlining the idea. The editor then writes or calls, and either turns down the idea or gives the assignment. If the article is assigned, the editor and writer discuss the payment terms and rights to be sold. The editor than sends a contract for the writer to sign.

Daily work / Pros and cons

Full-time freelance writers are self-employed and have home offices. All freelance writers use a computer and word processing program. The work requires self-discipline. The most difficult part of freelance writing is simply sitting down to write. Writers often set a goal of sending out two or three query letters per week. They should follow up on each if they haven't heard back in about four weeks. A system that keeps track of all their ideas, letters sent out, and replies received, as well as assignments and their due dates, is essential.

The beginning freelance writer has two hurdles to overcome. The first is to actually send out the query letter or sample article. The next is to get over the rejection slips and editorial changes. When it comes to editing, hold fast to being technically and medically correct, but be ready to give on stylistic editorial changes. It can be difficult to have someone reword your work; this is something you will have to get over if you hope to get your thoughts and expertise published.

Qualifications / To apply

To be successful, freelancers must be good at selling their work; being able to write is essential but insufficient. You many write the best article or book in the world, but if you can't sell it to a magazine or an editor, no one will ever know how great it was. Veterinarian writers don't have to be specialists to write well on a subject. Their veterinary degrees *make* them "experts" in most people's eyes when it comes to writing for pet or horse magazines. Also, whether their articles are directed at the lay public or veterinarians, they must use interviews with other experts to create a readable, credible, and interesting article. These interviews create the illusion of the author as "expert." Because of that, non-veterinarian freelancers who do a good job of interviewing experts may compete with veterinarian writers for the same market.

Writing successfully requires studying the *business* of writing. This is different from studying *how* to write. Successful freelance writers have a good understanding of how magazines are published, what editors do, and what readers like to read. They study magazines so that they know the style, word count, and complexity of each magazine's articles. They then match each of their article ideas to the magazine it fits best.

It is also useful to start networking within the small world of writing. Knowing someone at a particular magazine can be a big help in getting a "foot in the door" for publication. Although the article still has to be evaluated and accepted, having a contact helps to get an article to the right person. Use online social networks, writers' groups, and veterinary conferences to meet such people.

Serious beginning freelance writers should take these steps: join a local writer's group; read the book *Writer's Market*; and attend large writer's conferences (these are similar to large veterinary conferences, with seminars on the business of writing—from "what the magazines are buying" to "understanding electronic rights"). Also join a local writers' group that focuses on the business of writing nonfiction. To find such a group, search the Internet, or ask at your library, a local independent bookstore, or your local newspaper office.

Writer's Market is published annually; get the current year's edition. It contains the names and addresses of magazine editors, how to write a query letter, all about copyright, how to target your market, and all the basics of the business of writing. It lists hundreds of magazines, their pay scales, and the types of articles they accept. A new "Deluxe" edition includes access to an online database with thousands of listings and continual updates. *Writer's Market* is available from most bookstores or at the library reference desk. In addition, serious writers subscribe to *Writer's Digest* magazine (www.writersdigest.com).

Two national groups with many veterinarian members are the Cat Writer's Association (www.catwriters.org) and the Dog Writer's Association (www.dwaa.org). They each put out newsletters and hold annual meetings with educational seminars. Another group of interest is the National Association of Agricultural Journalists (www.naaj.net).

The American Society of Journalists and Authors (ASJA) is a national organization of independent nonfiction writers who have met the Society's standards of professional achievement (www.asja.org). The ASJA web site provides valuable free information to freelance writers, such as contract tips and current facts and fiction about electronic publishing.

Pay

Writing articles does not pay well, partly because pet magazines (e.g., *Cat Fancy*, *AKC Purebred Dog Gazette*, *Horse Illustrated*, *Western Horseman*) are accustomed to getting huge volumes of material from pet-loving writers who are willing to write for low pay. Most major pet magazines pay from $200 to $800 for an article.

It is unlikely that you will make a living writing magazine articles if you limit yourself to writing about pets or animals. Although you may be able to write an article in a day or two, you can't sell an article every day. The best you can hope for is that, at some point, you are hired to write a monthly column, so you get a regular but small trickle of income. (Once this happens, you are listed on the magazine's masthead as a "consulting" or "contributing" editor—a feather in your cap and something to put on your resume.)

There is more of a market for pet articles than just pet magazines, however. Many women's and home-type magazines also run articles about animals. The major women's magazines, such as *Good Housekeeping* and *Woman's Day*, pay well for an article ($1,000 and up). If you think you'll become a regular contributor, though, think again. Thousands of freelance writers try to break into these markets. No high-paying magazine will look twice at your work until and unless you have published many articles in smaller magazines *and* you have become very well known (even for those basic articles about fleas or worms). Start by writing articles for your local paper to accumulate a few "clips" (samples of your work) that you can send to magazines with your query letters.

One major reason to write is to help sell something else—another service or product that you provide. You can get a great deal of "free" advertising for your other products or services by writing articles on the same subject, and putting a plug in the author's bio (the short paragraph at the end of the article). For instance, the bio for an article in a veterinary business magazine about client relations could read: "Dr. Smith is the author of *Client Satisfaction Pays*." Another reason to write articles is to make a name for yourself, perhaps to augment your income as a speaker or as a consultant, or in some other way.

A brief overview of copyright for freelance writers

Freelancers are self-employed writers who sell the *right to use* their work—articles or books—to magazines, book publishers, or veterinary-related companies. Copyright law stipulates that a work is copyrighted as soon as it is recorded in tangible form—whether printed or on computer disk. As a freelance writer, the first thing to know about your writing is that you own it until you agree otherwise, in writing.

Once you write something, you can license or sell partial or all rights to use your material. "Rights" clauses include a time frame (or not); a format (printed, electronic); and the person or entity to whom those rights are granted. Unless specifically stipulated, "electronic" covers online, web, CD, and /or DVD. Many contracts ask for rights "in any format now known or ever to be invented."

Electronic publishing is changing the future of copyright. For more information, see the resources provided by the American Society of Journalists and Authors (www.asja.org), which include articles about electronic rights. The National Writers Union (www.nwu.org) provides analysis of electronic media and the future of copyright, and responds to concerns about access to information. Business forms and copyright information are available at www.copyright.gov or www.legalzoom.com.

Doing "work for hire" means that you are selling all rights to your material to the person who hires you. Once you do that, you no longer own the material and cannot use it without the buyer's permission. The buyer can combine it with other articles on the same subject, and create a book; they can reprint the same article in several magazines; and they can sell the article online to computer users, among other possibilities.

Many magazines attempt to get authors to sign a work for hire contract, agreeing only to something different if the author so requests. (It is common for writers to change the contracts they receive for writing an article or book.) Writers can ask for extra payment for every different form in which their work is published—including electronic forms. If the magazine insists upon a work-for-hire agreement, you can ask for a fee that is higher than what you'd get for the same article had you licensed more limited rights.

People who write as part of their jobs as salaried employees are always doing work for hire. However, freelancers may also agree to do work for hire. This makes sense with regard to technical writing (see discussion in the next section), and for articles that have no resale value (e.g., so specific and technical that you would never reuse it). Consider the potential for your own reuse of the material. One way around that problem is to authorize "shared" rights such that you also retain the right to use what you wrote.

Many first-time writers worry that someone will "steal" their ideas for articles or books. Although this can occur, it is rare. The difficult thing to realize is that none of your ideas are original. Chances are that someone, somewhere, has thought of the same idea. So, when you send out a query letter, your goal is to convince the recipient that you are better qualified than anyone else to write the piece and that you have a unique perspective that will make the article fresh and original. If you've done a good job of that, there is no reason for the recipient to "steal" the idea and have someone else write about it.

Note: Veterinary specialists who work in academia, conduct research, and publish papers based on that research are not freelance writers. This work is always done as work for hire, for two reasons. First, the writing is done as part of their full-time jobs, as employees of the institutions where they work. Second, most peer-reviewed, refereed journals buy all rights to ensure they are the first and only publication to "break the news," when or if that is important. Several international groups are working to share materials without fees or licensing, such as the International Veterinary Information Service (www.ivis.org).

Writing for web sites or electronic newsletters

Writing content for online use is just another type of freelance writing. Almost all the information about freelance writing applies to writing web site content. Pay for writing used online tends to be low, and many contracts stipulate that the writing is done as work for hire.

Veterinarians can write technical material or they can write informational material targeted at pet owners. They may also write regular columns, just as they would for a print magazine, or they may write informational articles that are indefinitely made available to pet owners searching for specific information online. They can write "blogs," (continually updated web logs), or they can use services such as Twitter ™ to disseminate information. The latter tend to be done as marketing tools, so veterinarians would either write these as a way to market their own service, or they could be hired as freelancers to write this material for another veterinarian or another company.

As part of a web site or online provider's services, veterinarians may answer questions posed by other online users (usually pet owners). It is important to define the number of questions that must be answered each week and the time frame in which questions must be answered. (Note that this is giving information, not medical advice.)

Web content may remain in the "virtual world" indefinitely unless you stipulate otherwise (and sometimes, even if you do so; beware of "archiving" clauses). Use caution with the material you release, since it may reappear at a future time or in a form you had not intended or anticipated.

Multimedia work

"Multimedia" is a term that refers to the use of print or electronic materials, video, computers, and television to convey information. Many veterinary-related companies create their own multimedia materials, whereas others hire an outside firm to do this work. With the increasing move from printed to electronic materials, "multimedia" is becoming the norm for many publications that were formerly print-only. Veterinarians can do this work as freelancers or as employees.

Lifelearn (www.lifelearn.com) is a multimedia company that serves the veterinary profession. The President of Lifelearn is a veterinarian. The company utilizes the services of veterinarians to create its media. The company's focus is production and marketing of veterinary continuing education and reference programs in electronic interactive multimedia format.

Advanstar (www.dvm360.com) is a company that produces well-read publications including *Veterinary Economics* and *DVM Newsmagazine*. Advanstar's materials are all available online, with only some of them also available in print. Veterinarian writers contribute much of their content, both as articles (see freelancing, above) and as short videotaped interviews (most interviewees are not paid).

Veterinary Learning Systems (VLS, www.vetlearn.com) is an example of a company that works to serve the multimedia needs of the veterinary profession. VLS creates videotapes, books, CDs, scripts, online journals, and other materials. They also organize meetings for companies, and assist companies with their customer service needs.

VLS employees have included veterinarians who perform a wide variety of tasks, from arranging space for meetings to editing technical material. Their jobs involve negotiating, working with people, and travel. They understand and are comfortable with marketing, enjoy writing and words, and spend much of their time on the telephone and answering mail. They constantly learn about new products and medications. More than half of their time is spent working at a desk.

Many other companies exist or will be created. Browse the exhibit hall at any national veterinary conference to find them, or search for them on the internet using search terms such as [veterinary] and [DVD].

Technical Writing

In contrast to the freelance writing described previously, it may be possible for veterinarians to make a living at technical writing. Technical writers may be self employed or employees. They may work for industry (e.g., pharmaceutical or pet food companies), or for people who work in academia (a form of ghostwriting of portions of textbooks, course manuals, or papers). With the rising costs of university textbooks, college professors are increasingly preparing their own course material, ranging from biology to physiology, sometimes hiring technical writers to help. Also, textbook publishing companies often look for science writers.

Copyright is less of a problem for technical writers than for magazine article writers. In contrast to other types of freelance writing, technical writing is usually done as work for hire, which means you do not own what you write. You may be writing confidential in-house materials for a company. The material you write is usually so specific that there is virtually no reprint market for it. Also, most of the technical background information is provided to you by the company for which you are writing. And finally, the pay is high enough to justify the work-for-hire agreement.

Technical writers may be asked to sign a confidentiality agreement that stipulates they will not reveal company internal information for a specified number of years. Those who are hired full-time as employees for a specific company also may be asked to sign a noncompete agreement. Some examples of technical writing assignments include the proceedings for a continuing education seminar; a booklet or brochure about a product, for use by sales staff; promotional materials for a new product; a publishable paper (for submission to a refereed veterinary journal), based upon raw data from a study; or materials for a company web site.

Essential books for any aspiring technical writer are the *Handbook of Technical Writing*, by G. Alred; *Technical Communication: A Reader-Centered Approach*, by P. Anderson; and *The Complete Idiot's Guide to Technical Writing*, by K. Van Laan.

Daily work / Pros and cons

The day-to-day work of a technical writer is similar to a magazine-article writer—basically sitting at the computer in a home office, typing away. Instead of sending query letters outlining an article idea, however, the technical writer responds to a company that calls and asks for a specific project.

A technical writer can theoretically work from any location. However, a computer with high-speed internet access is essential in this business, as well as access to overnight delivery services.

Technical writers must have a good understanding of the goals of the company for which they write. If they are writing a piece for publication in a refereed journal, for example, they must be able to match the material with the most appropriate journal. They then write the article so it fits that journal's requirements. At other times they may be writing material for a sales booklet or brochure, which must be understood by its intended audience. Writing for web sites requires adhering to length requirements as well as understanding the goal of the page once it is viewed by the reader.

Technical writers rarely get public recognition for their work. They don't expect to see their byline above a refereed article they helped write, since the official authors (the people who performed the study about which they are writing) will be the only ones listed (the writer may get a footnote of thanks).

A definite plus is that technical writing often involves interviewing lots of interesting people who are experts in their fields. Technical writers get to study and write about an incredible variety of fascinating subjects, some of which they would never otherwise explore.

Qualifications / To apply

The veterinary degree provides the knowledge base necessary for many of these jobs. Excellent grammar and spelling are required. Additional knowledge includes being aware of the author's guidelines for various publications or for the company's materials. Some will offer style guides that include the formatting of various items.

Many large companies use their own employees to do their technical writing, but the trend is for industry to hire outside freelancers (contractors) for some or all jobs. One way to break in is first to call the company and ask whether they do indeed hire freelancers; if so, ask who decides when they are hired. Then write a letter directly to that person, including your resume and any clips of your work. Do not expect to be called immediately; however, your letter will be filed and you may be surprised with a call months or even a year or more later (this is especially true if you have been contacting them a few times a year to ask if they have any work for you).

Look for jobs in the classified ads of newspapers of large cities; search general job web sites using the terms [science writer] or [technical writer]. The best way to get work is by networking. Follow the previous networking tips in this book. Get to know people who work in industry through these organizations:

- American Association of Corporate and Public Practice Veterinarians (AACPPV, www.aacppv.org), includes members who may want to hire you as a freelance technical writer.
- American Medical Writer's Association (AMWA, www.amwa.org), an important source for technical writers, produces a monthly job market sheet with lists of freelance, part-time, and full-time jobs for medical writers and editors. They also offer educational seminars about medical and technical writing.
- Canadian Animal Health Institute (CAHI, www.cahi-icsa.ca) is the trade association representing the developers, manufacturers and distributors of animal pharmaceuticals, biologicals, feed additives and animal pesticides in Canada.
- Council of Biology Editors, Inc. (CBE, www.councilscienceeditors.org), a joint action of the National Science Foundation and the American Institute of Biological Sciences, has a mission to improve communication in the life sciences by educating authors, editors, and publishers. You need not be an editor to join.
- International Association of Business Communicators (IABC, www.iabc.com.).
- Society for Technical Communication, whose 20,000 members (with 130 local chapters) includes technical writers, editors, and graphic designers, www.stc.org.

One sure way to make a living as a full-time technical writer is to get a job with the federal government (see Chapter 16). Any one of the government agencies, from the Fish and Wildlife Service, to the National Institutes of Health, to the National Technical Information Service, may hire technical writers. For more information, peruse the list of federal job vacancies at www.opm.gov or www.usajobs.gov.

Pay

Technical writing is far more lucrative than is writing magazine articles. It is customary to charge by the hour (from $50 to $150 per hour, depending on qualifications and the difficulty of the work) plus expenses, such as long distance telephone or computer research online charges. Some jobs are paid by a flat rate; this can be a problem with projects that are not clearly defined (which is common). It takes a long time to establish a clientele, so it's a good idea to keep another job on the side at first.

Informatics

The world of librarians and technical information specialists have merged into "informatics," with many job opportunities that include writing and researching (looking up information).

A variety of information services create indexes or abstracts of medical or veterinary literature. These services need people to review, index, or write abstracts of scientific literature; to do literature searches; and to gather database information.

Although library science professionals or technical writers are often used for this purpose, there is sometimes a need for a professional with the ability to understand medical terminology and complex studies. Veterinarians may be hired on a full-time or part-time basis, as employees or independent consultants. Employers include the government and industry (See Chapters 11, 15–18). Many groups, universities, and companies have ongoing needs for literature searching, abstracting, or indexing. Titles of full-time positions vary; they include *research literature analyst* or *technical information specialist.*

Daily work / Pros and cons

Specific examples of daily work follow this section. Regardless of the employer, these jobs have one thing in common: They involve sitting at a desk and using your brain. Informatics is necessarily an indoor job, which may be a drawback for some. The low level of contact with animals (and sometimes people) is desired by some veterinarians.

These jobs provide great mental stimulation and an easy way to keep up on the latest information in veterinary medicine. Tracking veterinary information has an impact not only on veterinary medicine, but also on public health and clinical care. Pay depends on the type of company or government job held.

Qualifications

While each position has its specific qualifications, they all have some factors in common. Excellent writing, typing and computer skills are essential, as is the ability to use online databases and conduct searches using a variety of approaches. The ability to read literature (sometimes in foreign languages) and distill it for a more general audience is also important. Some positions require data analysis and knowledge of statistics. This is great work for people interested in learning about the latest information in their fields. For those who are self-employed, access to your own computer and high-speed Internet is a must.

Informatics training is offered at many universities. The Association for Veterinary Informatics (http://avinformatics.org) keeps an updated list of courses in its newsletter.

Health informatics training is offered at the University of Missouri in Columbia. Short-term fellowships are available for veterinary students, and two- to three-year programs are offered for graduate veterinarians. The UM master's degree program in health informatics is designed to produce professionals who can lead organizations in the application of information technology to improve the delivery of health care; a certificate program is also offered. See www.hmi.missouri.edu; http://mudirect.missouri.edu > degrees and programs > graduate certificate programs > health informatics; and http://mudirect.missouri.edu > degrees and programs > degrees > health informatics.

The Stanford School of Medicine's Section on Medical Informatics offers a one-week introductory course on medical informatics each summer (www.smi.stanford.edu/shortcourse.html and www.smi.stanford.edu/community). Each day is devoted to a specific topic in medical informatics. Stanford offers morning lectures and afternoon hands-on computer laboratory sessions and project presentations and demonstrations of medical informatics research.

Informatics programs are also offered at the Virginia-Maryland Regional College of Veterinary Medicine (informatics.vetmed.vt.edu) and the University of California at Davis (www.ucdmc.ucdavis.edu/informatics).

In addition, the World Organisation for Animal Health has internships that stress informatics (www.oie.int; see Chapter 13), and the CDC offers an informatics fellowship (www.cdc.gov/phifp; see Chapter 16).

To apply

Search online job web sites using the terms [literature analyst], [information services], or [informatics]. Investigate federal government positions at www.opm.gov or www.usajobs.gov, looking for jobs in technical writing or information services. Potential hiring agencies might include the National Library of Medicine of the NIH; the National Agricultural Library of the USDA; or the National Technical Information Service (NTIS). NTIS is the official resource for government-sponsored US and worldwide scientific, technical, engineering, and business-related information.

Attend meetings of relevant associations:

- American Medical Informatics Association (www.amia.org) is dedicated to the development and application of medical informatics in support of patient care, teaching, research, and health care administration. It holds three meetings per year and publishes several journals.
- American Veterinary Health Information Management Association (www.avhima.org), works on information management, promotes patient care through health information, and advocates for the profession on governmental, educational, social, and business issues that affect the management of veterinary health.
- Association for Veterinary Informatics (http://avinformatics.org) provides information about informatics short courses and fellowships (for students as well as graduate veterinarians), as well as new software/computer resources.
- Information Technology Association of America (www.itaa.org) is a trade association for those involved with information technology. It offers newsletters, meetings, and seminars.
- Medical Library Association (www.mlanet.org) has a subsection for veterinary librarians and a job placement service (free for members; a fee is charged for nonmembers). The annual meeting is in May. The International Conferences of Animal Health Information Specialists was originally organized by members of the Veterinary Medical Libraries Section/Medical Library Association to enhance the flow of animal health information worldwide.
- National Federation of Abstracting and Information Services (www.nfais.org) is an organization of the world's leading publishers of databases and information

services in the sciences, engineering, social sciences, business, the arts, and the humanities, representing for-profit, nonprofit, and government sectors. NFAIS members are international leaders in information collection, organization, and dissemination.

- Society for the Internet in Medicine (www.internet-in-medicine.org) promotes education of the public and the medical community in the applications of the Internet and related technologies in the fields of the medical sciences, health care practice, and management. Events include MEDNET—The World Congress of the Internet in Medicine. This society publishes the journal *Medical Informatics*.
- Software and Information Industry Association (www.siia.net) represents companies involved in creating, distributing, and facilitating the use of information in print and digital formats. It has a subsection for veterinary librarians.

You can get on mailing lists for helpful online discussions. For example, Vetlib-L (http://listserv.vt.edu/archives/vetlib-l.html) is an online discussion list for veterinary librarians and those interested in the field.

An article by R. Smith in the *Bulletin of the Medical Library Association* defines informatics applications within the veterinary community. Also see the discussion of electronic medical records in Chapter 9.

The following specific examples of informatics work illustrate the kinds of jobs available. Dr. Kerri Marshall describes her work:

> Joining Banfield, The Pet Hospital was the single best career decision I made in my 25-year career in veterinary medicine. What I love best about my job is being involved in programs that help millions of pets each year, networking with more than 2,500 veterinarians and always having a new challenge. This job has allowed me to try out new career avenues, yet keep a career path with a single practice.
>
> Because of the large network of primary care veterinary hospitals and great systems that capture medical information, we have evolved to making our medical decisions based on evidence. Currently, I enjoy leading the Medical Informatics team and collaborating with both veterinarians and physicians who are working on electronic medical records. To satisfy my "softer side," I also have a chance to give back to the community through serving on the board of the Banfield Charitable Trust and helping with programs like delivering pet food to Meals on Wheels recipients.
>
> A large, well-organized practice offers so many ways to contribute to our society and truly make a difference both locally and globally. I have also developed friendships over the years at Banfield that will last a lifetime.

There's a Native American saying that describes teamwork in a large organization best: "If you want to go fast, go alone, if you want to go far, go together."—Kerri E. Marshall, DVM, MBA, Senior Director, Medical Informatics, Banfield, The Pet Hospital, Portland, OR.

National Agricultural Library

The National Agricultural Library (NAL) of the US Department of Agriculture (USDA) has a policy of hiring people with science backgrounds as *technical information specialists*. As one of the most comprehensive sources of US agricultural and life sciences information, the Agricultural Online Access (AGRICOLA) database serves as the document locator and bibliographic control system for the NAL collection, covering the field of agriculture in the broadest sense. The NAL hires technical information specialists for indexing. Veterinarians would be desired as indexers for the veterinary literature. NAL jobs are advertised through the USDA (these jobs are listed under "technical information specialist," not "veterinarian"). Foreign language ability is not required, but computer skills and the ability to use online databases are necessary. The NAL is located in Maryland; indexers can work out of their homes part of the time but must come into the office one or two days a week. Pay varies with experience; the scale ranges from GS-9 to GS-12 (see www.fedjobs.com for a list of pay scales in each government level). For details about applying for Federal government jobs, read Chapter 16.

Wisconsin National Primate Research Center

The Wisconsin National Primate Research Center (WNPRC) at the University of Wisconsin includes the Primate Info Net, with links to more than 5,000 pages of information about nonhuman primates, and is an access point to other Internet programs at WNPRC. One of those programs is Primate Lit, a free online database that indexes the scientific literature in primatology from 1940 to the present. This database of more than 225,000 citations is managed by the Jacobsen Library, and the article indexing is done by staff the Primate Information Center at WNPRC. Duties of the *research literature analyst* for the Primate Info Net include reading from a wide variety of journals, including those dealing with retroviruses and AIDS, then abstracting for the database all the veterinary and biomedical articles that mention nonhuman primates. See these web sites:
- Primate Info Net, University of Wisconsin, http://pin.primate.wisc.edu.
- Primate Lit, http:// primatelit.library.wisc.edu.
- Wisconsin National Primate Research Center, www.primate.wisc.edu.

Magazine or Journal Editor

A limited number of jobs are available in editing veterinary publications. There are basically two kinds of editing for a magazine or journal: copyediting and technical editing. *Copyediting* is editing for grammar, punctuation, and spelling; this is usually delegated to a nonveterinary person. *Technical editing* is often delegated to specialists or reviewers. For example, submissions to *JAVMA* and *AJVR* are sent to specialists in the field—the reviewers—for technical comments and suggestions for revision (these are volunteers). Copyeditors and technical editors work with the publication's editors-in-chief, who have the final say in whether an article is published. *Consulting editors, contributing editors,* and *editorial advisors* are usually freelancers, not staff. Full-time, paid positions include *Editor in Chief* and *Assistant Editor.*

Daily work / Pros and cons

Specific duties vary with the job title. The *Editor-in-Chief* is responsible for the content of an entire magazine or journal. This includes planning, coordinating, and organizing content for each issue, corresponding with authors and reviewing editors, working with copyeditors, and sending compiled content to the publisher.

Editing may include reading manuscripts that are submitted for publication; critiquing these and consulting with authors about changes and improvements (changes in style, sentence structure, scientific content, and so forth); deciding which articles to put in each issue, and how the issue should be organized; deciding about what types of columns or regular features to publish; reading letters to the editor, and deciding which of those to print; and doing some writing, too. That translates into time sorting through and reading mail; making phone calls; writing letters (such as to article authors explaining rejections and revisions); and marking up articles with questions, comments, and corrections for the author.

Editors spend most of their time at a desk, but their jobs are very much "people" jobs. Most editorial jobs require that the editorial staff live close to where the magazine is produced (usually a city). Few magazines or journals allow "telecommuting," or working from home.

Veterinarian editors use their knowledge of veterinary medicine to decide what information is important enough to print and thus to disseminate to other veterinarians. In the process of editing, they are exposed to all kinds of interesting information.

Drawbacks to the job include spending time reading unusable material, struggling to meet deadlines, and working with "difficult" authors. (Article authors sometimes have strong egos—especially when they are experts in their fields.) Magazines that rely on advertising income face a conflict of interest, in that there may be pressure not to print material that may be interpreted as denigrating to an advertiser.

Qualifications / To apply

Qualifications for editorial jobs include good writing skills, writing experience, love of words and reading, and an ability to interpret and analyze scientific studies for accuracy and logic. Editors must know how to use advanced features of word processing programs and to be able to work with documents via email and using collaborative web sites. The editor must be able to give authors tactful, constructive criticism and advice in a positive and helpful manner. Editors of scientific and technical publications may need a background in research or knowledge of statistics.

The *Journal of the AVMA* and the *American Journal of Veterinary Research* (both AVMA publications) have veterinarians on staff as editor-in-chief, associate editors, and assistant editors. The editor-in-chief is generally someone who has work experience as an assistant or associate editor. Therefore, the best initial approach may be to apply for a job as an assistant editor. Openings are advertised in *JAVMA*, but it's never a bad idea to get a resume on file, even if an opening is not advertised at the moment. All AVMA positions are located at AVMA headquarters in Schaumburg, Illinois.

See the sections on jobs with AVMA and AAHA in Chapter 12 for more information. For information about potential openings with any other veterinary publication, write to the publisher or editor-in-chief listed on the magazine's masthead. Be sure to write to the address listed for editorial offices, and not the ones for subscriptions or advertising. Also, the mastheads of veterinary and pet journals will indicate whether they have veterinarians on staff. Also investigate the International Committee of Medical Journal Editors (www.icmje.org).

Sample job announcement: Assistant editor, AVMA

> Do you want to ensure that veterinarians have the latest scientific information available? The American Veterinary Medical Association is seeking an Assistant Editor for the world's leading veterinary journals: the *Journal of the AVMA* and the *American Journal of Veterinary Research*. This full-time position, located at AVMA headquarters in Schaumburg, IL (a northwest suburb of Chicago), is a unique opportunity to be involved with the leading edge of veterinary medicine and biotechnology.

> The AVMA offers a supportive work environment and excellent benefits. Applications should include a letter indicating special qualifications and scope of experience, curriculum vitae, and a list of three references. Nominations of potential candidates are also encouraged.

> Qualified candidates must have a doctorate in veterinary medicine, with research and clinical experience, or have a PhD degree in a field relevant to veterinary medicine as well as research experience in applied or clinical veterinary medicine. All candidates must have a demonstrated proficiency in scientific writing or editing and be able to communicate and work effectively with contributors to the AVMA journals.

Publishing jobs

Publishing and editing go hand-in-hand. A very few veterinarians work in publishing—that is, the business of getting a book, magazine, or journal typeset, printed and bound (or electronically formatted), promoted, distributed, and sold. The publisher of a large magazine delegates work by hiring businesses that specialize in each of these areas. The publisher is the editor's boss, and works with the editor to make sure that there is content to fill each magazine. The publisher of a smaller magazine may be the editor-in-chief as well.

Another niche is to write and publish newsletters that individual practices can send to their clients. Publishers create these as a template with certain articles included, leaving space for the practice name or other personal touches.

Daily work / Pros and cons

Once a veterinarian has moved into the publishing field, the connection to veterinary medicine becomes abstract. This is an indoor job that includes managing people, attending meetings, computer/desk work, and attending to organization and planning. You will spend the majority of your time managing the business, coordinating printers, advertisers, and writers, and managing your editors—not reading or writing veterinary material. Publishers of veterinary-related material have the ability to affect the content and style of material that is seen by veterinarians. This can provide a great service to the profession.

Qualifications / To start

There are two basic ways to get into publishing. One is to begin a magazine or newsletter yourself. The other is to purchase a magazine from another publisher—that is, to buy the business. A strong background in editing and writing are necessary, as well as good business management skills.

For information about publishing, check out the trade publication, *Folio* magazine, a good source for information on magazine management (www.foliomag.com). Their web site also offers webinars on editing and publishing topics. Also investigate these groups:

- American Agricultural Editors Association, www.ageditors.com.
- Association of American Publishers, which conducts a course in publishing scholarly journals, www.publishers.org.
- International Committee of Medical Journal Editors, www.icmje.org.

Writing a Book

It is rare for a writer to start a career by writing a book. Few publishers will consider an idea presented by someone who has never published an article in a magazine. So, if you jumped to this section and skipped the first section in this chapter about writing magazine articles, go back and read that first.

Daily work / Pros and cons

Writing a book can be extremely fun and gratifying. Whether you will write a book about technical information, or a chapter for a textbook, or write for a larger audience about more general pet-related topics, the results will be rewarding.

For Justine Lee, DVM, DACVECC, writing a book was a lifetime dream. It took time, energy, persistence, hard work, and research. The end result was two very popular books: *It's a Dog's Life…But It's Your Carpet* and *It's a Cat's World…You Just Live In It*. As Dr. Lee puts it:

> Veterinarians play such a key role in public health and the human-animal bond, and writing books has allowed me to fulfill these roles, while also acting as a liaison to the public. In addition, becoming an author has opened up a lot of public relation roles and other press-

related opportunities for me. Writing two funny, humorous question and answer books for Random House was a great way for me to help people become the best consumer advocates for their pets, while providing important client education in an entertaining way.

Qualifications / To start

Many veterinarians have great book ideas. If you want to write a book, you must first answer this question: Do you want to *make money* with this book (i.e., write something that sells) or do you just want to produce a book for the joy of writing and to get the information out to those who need it (and you are willing to *pay money* to do so)? Your answer will totally change your approach to writing a book.

If you are interested in writing a book that will sell, you need to study the business of book writing and selling. Start by reading books such as *How to Write a Book Proposal*, by M. Larson and *Sell Your Book*, by G. Scott. Read writers' magazines such as *Writer's Digest* (www.writersdigest.com), which includes information about writer's seminars. Attend these just as you attend veterinary continuing education meetings. (This is essential, so don't skip it). Also, see the section on copyright earlier in this chapter. Business forms and copyright information are available at www.copyright.gov or www.legalzoom. com.

Many book authors have an agent, who represents the author by presenting a book proposal to a variety of publishers until it is sold, and helps the author negotiate the book contract. The use of an agent is optional. Learn details about agents from the resources listed above.

Another option is self-publishing a book. Successful self-publishing is done by experienced authors who have the time and knowledge to attend to all aspects of book production and marketing. It is most appropriate when the intended audience for the book is small or occupies a narrow niche. Authors who self-publish a book because no publisher will buy it often find that no one else will buy it either.

For self-publishers, the Independent Book Publishers Association (IBPA) publishes a newsletter that includes information about all aspects of book production (www.ibpa-online.org). Their annual "publishing university" is a two-day series of seminars on book editing, marketing, design, finance, law, sales, and publicity. Also check out the Small Publishers Association of North America (www.spannet.org). Read the *Self-Publishing Manual*, by Dan Poynter, whose business, Para Publishing, has many other resources for self-publishing (www.parapublishing.com).

"Writing a book" is rarely a career in itself, but just part of the freelance writer's or consultant's career. Once you enter the world of writing, attend writers' seminars, and read more about writing, the business of writing a book will become much clearer.

Media Work: Television and Radio

Although veterinarians do appear on or even host their own television or radio programs, few are able to make this a full-time job with a focus on veterinary medicine. Veterinarians who work with the news media do so for several reasons: to promote their other work (a book they're selling or their veterinary hospital); for the fun of it; to improve their speaking skills; to improve their image to the public or their clients; or to help educate the public. Veterinarians who make such appearances are viewed by some of the public as special or exceptionally talented. That statement is only partially true. The reality is that knowing the right people, making the right contacts, and being able to speak clearly, with animation, and in "sound bites" are important factors in getting on television or radio programs. For television, a good visual presence is important—professional-looking clothing, neat hair, and quiet body language (no fidgeting).

Qualifications / To start

Let's say you want to make some news media appearances. Because there are more radio than television stations, it may be easier for you to get on a radio show. The first question to ask is this: What programs are your potential customers watching or listening to? Unless you have written a pet care book that is directed at the general public, there's no point in appearing on the national news. Besides, they won't give you a second look unless your book is selling exceptionally well or is really different.

Start by either searching the Internet or going to the library and looking up the names and addresses of local or specialty television and radio shows. (Specialty shows include television and radio segments devoted to pets or livestock.) Send them a press release announcing your news (you must have some news or there's no reason to have you on). An example might be an announcement about your new housecall service or how you offer free classes on bird care at the local senior citizens' center. Another announcement might be that your new book just received an award, and you will be hosting a book signing at the local bookstore.

Follow up your press release with a phone call. If you're scheduled for an appearance, ask about what you will be expected to discuss and how long the interview will last. You can even volunteer to send a list of "typical questions" that they might ask (this is normal, and makes their work easier). During the show, remember that it will be impossible for you to say everything you want to say, so don't even try. Make sure the main receptionist has your contact information (listeners who want to contact you will call the station, so the person who answers the phone should have your name, address, and phone number handy). Record all your appearances or radio interviews, and listen to them to remember what sounded particularly good, or alternatively, to learn from your mistakes (if you hear yourself saying "um" more than once, join Toastmasters to improve).

Chapter 10 Resources

Groups and web sites

Advanstar, www.DVM360.com and www.advanstarvhc.com.

American Agricultural Editors Association, c/o Den Gardner, Executive Director, PO Box 156. New Prague, MN 56071; www.ageditors.com; phone: 952-758-6502; fax: 952-758-5813; e-mail: Ageditors@aol.com.

American Association of Corporate and Public Practice Veterinarians (AACPPV), 6060 Sunrise Vista Drive, Suite 1300, Citrus Heights, CA 95610-7098; www.aacppv.org; phone: 916-726-1560; e-mail: info@aacppv.org.

American Association of Corporate and Public Practice Veterinarians, www.aacppv.org; phone: 916-726-1560.

American Medical Informatics Association (AMIA), 4915 St Elmo Ave., Suite 302, Bethesda, MD 20814; www.amia.org/; phone: 301-657-1291; fax: 301-657-1206.

American Medical Writer's Association (AMWA), 40 West Gude Drive, Suite 101, Rockville, MD 20850-1192; www.amwa.org; phone: 301-294-5303; e-mail: amwa@amwa.org.

American Society of Journalists and Authors (ASJA), 1501 Broadway Suite 302, New York, NY 10036; www.asja.com; phone: 212-997-0947; fax: 212-937-2315.

American Veterinary Health Information Management Association, www.avhima.org.

Animal and Plant Health Inspection Service (APHIS-VS), USDA, www.aphis.usda.gov.

Association for Veterinary Informatics (AVI), http://avinformatics.org/avinform/); phone: 425-455-0727.

Association of American Publishers, Inc., 50 F Street, NW 4th Floor, Washington, DC 20001; www.publishers.org; phone: 202-347-3375; fax: 202-347-3690. New York Office: 71 Fifth Ave, New York, NY 10003; phone: 212-255-0200; fax: 212-255-7007.

Business forms and copyright information, www.copyright.gov and www.legalzoom.com.

Cat Writer's Association, www.catwriters.org; e-mail: comments@catwriters.org.

Centers for Disease Control and Prevention (CDC), Public Health Informatics Fellowship, www.cdc.gov/PHIFP.

Council of Biology Editors, Inc. c/o Drohan Management Group, 12100 Sunset Hills Road, Suite 130, Reston, VA 20190; www.councilscienceeditors.org; phone: 703-437-4377, fax: 703-435-4390; e-mail: CSE@CouncilScienceEditors.org.

Dog Writer's Association, c/o Secretary Pat Santi, 173 Union Rd, Coatesville, PA 19320, www.dwaa.org; e-mail: pat@dwaa.org.

Federal pay scale, www.fedjobs.com.

Independent Book Publishers Association (IBPA), 627 Aviation Way, Manhattan Beach, CA 90266; www.ibpa-online.org; phone: 310-372-2732; fax: 310-374-3342; e-mail: info@IBPA-online.org.

Information Technology Association of America (ITAA), 1401 Wilson Boulevard, Suite 1100, Arlington, VA 22209; www.itaa.org; phone: 703-522-5055; fax: 703-525-2279; Western Region Office, San Mateo, CA; phone: 650-357-7728.

International Association of Business Communicators (IABC), One Hallidie Plaza, Suite 600, San Francisco, CA 94102; www.iabc.com; phone: 415-544-4700 or 800-776-4222; fax: 415-544-4747.

International Committee of Medical Journal Editors (ICMJE), www.icmje.org.

Medical Library Association (MLA), 65 East Wacker Place, Suite 1900, Chicago, IL 60601-7246, www.mlanet.org; phone: 312-419-9094; fax: 312-419-8950; e-mail: info@mlahq.org.

National Agricultural Library (NAL), USDA, www.nal.usda.gov.

National Association of Agricultural Journalists (NAAJ), www.naaj.net; e-mail: ka-phillips@tamu.edu.

National Federation of Abstracting and Information Services (NFAIS), 1518 Walnut Street, Suite 307, Philadelphia, PA 19102; www.nfais.org; phone: 215-893-1561; fax: 215 893-1564; e-mail: nfais@hslc.org.

National Technical Information Service (NTIS), Technology Administration, US Department of Commerce, Springfield, VA 22161; www.ntis.gov/about/form.aspx; phone: 703-487-4650.

National Writers Union (NWU), www.nwu.org.

Office of Personnel Management, www.opm.gov.

Para Publishing, PO Box 8206-222, Santa Barbara CA 93118-8206; www.parapublishing.com; phone: 805-968-7277; fax: 805-968-1379.

Small Publishers Association of North America, 1618 W. Colorado Ave, Colorado Springs, CO, 80904; www.spannet.org; phone: 719-475-1726; fax: 719-471-2182; e-mail: info1@spannet.org.

Society for Technical Communication (STC), 901 N. Stuart St., Suite 904, Arlington, VA 22203-1854; www.stc.org; phone: 703-522-4114; fax: 703-522-2075.

Society for Veterinary Medicine and Literature, www.vetmedandlit.org; e-mail: information@vetmedandlit.org.

Stanford University School of Medicine, Medical Informatics Short Course, www.smi.stanford.edu/shortcourse.html; phone: 650-723-6979; e-mail: short-course@smi.stanford.edu.

Toastmasters, 23182 Arroyo Vista, Rancho Santa Margarita, CA 92688, www.toastmasters.org; phone: 949-858-8255; fax: 949-858-1207.

University of Missouri master's degree program in health informatics, www.hmi.missouri.edu or http://mudirect.missouri.edu/degprog/hmi-infor/inddex.shtm; phone: 573-882-3598 or 800-877-4764; e-mail: MUdirect@missouri.edu.

USA Jobs, www.usajobs.gov.

Vetlib-L, http://listserv.vt.edu/archives/vetlib-l.html; e-mail: listserv@listserv.vt.edu.
World Organisation for Animal Health, www.oie.int.

Books and articles

Alred, G. J., *Handbook of Technical Writing*, 8th edition (Bedford/St. Martin's, 2005).

Anderson, P. V., *Technical Communication: A Reader-Centered Approach*, 6th edition (Wadsworth Publishing, 2006).

Crawford, T, *Business & Legal Forms for Authors and Self-Publishers* (Allworth Press, 2005).

Folio: The Magazine for Magazine Management, www.foliomag.com; phone: 203-358-9900.

Harper, T., ed., *ASJA Guide to Freelance Writing: A Professional Guide to the Business, for Nonfiction Writers of All Experience Levels* (St. Martin's Griffin, 2003).

Larsen, M., *How to Write a Book Proposal*, 3rd edition (Writers Digest Books, 2004).

Poynter, D., *Self-Publishing Manual* (Para Publishing, 2007).

Scott, G., *Sell Your Book, Script or Column* (ASJA Press, 2007).

Smith, R., et al., Applications of Informatics in Veterinary Medicine, *Bulletin of the Medical Library Association*, January 2000; available at: www.pubmedcentral.nih.gov.

Van Laan, K., and C. Julian, *The Complete Idiot's Guide to Technical Writing* (Alpha Books, 2001).

Writer magazine, www.writermag.com.

Writer's Digest, www.writersdigest.com.

Writer's Market (Writer's Digest Books, published annually).

11 VETERINARY INDUSTRY AND THE CORPORATE WORLD

During one of my presentations on veterinary industry, I asked the audience what motivated them to enter a career in industry. Several pursued their strong interest in business and seized the opportunity to work with other veterinarians in a corporate setting of long-term goals and objectives. Veterinary industry offers a way to combine veterinary education and business skills in order to improve animal health, solve problems and educate other professionals. Some found that private practice was not challenging or interesting enough for them. Others expressed very practical reasons for choosing a career in veterinary industry. Some of them had health concerns that kept them from practicing with animals and others needed better health insurance and more lucrative salary than they could receive with private practice. Many of them mentioned that a career in industry allowed them to enjoy a more balanced lifestyle. Finally, some just happened to be in the right place at the right time, even if they were not actively looking for a job in industry.— Deb Nickelson, DVM, Marketing Manager, Veterinary Products Laboratories, Phoenix AZ

Veterinarians and students often hear the words "veterinary industry" and visualize a negative picture of a pet food or drug sales representative. That unfortunate stereotype could not be more wrong. Let's start by being more specific about these jobs, which are careers that simply serve veterinary professionals and animal owners.

A wide variety of companies make products or perform services for veterinarians and pet owners. These include:

- Medications
- Medical supplies
- Medical equipment
- Pet foods (regular, "diet," therapeutic)
- Laboratory supplies and equipment
- Pet and livestock insurance
- Laboratory and diagnostic services

Veterinarians are hired in every business that manufactures, provides, or distributes these products and services. Because of mergers and acquisitions, as well as continual development of new companies, this book does not list the many potential employers in the industry segment.

Industry veterinarians may hold a veterinary degree alone, or they may also hold additional degrees. Some schools have programs to help prepare students for jobs in industry. For example, the Virginia-Maryland Regional College of Veterinary Medicine has a Department of Corporate and Public Practice to prepare those interested in public and corporate areas of veterinary medicine. The association that represents veterinarians in industry is the American Association of Corporate and Public Practice Veterinarians (AACPPV; www.aacppv.org).

Approximately 3,000 veterinarians are employed in veterinary industry, with that number growing slightly each year in spite of corporate mergers and cutbacks. Pay is generally good, and benefits are excellent.

Daily work / Pros and cons

> In my experience it is rare for a veterinarian who enters industry to go back into practice, because there is a reason they left practice in the first place. Some of them come to me because they feel they have learned everything there is to learn in practice and they want to broaden their experience and learn something new or they are tired of being in practice and want a different experience. Some of them have other areas of interest such as marketing, technical support, public speaking or university relations and they want to combine other business interests with their clinical practice experience.

> Travel is often required, especially in sales technical supporting roles, often as much as 75–80% of the time. In my experience, just as many women as men will take on heavy travel schedules; some are women with families and children. They make it work with spouses and outside help.

> The area of Regulatory Affairs seems to have a shortage of qualified professionals. Some companies that would prefer to hire a DVM are accepting non-DVMs because they cannot find a qualified veterinarian to fill that role.

> Another role is a Marketing Liaison Veterinarian. This is someone who works with R&D, sales, marketing and technical services. This position requires strong communication skills and the ability to translate information across departments. To qualify you might start in Technical Services. Some companies will cross train so that you can gain other

experience such as marketing and sales. Someone who has had industry experience across multiple areas might qualify for this type of role—Stacy Pursell, Founder and President, The VET Recruiter®

Some industry jobs allow you to continue to work with animals or pet and livestock owners; others allow you to interact with other veterinarians. All require that you use the knowledge you gained in veterinary school, even if it does not involve hands-on animal work. Job duties range from technical support (providing information about the company's products to veterinarians) to management (directing other veterinarians or researchers in the company) to clinical research. Positions are available in several departments or areas, and you can sometimes transition between areas within a company.

Typical industry departments that employ veterinarians include:

- Technical service
- Quality control
- Business development
- Research and development (R&D)
- Regulatory affairs and product development
- Sales and marketing
- Production
- Product registration

No matter what your specific job, you represent the company for which you work—so you should have a positive opinion of their products, services, and business goals. Many jobs allow you to continue to work with animals or to have contact with practicing veterinarians. Pay and benefits are excellent, and there is plenty of opportunity for advancement.

All veterinary industry jobs require an ability to work within the structure of a business organization, including following all the company policies and procedures. Coming from private practice, where often there are few rules and regulations, this can be a tough transition. There can be a lot of bureaucracy associated with working for a large company.

All corporate employees are evaluated periodically by measurable performance criteria. For instance, you may be required to write a list of goals for each year, and your raises, bonuses, and promotions are based on whether you achieve your goals (often these are financial goals such as total sales). Since there is always more than enough to do, you must learn to focus on the important tasks.

Mergers and acquisitions may take a toll on some industry veterinarians. Mergers can both create opportunities and decrease jobs. However, the AACPPV annual salary survey for 2008 (published in 2010) showed that 80 percent of respondents had *not* changed employers in the past two years (down from 84% in 2007). The timing of a merger or acquisition can range from months to years. Dealing with the uncertainty, cultural changes, and personnel changes requires flexibility, keeping options open.

Qualifications

Working for any veterinary-related company will invariably mean that you must already live in, or are able to move to, the city where your services are needed (that is not always the company's headquarters, though, especially for technical services jobs).

You should enjoy working as part of a team, and be interested in keeping up your knowledge of company (and competitor) products and the associated diseases or management problems. Basic computer skills and good writing and speaking skills are necessary. Experience with a wide variety of animal species and a background in statistics are helpful. Knowing how to interact with the media is useful. Companies often send their employees to speaker training or media training workshops.

Some jobs require a few years of experience in practice, whereas others require sales, managerial or research experience. If a position looks good to you, but you lack the experience, take a lower-level job and gain the experience as you work. Good communication skills (telephone, interpersonal and group speaking, and writing) will increase an inexperienced person's chances of being hired.

One thing that veterinary industry is *not* looking for is a veterinarian who just wants to "get out of private practice." What company would hire someone because they want to get *away* from something else? Instead, they're looking for people who want to get into the business (those who have a positive reason for change). They want people who may still like private practice, but who are looking for a greater challenge. An interest in the specific company also helps.

To get promotions and advance your career, you should, over time, take jobs in more than one area and should be willing to move between companies or to other locations. Often, a higher salary or promotion means advancing into a management position, farther away from working with animals, animal owners, or veterinarians. Many veterinarians elect not to pursue promotion because they prefer to live in one place and are happy with their jobs. Additional qualifications for specific positions are described below.

To apply

Jobs in industry are filled through a network. Who you know is important. This needn't be a roadblock—just because you don't know anyone today doesn't mean you can't meet people. Go to any large veterinary meeting, and chat with the people working in the exhibit area (when they're not busy with customers). How do they like their jobs? What other jobs are available in their company? Where do they live, and how much do they travel? Tell everyone you know that you are investigating jobs in industry.

Knowing the right person can make all the difference. For example, Dan Green, DVM, took a position in industry completely by chance. A company representative was going on maternity leave and asked him to "run her route" for her for six weeks until she returned. Dan said yes, and he spent the next six weeks teaching veterinarians about congestive heart failure in the dog as a part of a campaign launching a new drug. Dr. Green went on to a permanent position and has been with industry ever since, helping animals on a daily basis. His work has even taken him overseas to work in Germany. In his own words:

I realized I could do more good, and help more animals, by spreading the information about new treatments in veterinary medicine than I had done in 18 years of emergency medicine. I touch so many veterinarians, and hopefully inspire them to do better quality medicine.

Join the AACPPV (www.aacppv.org). Attend their annual meetings, breakfasts, or luncheons which are held at various national-level veterinary conferences. This association is also involved with the creation of programs in corporate and public practice that are held at various veterinary teaching colleges. Their web site includes a career center with links to many companies, recruiters and web sites with job announcements.

Two other useful associations are the American Pet Products Association (APPA), which presents information, surveys, and economic reports of interest to the industry (www.americanpetproducts.org); and the Drug Information Association (DIA, www.diahome.org), which includes many veterinarian members. Their web site includes a career center.

If you currently have a job in private practice, take time to visit with all the sales reps who come in, and ask them when they will have a technical services veterinarian riding with them. Then, talk to that veterinarian. Say yes to offers to go out to lunch. Offer to do clinical research in your hospital for the company.

Focus on companies you consider to be reputable and strong, carry good products, and whose veterinarian employees you would like as colleagues. Find out as much as you can about the company before you make your approach. Get their literature, brochures, and annual report. Look up their financial data online or in your library's reference department.

For an overview of companies, view the *Veterinary Economics* supplement, *Vetguide*, (http://marketplace.dvm360.com), an illustrated buyer's guide to a large array of equipment and supplies. *Veterinary Pharmaceuticals and Biologicals* and the *Compendium of Veterinary Products* are books that include the names and addresses of companies that manufacture and sell veterinary modifications, supplies, and pet foods. They are updated at irregular intervals, so find the most recent edition possible.

Peruse veterinary journals and online job sites for advertisements (see Chapter 1 on getting started and how to apply for any job). All of the major companies will have "careers" or "jobs" links on their web sites. Most larger job databases are free of charge and will list positions as well. Veterinary journals will also have job openings listed for positions in industry.

Don't turn down a job just because it's not the exact one you want. Once you have "industry experience," your choices are much wider. Why not work for a year or two as a technical services rep, for example, if it gives you a leg up when you want to apply for a job in R&D? Once you're "in," opportunities increase.

Every company will have slightly different job descriptions, duties, and titles. One job in company A may have an entirely different title in company B and be divided into two jobs in company C. The descriptions that follow are included to give you a peek at the potential choices and some sample job announcements.

Pay

Veterinarians working in industry consistently earn higher salaries than do veterinarians in any other category of work. Board-certified veterinarians or those with additional degrees also see the most financial benefit from their training if they work for industry.

The AACPPV annual survey showed that the average base salary for industrial veterinarians with a veterinary degree was $135,000 (see Table 11.1). Salaries tended to be higher in companies focusing on human pharmaceuticals and medical devices, contract research, animal health products, and pet foods, and lower in companies focusing on animal feeds. Salaries are higher for management positions, but those with an MBA did not earn more than average. Most jobs in industry provide exceptional benefits, which add a significant sum to the total income. The AACPPV survey provides details on benefits and other items of interest. Pay and benefits received by veterinarians working in Canada may be found in the Report on Veterinarians in Alternate Career Paths, available from the Ontario Veterinary Medical Association (www.ovma.org).

Table 11.1: Mean salaries of veterinarians working in industry

Job Title	Mean Salary*	% of Respondents
Technical services	$122,000	29%
Director	$155,000	25%
Manager	$126,000	20%
Primary Nature of Job		
Technical services	$120,000	29%
Management	$178,000	18%
Research/product development	$115,000	9%
Sales/marketing	$131,000	7%

Source: AACPPV annual survey for 2008, released Feb 2010 (www.aaccppv.org). *All values rounded.

Technical or Professional Service

Technical services is a good place for a veterinarian to start in a career in industry. From here, you can advance to other jobs. A *technical service representative* (TSR), regional technical manager, or professional services manager learns the technical details about a company's products and uses that knowledge to answer customer questions or to train sales people for the company. A *technical affairs manager* is responsible for a budget, strategic planning, and supervising other people. The job involves less travel than does the TSR position. The *director of professional services* is in charge of the technical services department.

Daily work / Pros and cons

TSRs give seminars for sales staff and for practicing veterinarians, where they speak about their company's products or services, usually speaking in a broader sense of the disease, disorder, or injury that creates a need for that product or service. For example, pet food company TSRs give talks about nutrition in relation to health and disease.

The TSR may "ride along" with sales representatives on their daily rounds to veterinary clinics, helping them to answer questions and teaching them about the veterinarian-customer's concerns. They also represent the company to schools and colleges and at veterinary meetings.

TSRs spend 50 percent or more of their time traveling; a company car is sometimes provided. Many give more than 50 lectures per year. The company may provide information to be given in a talk, but TSRs often rearrange the material to suit their needs. TSRs must become experts in the medical or surgical area in which their company's products or services are used. They may be in charge of handling complaints about a product, including the follow-up for each.

Answering telephones (as a telephone consultant) can be a big part of technical services. Non-veterinarians are assigned to telephone duty to screen calls, so the veterinarians handle only the calls that require their expertise. The veterinarian telephone consultant provides information to pet owners, veterinarians, journalists, breeders, and universities about the company's products or services, and may mail out printed information after a telephone conversation.

The telephone consultant may interact with company workers in R&D, marketing, or the packaging/labeling department to help answer caller's questions. In some companies, veterinarians may be assigned to do only phone duty (at least one pet food company hires veterinarians part-time on a contract basis for this purpose). Other companies have their regular TSR staff rotate through phone duty (e.g., one week on phone duty, then several weeks traveling).

Qualifications

Qualifications include willingness to travel and interest in, and preferably experience with, sales, marketing, and customer relations. (Veterinarians who have been in private practice usually have this experience.) The ability to write and speak well is a basic requirement, as is computer literacy (being comfortable using computers; extensive knowledge is not generally required). Many of the calls that are managed involve complaints or problems, so strong client relations skills, remaining calm and professional, are key attributes.

Sample job announcements

Companion animal technical services veterinarian

> Pharmaceutical company. Provide technical support to marketing. Design, implement, and report market support trials. Generate written and oral technical communications, including scientific papers and presentation at professional meetings. Provide technical training (internal and external). Requires DVM, minimum 3 yr experience in animal health industry, exposure to trial design and statistical analysis.

Professional services veterinarian—swine

> Pharmaceutical company. Communicate with veterinarians, distributors, swine producers, and other customers concerning products. Assist in

handling suspect adverse events, assist on marketing projects. Perform public speaking. Requires DVM, knowledge about swine production medicine, computer skills, ability to effectively communicate and effective interpersonal skills.

Veterinary affairs manager

As a Veterinary Affairs Manager, you will be responsible for positioning us as an important leader among the academic community and practicing veterinarians in a given geography. This position provides regional responsibilities including coverage of universities. Duties: technical training and development of sales and distributor staff, assisting on direct call with key accounts, and the delivery of technical presentations. Your home office can be based anywhere within the assigned region. Requires: veterinary degree; 2–5 yr practice or academic experience. Preferred: current DVM license/MBA/Advanced training/ Board Certification/ 1–3 years industry or equivalent experience with a professional veterinary medicine organization /1–3 years of public speaking experience. Previous experience in sales, communications, or a marketing role specifically associated with our product type is highly desirable. Excellent communication skills, presentation skills and computer proficiency (Excel, Word, PowerPoint, and Lotus Notes) are required. Requires up to 80% travel, including overnight and some weekends.

Research and Development (R&D)

Research and development is the area to explore if you still want hands-on work with animals and have an interest in clinical medicine. Many positions are open to veterinarians, although some require additional training. Some R&D jobs allow you to stay in one place, but others require travel. Compared with some other industry jobs, the hours of some R&D jobs can be long due to frequent deadlines. Veterinarians with these jobs must be comfortable with the company's use of animals in research.

Daily work / Pros and cons

The *R&D facility veterinarian* manages the animal facility, including care and feeding of a large number of animals, treatment of sick or injured animals, and practicing preventive medicine (exams, vaccinations, and so forth). The facility veterinarian monitors the use of animals in research projects to be sure that experiments are both necessary and appropriate, and makes sure the facility passes inspection by meeting federal requirements. In most cases this person has advanced training in laboratory animal medicine. (See Laboratory animal medicine in Chapter 6 and the section on the FDA in Chapter 16.)

The *biological staff veterinarian* is involved in project planning and monitoring, including deciding what animal species is best to use for a study, how many animals should be used, what special conditions should be provided, and the best way to perform an experiment. Duties might include looking for adverse signs, drawing blood samples, or performing necropsies.

A *clinical research coordinator's* job can include designing a study and then soliciting private practitioners, who then enroll their own patients. The work includes traveling to the practitioner's clinics to educate them about their roles and to monitor the study; negotiating contracts with those practitioners; handling problems (side effects in patients) that arise during the study; and then compiling and analyzing the data and generating a final report. The job can involve travel from 25 to 75 percent of the time. The rest of the time is spent on the telephone and at the computer. Knowledge of various regulatory requirements is essential.

The *director of research* manages a group of researchers dedicated to finding new products for animal health. Many companies will hire a veterinarian because of the practical, "real life" point of view this person brings to the research setting. The director makes management decisions, writes budgets, and directs research (specialists do the actual research)—focusing on the business feasibility and common sense of each project. The director tells the researcher what's needed, and the researcher tells the director how they can best achieve that goal.

Qualifications

Basic research often requires specialists such as veterinary pathologists, toxicologists, and laboratory animal veterinarians. However, clinical research can be done by a veterinarian with clinical practice experience. The veterinarian in R&D should have a working knowledge of statistics and study design, obtained via an MS degree, research work during veterinary school, or even on-the-job training by starting out as an assistant on another research project.

Sample job announcements

Research veterinarian

> Pharmaceutical company. Discovery and evaluation of animal health products for food and companion animals; conducting safety and efficacy studies; working with infectious disease models; and providing veterinary services for animals at the research center. Requires DVM with large animal research experience, knowledge of experimental design, statistics and regulations, and excellent communication skills.

Animal care center veterinarian

> Pet food company. Provide veterinary care for research animals, including exams, surgical, medical, wellness, emergency, and dentals. Visit and monitor studies performed by outside research facilities; give presentations; write summary reports, technical training material/papers. Requires 2 yrs of clinical practice and 1–3 yrs of applied experience in animal research.

Regulatory Affairs and Product Development

The regulatory affairs department is in charge of all communication with the appropriate regulatory office (usually the Food and Drug Administration).

Daily work / Pros and cons

The *regulatory affairs veterinarian* or *product development (PD) manager* takes a new drug concept to the FDA and negotiates with that agency about the work that must be done to get it approved (including the types of studies—toxicity, field efficacy, or dose titrations; how many animals must be used; and duration of the study). They also perform any work necessary to keep existing products on the market; for example, documentation or studies may be necessary if adverse events about a product are reported. Additional studies may also be needed to extend the life of current products or to expand their use.

The regulatory affairs department gives their information to the clinical research department, which writes a study protocol that meets the FDA requirements. The FDA then reviews these protocols, which must be renegotiated to everyone's satisfaction before the study can begin. FDA approval also depends on developing package insert information and a label for the product. (See the section on the FDA in Chapter 16.)

Product development managers oversee the entire process. They work with the formulations chemist to make the drug conform to the stringent regulations the government requires. In order for the product to meet specifications, the analytical group develops tests to analyze its content. The PD manager works with the toxicology group to determine safety for animals receiving the drug as well as for people handling the drug. Some companies have a team that may include a manager and field investigators. They may contract out a study to a university, with supervision by the field manager.

Regulatory affairs jobs involve mostly desk work (writing, computer, telephone). These veterinarians must keep up on developments in government regulations and in new products similar to the ones they are bringing to market. As with R&D, meeting strict deadlines may involve long working hours.

Qualifications

Knowledge of laws, medicine, R&D, and the needs of practicing veterinarians are important, as is the patience to deal with government regulations and government workers. One route to jobs in regulatory affairs is by working in R&D.

The PD manager is not an entry-level position, but a field product coordinator or field monitor could be. A variety of backgrounds would be appropriate for these positions, since the work differs with every project.

Sample job announcements

Manager of regulatory affairs

> Animal Health. Involved in the preparation and execution of regulatory submissions, including communicating with regulatory agencies to expedite the approval process, assisting preparation of regulatory

strategies, and assisting in regulatory support for clinical development. Requires DVM, excellent oral and written communication skills, computer proficiency. Prefer 2 yr experience in regulatory affairs.

Product development manager

Pharmaceutical company. Involves coordination of several projects involving cattle, swine, and poultry products. Duties include designing efficacy and safety studies, coordinating efforts with product development and marketing departments, providing technical advice on assigned projects, and monitoring studies required in an animal drug submission. Postdoctoral experience and knowledge of US registration procedures are desirable.

Diagnostic Laboratory Work

Melissa Blauvelt, DVM, MS, holds a job as a clinical pathologist with a private diagnostic laboratory in addition to teaching veterinary students. She shares her thoughts on her role as a staff clinical pathologist:

Clinical pathologists are more distant from the patient than are the attending clinicians, but the opportunity to serve them is not lost by this distance. Clinical pathology lends unique and significant insight. I think I have always been a visual person, and this coupled with kind mentors and years of experience has allowed me to recognize the often subtle declaration of pathology that passes under my microscope so frequently. I am very grateful that I can focus in this specialization that makes me happy, and still serve the patients that had initially drawn me to veterinary medicine.

Jobs for veterinary pathologists are in high demand in industry. Veterinary diagnostic laboratories are major employers of veterinary pathologists. Other employers include universities and state-run diagnostic laboratories. A survey conducted by the American College of Veterinary Pathologists found 150 open positions for both anatomic and clinical pathologists, with half of those being in the industrial sector (private laboratories, not academic labs). Although that was some years ago, this is a significant number of openings given the total number of board certified pathologists (see Table 4.1). The number of openings is rising due to a combination of increased demand and increased retirement of the current generation of pathologists. (See www.acvp.org > career opportunities > employer demographic survey).

Daily work / Pros and cons

Much of a veterinary pathologist's day is spent reviewing blood and urine samples, examining cytology submissions (such as cells from suspected infections, bone marrow biopsies, and so on), or performing specific tests with specialized equipment. This can vary based upon the clinical pathologist's specific training. The pathologist may also consult by telephone with veterinarians who have questions about submitting samples or interpreting test results.

A major benefit of this job is the opportunity to help submitting veterinarians and their patients in whatever way possible. Sometimes that may be through an obvious answer obtained via cytology or hematology; at other times, negative test results help narrow the diagnostic possibilities. The lifestyle is great, with good work hours and no emergency work required, and only an occasional weekend or late night.

A clinical pathologist has limited contact with live animals or with clients, as well as limited feedback; without follow-up, contact with veterinarians who submit samples is limited to a few words on the submission form. This isolation may not appeal to some.

Also see Forensics in Chapter 13.

Qualifications

Pathologists may have an additional degree beyond the DVM, such as an MS or PhD or both. The majority working in the field are board-certified, usually in clinical pathology or anatomical pathology (see Chapter 4). However, a few larger laboratories do hire non-board-certified veterinarians as clinical pathologists or histopathologists. Pathologists may be members of the American Association of Veterinary Laboratory Diagnosticians (www.aavld.org). A list of some veterinary diagnostic laboratories may be found at www.aphis.usda.gov > animal health > NAHLN Home > NAHLN Laboratories.

More Choices

Business development or international positions

Business development workers look for potential new products, make deals with other companies for cooperative ventures or buyouts, and perform other business services. Usually, these people have business degrees, but a technical background is also necessary.

Companies with offices overseas may have openings for veterinarians. Qualifications for these positions include experience in a multinational company; an understanding of the international differences in animal health markets, product development requirements, and scientific approaches; and exposure to colleagues in other countries. Foreign language skill is often not required. To gain the necessary experience, get any job in the US (or your home country) working for a company that has offices in other countries, so you can learn their goals and methods of operation, and later move to an international position. Or take a temporary position with an international assistance group (see Chapter 13 for more on international opportunities).

Computer software

Veterinarians may work with computer software in two main ways: writing programs or performing sales or technical assistance for a software company. Veterinary software includes diagnostic programs, business management programs, herd health monitoring programs (e.g., dairy production, nutritional analysis), and database programs for journals, abstracts, or seminars.

Software programs made specifically for veterinary practice are usually created by people with a background in computer language, but knowledge of the needs of the veterinary practice can be an asset, and veterinarians with both kinds of knowledge may find a niche in this field.

Companies that write computerized diagnostic programs may hire veterinarians to write some of the program content. Entrepreneur veterinarians may also write their own software programs for sale to veterinary hospitals. Online vendors may hire veterinarians to answer pet owners' questions or to write columns (see writing jobs in Chapter 10). Finally, software companies are integrating electronic medical record codes into their systems (Chapter 9).

Up through the 1990s, most veterinarians doing computer software work were self-taught. As the area becomes more specialized and the amount of technical expertise becomes greater, it is likely that many veterinarians will have additional training; to work on designing new software, a degree in computer sciences is preferred. One useful resource is the Software and Information Industry Association (www.siia.net).

Sales and marketing

Sales jobs involve traveling to potential buyers (veterinary clinics) to present product information and to take orders. Additional marketing staff members work to present a company's product or services to the veterinary profession as a whole. This work may include advertising and promotion, or presentations to veterinary students or veterinary technicians. Although veterinarians can fill these positions, most sales and marketing people are non-veterinarians. These jobs are suited to people who are interested in organizational tasks, working with people, and traveling. They do not involve clinical medicine, but do require interacting with practicing veterinarians. Jobs in marketing require experience or additional education in that field.

Chapter 11 Resources

Groups and web sites

American Association of Corporate and Public Practice Veterinarians (AACPPV), 6060 Sunrise Vista Drive, Suite 1300, Citrus Heights, CA 95610-7098; www.aacppv.org; phone: 916-726-1560; e-mail: info@aacppv.org.

American College of Veterinary Pathologists, Veterinary Pathologist Survey: Final Report, 2002, available at www.acvp.org/career/employsurv.pdf.

American Pet Products Association (APPA), www.americanpetproducts.org; phone: 203-532-0000.

Drug Information Association, www.diahome.org.

Books and articles

AVMA Report on Veterinary Compensation, 2009 (AVMA, 2009).

Compendium of Veterinary Products (North American Compendiums, 2008).

Ontario Veterinary Medical Association, *2010 Report on Veterinarians in Alternate Career Paths,* www.ovma.org; 1-800-670-1702.

Vetguide, Veterinary Economics supplement, http://marketplace.dvm360.com; phone: 800-255-6864.

Veterinary Pharmaceuticals and Biologicals (Medical Economics and Veterinary Healthcare Communications, 2001).

12 ASSOCIATION AND ORGANIZATION JOBS

There are good opportunities for veterinarians to work in "organized veterinary medicine." This term refers to the professional associations that are related to veterinary medicine. In addition to those groups with direct ties to veterinary medicine, many other livestock or animal-related groups may have jobs that a veterinarian could fill.

A few association jobs are detailed in this chapter as examples of the kinds of possible work. Examples of potential employers include animal welfare organizations; state licensing boards (board members are usually volunteers, but the director or chair is often a paid position); the American Kennel Club (AKC); the Orthopedic Foundation for Animals (OFA; certifies dogs of certain breeds to be free of signs of joint disease, and employs board-certified radiologists); the Delta Society (devoted to the human-animal bond); the National Cattleman's Beef Association; and the Morris Animal Foundation (where veterinarians currently serve as the President and as the Chief Scientific Officer). For information about jobs with animal shelter and rescue organizations, and with international assistance organizations, see Chapter 13.

Some of these groups are listed on the AVMA web site (www.avma.org > My AVMA > Member Resource Directory > Veterinary Associations and Specialty Boards). However, since the AVMA switched from a printed directory to an online version, it has decided to not list all veterinary-associated groups, so it is no longer a centralized information source as was the printed the directory.

Daily work

Most association jobs are primarily indoor jobs that include telephone communication, reading, writing, supervising, and managing. Some positions require extensive travel and involve attending numerous meetings (in-house as well as conventions). Many jobs allow for continual contact with veterinarians. Some include extensive contact with students at the veterinary schools and colleges. Details are described in subsequent sections of this chapter.

Pros and cons

Pros include working with motivated and outstanding members of the profession, working on a wide variety of tasks and issues, and keeping current on important issues facing the profession. Working hours vary with the organization; hours often are well-defined, although overtime and weekend work may be necessary, particularly with travel to meetings. There is no direct work with animals. Work can be stressful due to project deadlines, particularly when volunteers are involved. Another stress is dealing with conflicts among constituents or between groups.

Organizational work dictates that you must always balance your personal opinion with the official position of the group, and you may have to work closely with people with whom you disagree on a particular issue. Meetings can become tedious, juggling many projects at once can be difficult, and the amount of time it takes to resolve issues can be frustrating.

Many associations have both a paid staff and a separate, parallel board of directors who are elected volunteers. Additional volunteers form various committees and working groups within most associations. Working with all these groups can be challenging.

To apply

Specific organizations are described in this chapter, but many more exist. Although some state veterinary associations work with volunteer veterinarians (hiring a secretary or office worker full- or part-time), others have a full-time veterinarian on staff, usually as the director. Many state associations currently have a non-veterinarian as director, but the position could easily be filled by a veterinarian. Some positions that would be ideal for a veterinarian may not necessarily be advertised that way; many times, the person responsible for hiring has a typical stereotypic view of "veterinarian," which may result in misinformation that the group doesn't have any jobs for a veterinarian. Modify your approach to ask about any job openings at all, then see for yourself whether any are suitable for your talents.

Several societies can assist in a quest for association and organization jobs:

- American Society of Association Executives, conducts Association Management Career Seminars; sponsors continuing education meetings for association executives; certifies association executives; publishes *Career Opps*, a biweekly newsletter listing nonprofit openings nationwide, and *Career Starters*, listing openings with entry-level salaries; and has a resume critique service (www.asaenet. org).
- American Society of Veterinary Medical Association Executives, promotes cooperation and learning among administrative executives of veterinary organizations (www.vmaexecs.org). It publishes a newsletter, a member profile book, and a membership directory; hosts an annual public relations workshop; and holds an annual continuing education session.
- AVMA, has current and updated addresses of many of the groups or associations listed throughout this book (www. avma.org > Advocacy > State legislative resources > Allied associations).
- Meeting Professionals International, made up of professionals who plan or manage meetings for associations (www.mpiweb.org).

Association Director

Veterinarians fill the executive director position of many groups, including:

- American Animal Hospital Association, www.aahanet.org.
- American Veterinary Medical Association, www.avma.org.
- Association of American Veterinary Medical Colleges, www.aavmc.org.
- National Board of Veterinary Medical Examiners, www.nbvme.org
- North American Veterinary Conference, www.navc.org.
- Western Veterinary Conference, www.wvc.org.
- VetPartners, www.vetpartners.org.

The first three of these groups are discussed in detail in this chapter.

Daily work / Pros and cons

The director oversees management, finances, budget, association meetings, publication of newsletters or other items, and much more. Whether the director does this work alone or manages others who perform the tasks varies with the size of the organization. The "others" who perform the work or assist with the necessary tasks may be paid staff or volunteers. The director often reports to an elected president and/or board of directors.

Day-to-day tasks for an association director include working on the computer, using the telephone, and conducting meetings. A lot of time is spent communicating with people (group members, journalists, members of related groups)—on the phone, by mail, by fax, by e-mail, and via web conferencing or in person at meetings. Travel is required (up to 50 percent of the time), both to conduct meetings for the association as well as to represent the association at various other meetings. Some paid directors have a background in management or are Certified Meeting Professionals (www.conventionindustry.org) or Certified Association Executives (www.asae.org).

Qualifications / Pay

The salary for directors' jobs varies widely. States with a low population may hire a part-time director for as little as $15,000 per year; full-time positions with very large associations could pay from $100,000 to $200,000 per year. Benefits are usually excellent.

Qualifications include experience in some kind of practice; excellent verbal and written communication skills, including public speaking and the ability to work with people on complex and often controversial issues; excellent interpersonal skills; and the ability to develop and maintain professional relationships with constituent groups. A director must have staff management and administrative skills (usually gained by performing those tasks in private practice, through volunteer work with associations, or other work experience). Leadership skills are essential. Facilitation skills are a bonus.

The director generally lives in the city where the association or group has its headquarters. The director of a state association should have a history of working within the association in volunteer positions; the director of a conference should have experience working on the conference board.

To learn more, talk to veterinarians who are on state association committees or on a conference's board of directors. Getting on a board or committee is a good way to gain experience; these are part-time, volunteer positions. Once you are involved with a particular association, you will have a better idea of how to advance to a paid position.

The American Animal Hospital Association

The American Animal Hospital Association (AAHA) is a group whose mission is to provide veterinary professionals with the resources they need to effectively manage their businesses and deliver the best in companion animal care. AAHA works to enhance the abilities of veterinarians to provide quality medical care to companion animals and to maintain their facilities with high standards of excellence. Member veterinary hospitals are certified by the association if they meet stringent criteria for excellence. Certification is based on a number of factors including quality medicine and business practices.

AAHA has numerous openings for volunteers on its board and on various committees. Working in this capacity can help you learn more about how the association functions. The AAHA Board of Directors is a group of selected volunteers who serve two-year terms. This is a great leadership position that provides opportunities to learn and to meet with other leaders. AAHA employed three veterinarians in their Denver office as of 2009: the *executive director; deputy executive director,* and *veterinary and professional education manager.*

Daily work / Pros and cons

The *executive director,* who is appointed by the board of directors, is the chief executive officer of the association with the responsibility to oversee the affairs of the association in keeping with the policies, programs, and budget as established by the board of directors. The executive director collaborates with the chief operating officer and deputy executive director, recommends and participates in the formulation of new policies and makes decisions within the existing policies as they have been approved by the board of directors. The executive director is the consistent strategic leader and the voice and presence of AAHA.

The *deputy executive director* has responsibility for all external programs, relationships and functions required to operate the association and its programs and services efficiently and effectively. Following establishment of priorities by the board and the executive director, and on approval of the budget, the deputy executive director is responsible with the chief operating officer for implementing all approved activities and overseeing programs and services.

The *veterinary and professional education manager* duties include representing AAHA on various veterinary issues to the association's staff, its members, and to the public. This person may serve as a liaison to other veterinary professional organizations, manufacturers, outside consultants, and prospective members in order to develop and strengthen relationships in support of AAHA's mission. In addition, this person is responsible for managing the development of the association's professional education programs.

In the past, veterinarians have also held the position of *practice consultants.* These positions, although appropriate for veterinarians, do not require a veterinary degree. The national *field operations manager* (currently a credentialed technician) plans and directs the hospital survey program, supervises practice consultants, informs AAHA members of standards and assists them in compliance, and performs hospital surveys. The practice consultant works in various areas of the country and conducts AAHA's on-site hospital evaluations to assure adherence to the AAHA standards, acts as an ambassador of AAHA, and provides practice management assistance to members.

AAHA consults with a veterinarian for work on the *Journal of the American Animal Hospital Association*. See Chapter 10 for details about such a position.

The American Veterinary Medical Association

The American Veterinary Medical Association (AVMA), with more than 80,000 member veterinarians, is the national professional organization of veterinarians in the US. Its objective is to advance the science and art of veterinary medicine through programs of member service and public education. The AVMA runs on a lot of volunteer labor, but some paid positions are available in various AVMA divisions.

Elected and appointed volunteers include councils, committees, and the House of Delegates (volunteer representatives of 68 state and allied veterinary medical groups, which elects association officers; see www.avma.org > About the AVMA > Governance). The President is the chief representative of the association.

The AVMA Executive Board consists of veterinarians elected for six-year terms. These people are reimbursed for expenses, but they are not paid a salary or fee. Committee and council recommendations are sent to the board for approval and are then given to one of the AVMA divisions for action. Here is where the veterinarians and other professional staff employed by the AVMA take up the work.

Veterinarians working for the AVMA must work on-site (with rare exceptions). Most of the AVMA divisions are centered at AVMA headquarters in Schaumburg, IL. The Governmental Relations Division has its own office in Washington, DC.

About 25 percent of the approximately 140 staff positions do require a veterinary degree. Some positions require a specific advanced degree (e.g., MBA); others require a DVM but also require specific experience and training (not necessarily a specific degree).

Daily work / Pros and cons

The AVMA staff includes veterinarians in a variety of roles that allow them to influence and advance the profession on a national and international basis. Most of these positions require some travel; all require working within a large organization, and communicating with a variety of other divisions and outside groups every day. Most positions involve writing reports and formal response letters on behalf of AVMA members based on AVMA policy; attending meetings; and spending quite a bit of time on the telephone and communicating with numerous individuals and groups through e-mail. Each division must organize meetings of its assigned AVMA committees and councils, and then carry out the directives as determined during each meeting. This could involve writing letters, setting up new meetings, arranging for speakers, or setting up symposia.

Qualifications / Pay

Among elected officers, the president and president-elect receive a stipend, whereas the remaining officers are simply reimbursed for travel expenses.

Salaries of association employees are confidential and are not made available by the AVMA. The qualifications and salary ranges for each position vary based upon the responsibilities, level of experience, and educational requirements for the position. Benefits are good.

All of the positions are listed on the Veterinary Career Center (VCC) on the AVMA web site (www.avma.org > Jobs > AVMA employment opportunities) and are listed in the *Journal of the AVMA*. You can also contact the director of each division, or the Human Resources Department at the AVMA, if you don't see an ad.

AVMA divisions and their employees

The AVMA includes 10 divisions, plus the Office of the Executive Vice President. Brief descriptions are presented in the following subsections. These descriptions are not all-inclusive, and they sometimes change.

Office of the Executive Vice President

The executive board selects the *executive vice president* and *assistant executive vice president*, who are full-time employees of the association. The executive vice president is the chief executive officer (CEO) of the AVMA and works with the executive board and executive management team to establish long-range goals, strategies, plans, and policies.

Animal Welfare Division

The Animal Welfare Division is charged with monitoring the science of human-animal interactions and assisting the AVMA in proactively addressing animal well-being and the human-animal bond. This applies to animals used for companionship, biomedical research, education, food and fiber production, work, recreation or exhibition. The division regularly interacts with organizations, educators, various industries, the public and the media. Activities aim to fulfill the AVMA's goal to be "a leading advocate for, and an authoritative, science-based resource on animal welfare." Paid positions include the *director* and three *assistant directors*.

Communications Division

This division is responsible for media relations, crisis communications, and professional and public information. The position of *assistant director for professional and public affairs*, which requires a veterinary degree, develops and implements professional and public communications programs. The assistant director is responsible for making sure that information and products generated by the Communications Division are accurate and relevant to veterinary medicine and AVMA policies.

Scientific Activities Division

Positions held by veterinarians in the Scientific Activities Division include the *director* and five *assistant directors*. This division represents the AVMA in the areas of public health and food safety, regulatory veterinary medicine, animal disease prevention and control, animal agriculture, aquaculture, antimicrobial resistance, environmental issues, and disaster/emergency preparedness and response. It also develops cooperative projects with national organizations, and maintains contact with government agencies such as the FDA and USDA.

Publications Division

The Publications Division oversees publication of the *Journal of the American Veterinary Medical Association* (*JAVMA*) and the *American Journal of Veterinary Research* (*AJVR*) in print and online; and publishes news of the association and veterinary profession as well as a variety of other materials. The nine veterinarians in this division include eight *scientific editors* responsible for peer review and editing of manuscripts submitted to the journals, and an *online professional services editor*. All of the scientific editors hold advanced degrees beyond the veterinary degree, and there is a trend toward requiring that all scientific editors be veterinarians with a PhD or board certification. In addition, scientific editors are generally expected to have experience both in clinical practice and research. See Chapter 10.

Membership and Field Services Division

The Membership and Field Services Division is responsible for the recruitment and retention of AVMA members, student outreach and veterinary career assistance. Division services include maintaining online resources such as the Member Resource Directory, the Veterinary Practice Resource Center, and the Veterinary Career Center (see Chapter 1). Three positions in this division are held by veterinarians—the *director*, who oversees the activities of the division, and two *assistant directors*. One assistant director works with the AVMA Career Center. The other works with the Student Chapters of the AVMA (SCAVMA) and travels to each campus to support student activities and educate them on the benefits available through AVMA membership.

Education and Research Division

Positions held by veterinarians include the *director* and three *assistant directors*. The assistant directors implement AVMA policies and projects concerning the accreditation of veterinary and veterinary technician education programs, certification of foreign veterinary graduate equivalence, animal health research and specialty board certification. They conduct accreditation site visits for veterinary colleges and veterinary technology programs. Travel is required. A recently-created position in this division is the *coordinator of international affairs*.

Governmental Relations Division

The Governmental Relations Division (GRD, www.avma.org > advocacy) located in Washington, DC, advocates for the association on federal legislative and regulatory issues that influence animal and human health and advance the veterinary medical profession. The GRD currently employs 10 staff members. The *director* and two *assistant director* positions require a veterinary degree, while the third assistant director position is open to veterinarians and non-veterinarians. All directors are registered federal lobbyists and spend a majority of their time lobbying Congress and the Executive Branch on issues of importance to the AVMA. They also act as liaisons for the profession to other stakeholder groups based in Washington, DC. The GRD office manages the AVMA's Political Action Committee (PAC), and works closely with the AVMA-PAC Policy Board.

The GRD also coordinates the AVMA Fellowship Program, which offers selected veterinarians the opportunity to spend one year working as science policy advisors in the personal offices of members of Congress, congressional committee offices or federal agencies. See www.aaas.org and www.avma.org > advocacy > federal.

The AVMA-GRD Veterinary Student Externship Program provides third- and fourth-year veterinary students the opportunity to experience the development of public policy concerning regulatory and legislative activities of importance to veterinary medicine (www.externsonthehill.com).

The Association of American Veterinary Medical Colleges

The Association of American Veterinary Medical Colleges (AAVMC) provides leadership for and promotes excellence in academic veterinary medicine (www.aavmc.org). It represents its member institutions in its collective dealings with governmental bodies, veterinary medical organizations, the animal and human health industry, educational and scientific organizations, and the public. The association also promotes the priority areas of academic veterinary medicine. Member institutions include not just veterinary medical colleges, but also the departments of comparative medicine at leading medical colleges.

Several positions at the AAVMC are filled by veterinarians: the *executive director, deputy director, associate executive director for academic and research affairs*, and the *editor* of the *Journal of Veterinary Medical Education*. A veterinarian was also hired as the *project manager for the North American Veterinary Medical Education Consortium* (NAVMEC), established by the AAVMC board of directors in 2008 with the objective of developing a plan to enhance the efficiency and effectiveness of veterinary medical education to meet societal needs.

Animal Welfare Organizations

Several humane societies or animal welfare organizations employ veterinarians on staff, including the Humane Society of the United States, the American Society for the Prevention of Cruelty to Animals, and the American Humane Society. Both administrative and hands-on animal work are possible. See Chapter 13.

Chapter 12 Resources

Groups and web sites

American Animal Hospital Association (AAHA), 12575 West Bayaud Ave, PO Box 150899, Denver, CO 80215-0899; www.aahanet.org; phone: 303-986-2800.

American Association for the Advancement of Science fellowships, http://fellowships.aaas.org.

American Association of Veterinary Medical Colleges (AAVMC), 1101 Vermont Avenue, NW, Suite 301, Washington, DC 20005; www.aavmc.org.

American Humane Association, 63 Inverness Dr East, Englewood CO 80112-5117; www.americanhumane.org.

American Kennel Club, www.akc.org.

American Society for the Prevention of Cruelty to Animals (ASPCA), www.aspca.org and www.aspcapro.org; phone: 800-628-0028.

American Society of Association Executives, 1575 I St NW, Washington, DC 20005-1168; www.asaenet.org; phone: 202-626-ASAE; fax: 371-8825; e-mail: asae@asae.asaenet.org,

American Society of Veterinary Medical Association Executives, PO Box 280425, Lakewood, CO 80228, www.vmaexecs.org; e-mail: tesha.hoff@att.net.

Amercan Veterinary Medical Association (AVMA), 1931 N Meacham Rd, Suite 100, Schaumburg, IL 60173-4360; www.avma.org; phone: 800-248-2862, e-mail: avmainfo@avma.org.

AVMA,GRD, Governmental Relations Division, 1101 Vermont Ave NW, Suite 710, Washington, DC 20005-3521; fellowships, www.avma.org > advocacy > federal > legislative activities; externs, www.externsonthehill.com phone: 202-789-0007 or 800-321-1473.

AVMA listing of veterinary medical associations, www. avma.org > Advocacy > State legislative resources > Allied veterinary medical associations. For position announcements online, use www.avma.org/jobs/default.asp.

Certified Association Executives, www.asae.org; phone: 269-429-0300.

Certified Meeting Professionals, www.conventionindustry.org; phone: 517-527-3116.

Delta Society, 425-679-5500; www.deltasociety.org.

Humane Society of the United States, www.hsus.org.

Meeting Professionals International, 3030 Lyndon B. Johnson Freeway, Suite 1700, Dallas, TX 75234-2759; www.mpiweb.org; phone: 972-702-3000; fax: 972-702-3070; e-mail: feedback@mpiweb.org.

Morris Animal Foundation, www.morrisanimalfoundation.org.

North American Veterinary Medical Education Consortium, www.navmec.org.

National Cattlemen's Beef Association, www.beef.org.

Orthopedic Foundation for Animals, www.offa.org.

13 HUMANITARIAN WORK WORLDWIDE

People who want to broaden their horizons, help others, work in another country, or travel, may find a niche working for nonprofit groups and service organizations. These jobs are "lumped together" in this book because they often overlap—many service and volunteer opportunities exist all over the world. Work may include clinical veterinary medicine, public health, animal production and health, sustainable agriculture, economics, and research. Positions may be paid or unpaid, part-time or full-time, and temporary or permanent.

Daily work / Pros and cons

Daily work is as varied as the many opportunities that exist. Most of these jobs do require working with groups of people. Working and living conditions vary depending on the situation.

Many positions are filled by volunteers and are not paid. Some volunteers have expenses reimbursed. Volunteering is a great way to "give back," to meet people, to expand your skills, and to investigate new career paths without risk. Among paid positions, although there are exceptions, pay is generally lower than in other positions for veterinarians.

Service work can be emotionally draining, but it has many positive aspects. It is extremely rewarding to help people and animals in difficult circumstances. The skills and experience you gain may fill a void in your resume. Connections made during service work can help with future job opportunities. Skills and knowledge gained may apply to many other jobs, including fascinating projects in international development.

Some veterinarians find their long term career niche in working with nonprofit or service groups. Others find that participation in short-term projects adds variety and interest outside of their regular jobs. A short-term position may also provide a temporary break from your current job without taking the leap of leaving that job. You can use the time to reflect on your future goals.

Opportunities in the United States

A wide variety of opportunities exist for veterinarians within the US. Many of those options are described in various chapters of this book, such as the sections about wildlife and wildlife conservation in Chapter 6. See also Chapter 16 on government jobs, including jobs with APHIS, USAID, EPA, and FWS. Chapters 9 (Consulting), 11

(Industry), and 18 (Uniformed Services) may also be helpful. One of the major niches for veterinarians who want to serve their communities is in shelter work, which is described in this chapter.

Serving the disadvantaged

Veterinary services for disadvantaged people usually focus on basic health care. Veterinarians in private practice often volunteer their services for low-cost spay/ neuter or vaccination days or clinics. Students may participate in such clinics offered in the inner city or in underserved rural areas. One such program is Native American Veterinary Services (NAVS), a division of the Pennsylvania Veterinary Foundation. NAVS provides free veterinary care for Native Americans living on reservations throughout the US (www.pavetfoundation.org).

Rescue and disaster response

Rescue and disaster recovery are becoming areas of special expertise. The incidents of September 11, 2001, reminded the world of the crucial role that service dogs play in disaster recovery. After the fiasco in the wake of Hurricane Katrina in 2005, the recovery of pets from natural disasters has also become an important focus. The Pets Evacuation and Transportation Standards Act, signed into law in 2006, requires state and local preparedness offices to take into account pet owners, household pets, and service animals when drawing up evacuation plans.

Veterinary teaching hospitals in Louisiana, Texas, and other southern states have first-hand experience with responding to hurricanes. Human-caused disasters such as the 2010 oil spill also create a need for veterinarians (see Chapter 6, Wildlife Rehabilitation).

Qualifications / To apply

Colorado State University offers the American Academy on Veterinary Disaster Medicine (www.cvmbs.colostate.edu/clinsci/wing/aavdm/aavdm.htm).

The National Animal Health Emergency Response Corps (NAHERC) and the National Veterinary Response Team (NVRT) operate under the federal government. Both teams consist of private citizens who have been approved as intermittent federal employees and are activated in the event of a disaster.

The NAHERC is a program of the USDA Animal and Plant Health Inspection Service (APHIS), which responds to exotic disease outbreaks and other disasters that affect livestock, poultry, companion animals, and wildlife. (See Chapter 16 and www. aphis.usda.gov > animal health > emergency management > NAHERC).

The NVRT, part of the National Disaster Medical System of the Department of Health and Human Services (DHHS), consists of individuals who have professional expertise in areas of veterinary medicine, public health, and research. (See www.hhs. gov > Assistant Secretary for Preparedness and Response > National Disaster Medical System > NDMS Teams).

The AVMA's Veterinary Medical Assistance Teams (VMAT) serve as first respond-ers to ensure high-quality care of animals during disasters and emergencies. These teams bridge the gaps among local, state, and national disaster programs. When requested by a state, VMAT volunteers provide operational emergency response programs to state animal health authorities, as well as preparedness programs to animal health authorities, veterinary medical associations, and other relevant organizations.

Veterinarians also have a potential role in *human* health care following catastrophic events. The American Medical Association's Basic Disaster Life Support course includes a curriculum for veterinary professionals. (See www.ama-assn.org > physician-resources > public-health > preparedness and disaster response). The AVMA has created a policy on the veterinarian's role. (See www.avma.org > issues > policy > Addressing the Role of Veterinary Medicine in Human Health Care Following Catastrophes Involving Mass Human Casualty).

Disaster preparedness resources include:

- AAEP, American Association of Equine Practitioners Emergency and Disaster Preparedness, www.aaep.org/emergency_prep.htm.
- AVMA disaster resources, www.avma.org > public resources > disaster preparedness.
- ASPCA, American Society for the Protection of Cruelty to Animals disaster preparedness resources, www/aspca/org and www.aspcapro.org.
- HSUS, Humane Society of the United States Disaster Center (holds an annual conference on animals in disaster), www.hsus.org.
- National Alliance of State Animal and Agricultural Emergency Programs, www.nasaaep.org.
- National Incident Management Center, www.fema.gov/emergency/nims.
- State Animal Response Teams, www.sartusa.org.
- Veterinary Medical Assistance Teams, www.avma.org/vmat.

Forensic veterinarians

Veterinary forensics is most often involved in animal cruelty cases, but can be involved in other cases, including murders. Evidence gathered can help gain a conviction. This means traveling to crime scenes and having knowledge regarding obtaining and submitting evidence. It doesn't end there, though; next, you must work with a prosecutor who will bring charges, and you will likely have to testify at trial.

Melinda D. Merck, DVM, Senior Director of Veterinary Forensic Sciences at the American Society for the Prevention of Cruelty to Animals (ASPCA), has been studying and investigating animal cruelty cases since her career began. To develop her expertise in this emerging field, she worked closely with medical examiners and studied human forensics textbooks. She now works full-time as a national and international consultant on animal cruelty cases. Dr. Merck provides expert witness testimony and gives seminars about forensics at veterinary meetings and veterinary schools. She has also helped create a DNA database ("canine CODIS" or Combined DNA Index System), a computerized archive that stores DNA profiles from criminal offenders and crime scenes and is used in criminal investigations.

Dr. Merck's web site on veterinary forensics offers links and resources for learning more (www.veterinaryforensics.com), including articles such as The Veterinarian's Role in Handling Animal Abuse and Animal Cruelty: Prosecution Opportunities for Early

Response to Crime and Interpersonal Violence. See also her book, *Veterinary Forensics: Animal Cruelty Investigations*, as well as *Investigation of Animal Cruelty: A Guide for Veterinary and Law Enforcement Professionals*, by L. Sinclair et al.

The University of Florida's College of Veterinary Medicine has partnered with the ASPCA and Dr. Merck to set up a program in veterinary forensics. The University of Florida offers student courses and veterinary continuing education in shelter medicine, veterinary forensics, and disaster response (www.ufsheltermedicine.com > Animal Forensics).

While performing basic forensics may be possible with a DVM degree and taking short courses, more advanced work might require a Master's or Board Certification in pathology. (See Chapter 4, Specialists.)

Animal shelters and animal rescue

> We have five doctors on staff. Each day, one is dedicated to shelter medicine and two work with public practice clients. I do the shelter medicine work full-time (40-50 hours per week). The shelter serves about 9,000 animals annually.
>
> We use a shelter specific computer program. When entering notes there are many fields that need to be dated to ensure rechecks are done, medication are entered to be administered and medical disclosures printed, copied and pasted in specific places. This is to ensure that animals aren't overlooked and that the adoption process goes smoothly. It requires a lot more time before the adoption to help reduce client concerns post-adoption.
>
> There are great opportunities for relief veterinarians in shelters, particularly in performing spay and neuter surgery. For those shelters using relief or community doctors for treating illness or injuries, I think it is important to have specific guidelines and clear communication between those doctors and the shelter about what resources are available, such as time, money, staff, and equipment.—Lesli Groshong DVM, Chief Shelter Veterinarian, Humane Society of Boulder Valley, CO.

Veterinarians are employed by humane societies, animal control facilities, animal shelters, and rescue groups to provide veterinary services for animals in their care. Animal shelters are operated by nonprofit groups or by city and county governments. Some cities have both nonprofit shelters and animal control facilities. There are no data collected about the total number of, or attributes of, animal shelters or animal control facilities. Also see Chapter 15, City/county government jobs.

Shelters vary in size and complexity, from small foster or rescue shelters to large-volume animal control facilities in larger cities.

Foster or rescue Shelters

Foster or rescue shelters can range from informal, home-based efforts with no fundraising or outside revenue source to free-standing facilities with nonprofit status, staff, and significant revenue and expenses. Depending on the size and sophistication, veterinary services may range from physical examination and rudimentary treatment to extensive rehabilitative treatment and care.

A typical suburban shelter is run by an independent nonprofit organization. These suburban shelters typically perform a wider variety of roles to the community, including stray and unwanted animal intake, animal adoptions, and humane law enforcement. Often these agencies provide animal control on a contractual basis with towns, boroughs, and municipalities on a fee-for-service basis. Veterinary services typically include shelter wellness, injured animal triage, examination of humane cases, and pre-adoption spay or castration. Post-adoption wellness, community vaccination, microchip clinics, and support of adoption events ("Ask the Vet" booths, for example) may also be provided.

Large volume animal control facility

In urban areas, animal control (stray animal pick-up, code enforcement, animal surrender) is often funded through a municipal contract to a nonprofit group expressly formed for the purpose of administering the contract. Some of these facilities handle 30,000–40,000 dogs and cats per year. Veterinary care in these environments is challenging. Kennel wellness protocols, disease surveillance, triage care, treatment, public vaccination and wellness clinics, and spay or castration services are typical. Municipal shelters are often part of a community animal disaster preparedness plan, so veterinarians may be engaged in county- or state-level animal response team planning and exercises.

Daily work

The scope of services in any shelter may range from triage and basic supportive care (which might be found in a typical animal control facility) to tertiary care of complex cases (as is seen in large specialty hospitals affiliated with some of the more sophisticated shelters). Veterinary positions can range from volunteer board member or occasional clinical volunteer, to paid part-time, consulting, and full-time job opportunities.

Technical roles include the development of wellness and treatment protocols, oversight and training of the animal care staff, oversight of the surgical (spay/castration) services, and public wellness and vaccination clinics. Long-term or complex care is usually not performed, since resources must be concentrated on animals most likely to be adopted.

Nontechnical roles, although less common, are opportunities for veterinarians to contribute to the humane organization in strategic or "big picture" ways—as board members, officers, or as an executive-level managers (e.g., chief executive officer, chief operating officer, chief of veterinary services, or director of development/fundraising).

Pros and cons

Michael Moyer, DVM, has years of experience in shelter medicine and now is the Rosenthal Director of Shelter Animal Medicine at the University of Pennsylvania. He also teaches fourth-year veterinary student rotations in shelter medicine, and serves on the board of directors for local shelters. He observes:

> In my small animal practice, it would take me years to reach the impact of just one year of work with a busy shelter. As an instructor of a shelter medicine residency I am able to ensure that others have this same opportunity in the future.

Shelter veterinarians can find the dynamic environment of sheltering to be challenging, compelling, inspiring, and rewarding. The number of animals whose lives are in the balance is remarkable, and the skilled veterinary clinician can save lives every day. Compensation packages are often very competitive with private practice, and there may be significant managerial opportunities within the organization. The successful shelter veterinarian can become a much admired and recognized member of the community.

The National Animal Control Association publishes a list of "Pros and Cons of Working in the Field of Animal Control" (www.nacanet.org/careeropps.html). Pros include the ability to protect pets and people; the joy of seeing animals adopted by loving, responsible people; the gratification of assuring that impounded animals are being provided shelter and care; the peace of knowing that unwanted animals are at least provided a humane and dignified death; the excitement of unusual animal calls; and the friendships developed with other shelter workers all over the country.

Cons include frustrations with irresponsible pet owners; lack of understanding by the public of the need for animal control and of the problems of animal overpopulation; stress from seeing neglected or abused animals, and depression because of animal euthanasia; exposure to communicable disease and injuries by animals and humans; and sometimes long hours or being on call.

Some veterinarians may find shelter employment to be overwhelming and frustrating. The facility may be ill-suited for the purpose, the budgetary constraints may preclude all but triage care, and staff support insufficient. The level of cooperation or antagonism among veterinarians in the community and those working in shelters varies markedly among different communities.

Qualifications / To apply

Most shelter veterinarian positions require a state veterinary license, but no formal or advanced veterinary training. The Association of Shelter Veterinarians is a good resource for the prospective or active shelter veterinarian to find information and network with others in the field (www.sheltervet.org). To add to your expertise, find out whether your local community college offers classes in human relations, city management, municipal law, or public relations. Read the literature about animal behavior. Join Toastmasters to improve your public speaking skills.

Apart from knowledge, it is vital that the successful shelter veterinarian understand the environment, the type of shelter, the sources of funding, and any sources of friction. Veterinarians are, as licensed professionals, ultimately responsible for the standard of practice. Accordingly, they should be comfortable with the equipment, facility, staff, protocols, and emergency resources, and have the ability to see the big picture and not get too stressed about the daily problems, such as the barking and the sadness of abandoned animals.

Veterinary examination of animals in cruelty or neglect cases or dog-fighting investigations require more specialized, additional knowledge of crime scene management and techniques, chain of custody, appropriate documentation, and the ability to effectively testify to the evidence in legal proceedings. (See "forensics" in this chapter.)

The following are sources of information, education, and/or job announcements:

- American Humane Association, www.americanhumane.org.
- American Society for the Prevention of Cruelty to Animals, www.aspca.org and www.aspcapro.org.
- Association of Shelter Veterinarians, www.sheltervet.org.
- Humane Society of the United States, www.hsus.org.
- National Animal Control Association, www.nacanet.org.
- Society of Animal Welfare Administrators, www.sawanetwork.org.

Also check university offerings; for example, the UC Davis shelter medicine program runs Shelter Veterinarian (www.sheltermedicine.com), and the University of Florida offers shelter medicine and forensics continuing education (www.ufsheltermedicine.com). Several veterinary teaching hospitals also offer externships or programs for students. The website for "Maddie's Fund" describes the program at the University of Pennsylvania and also has links to programs at other veterinary teaching hospitals. (See www.ufsheltermedicine.com > training programs > students; and www.maddiesfund. org > Funded Projects > Colleges). Shelter externships are also available for veterinary students at many nonprofit and public shelters.

A number of veterinary schools have residency programs for shelter medicine (Colorado State, Cornell, UC Davis, Florida State, University of Pennsylvania), and more such programs are in the development stage at other schools. These programs are designed to train veterinarians in skills that can maximize the lifesaving efforts of shelters of all descriptions. Infectious disease, epidemiology, vaccine protocols, population medicine and management, anesthesia and surgical principles, and emergency medicine are a partial listing of the skills required. Board certification in shelter animal medicine is not yet available, but is being developed (see Chapter 4).

Pay

Pay varies by geographic area, but is generally as good as that of the average veterinarian employed in private practice. For example, one veterinarian working for a county animal shelter earned $90,000 (2009), with excellent benefits including a retirement plan, vacation leave, sick leave, health insurance, continuing education, licenses, and professional liability insurance; as the only staff veterinarian, this person works 4 days a week but is on call at all times. Additional possible benefits received by shelter veterinarians include dental care, life and disability insurance, tax-deferred child care expenses, professional memberships, and discounted retail purchase and other services.

Full-time and part-time veterinarian wanted. Low-cost, high-volume spay/neuter clinic run by a no-kill cat shelter/sanctuary serving the general public. We are looking for community-minded individuals to help this clinic be a huge success. We believe in a happy working environment. Our salaries are very competitive and we have excellent benefits! This job is ideal for vets wishing to practice medicine without all of the headaches that come along with managing a clinic. We pay 100% of your health, dental, vision, and disability. All employees will receive bonuses if the clinic exceeds expectations.

Humane Society of the United States

The Humane Society of the United States (HSUS; www.hsus.org or www.humane-society.org) is the nation's largest animal protection organization, established in 1954. It seeks "a humane and sustainable world for all animals—a world that will also benefit people."

HSUS veterinarians provide medical assistance to animals at each of five animal care centers. Three centers handle wildlife rehabilitation (see Chapter 6). These wildlife centers see over 16,000 animals a year and assist a wide variety of species that would not be seen in a traditional veterinary hospital setting. HSUS sanctuary programs house over 500 equines and other animals that need constant medical attention. HSUS offers a variety of veterinary internships at these centers.

HSUS emergency services division provides opportunities for veterinarians to respond to human-caused disasters (such as animal hoarding and cruelty) as well as natural disasters. Veterinarians provide medical treatment on site and serve as expert witness. In hurricane Katrina alone the HSUS assisted in bringing in over 100 veterinary professionals to assist with the response.

The HSUS employs approximately a dozen veterinarians in its HSVMA, Animal Care Centers, and its Emergency Services divisions. They also employ veterinarians who are advocating for better public policies for animals and advancing humane alternatives in veterinary education. A wide variety of internships are available. The HSUS offers the "Humane Society University," which provides leadership training for shelter owners, managers, and other leaders. HSUS job openings and internships are posted at www.humanesociety.org > about > employment.

Humane Society Veterinary Medical Association

The Humane Society Veterinary Medical Association (HSVMA; www.hsvma.org) is a professional veterinary membership organization formed from the merging of the Humane Society of the United States and the Association of Veterinarians for Animal Rights.

HSVMA gives veterinarians, veterinary technicians, and veterinary professional students an opportunity to participate in animal welfare programs, including disaster response; expanded hands-on animal care; spaying and neutering programs; and advocacy for legislative, corporate, and veterinary medical school reforms.

HSVMA's Field Services—formerly Rural Area Veterinary Services—is a non-profit veterinary outreach program. HSVMA Field Services provides veterinary services to rural communities worldwide where regular veterinary care is not available. Accompanying the veterinarians are over 400 veterinary students a year who assist each year in the program. Most trips are within the US, but they also visit several locations in Latin America, such as Peru. Volunteer opportunities are available for veterinary students, technicians, and licensed veterinarians. Trips range in length from a weekend to two weeks and require a fee to participate, which covers room and board.

International Opportunities

International opportunities are available in almost any niche. Some jobs are with nonprofit, service, educational, or religious organizations. For other international positions, see the sections in Chapter 9 (consulting), Chapters 15–17 (government), and Chapter 18 (military jobs). Notice the description in Chapter 17 about the veterinarian working for the Ontario Ministry of Health, in international diplomacy. There are a variety of job openings in industry for veterinarians with language skills and an interest in travel. Industry jobs are typically with a US-based company that has offices in another country (see Chapter 11).

A survey of international employment opportunities published in *JVME* by M. Correa showed that about 75 percent of international jobs paid a salary, 15 percent relied on volunteer services but paid some expenses, and the rest paid no expenses at all. The survey also showed that about 20 percent of the positions required only a veterinary degree, but the rest desired an additional degree (MS or PhD, often in public health or epidemiology). About half required fluent language skills and 20 percent required minimal language skills.

General information

For a wide variety of new opportunities, do a search on the Internet using the words [veterinarian], [international], and perhaps [volunteer]. Numerous opportunities are listed on web sites such as Volunteer Abroad (www.volunteerabroad.com).

Attend meetings of the World Small Animal Veterinary Association and World Veterinary Association to network on an international level (www.wsava.org and www.worldvet.org, respectively). Other large conferences that attract an international crowd include the North American Veterinary Conference (www.navc.com, held in Orlando each January); the Southern European Veterinary Conference (www.sevc.info, held in Barcelona each October); the Latin America Veterinary Conference (www.tlavc-peru.org, held in Peru each October); and the Federation of Asian Veterinary Associations Congress (www.favamember.org, held in February).

The American Scandinavian Foundation coordinates educational and cultural exchanges, fellowships, grants, and intern/trainee sponsorships (www.amscan.org). Similar organizations may exist for other countries.

The Alliance of Veterinarians for the Environment helps veterinarians find work related to conservation and environmental health (www.aveweb.org). See also the section on jobs related to the environment in Chapter 6.

For those interested in international development work, FRAMEweb (www. frameweb.org) is a peer-to-peer network of Natural Resource Management practitioners that focuses on knowledge sharing.

Practicing veterinarians can host an international student through the International Veterinary Student Association (IVSA; www.ivsa.org), which may lead to an opportunity to visit that student's home and learn about the country (contact your area's veterinary school for information). As SCAVMA members, students are also automatically IVSA members. IVSA hosts symposiums and congresses yearly around the world.

For information related to living and working overseas, consult books such as *Do's and Taboos* by R. Axtell; *Survival Kit for Overseas Living* by L. Kohls; and *Global Business Etiquette* by J. Martin.

International programs at US veterinary schools

So far, international programs at veterinary schools are directed at students; however, opportunities for graduate veterinarians may become available, including distance learning and short courses. Through the efforts of Washington State University (WSU), a consortium among the colleges of veterinary medicine at Purdue, Texas A & M, Tufts, and WSU has been formed with the goal of enhancing foreign language and cultural abilities of veterinary students so they can effectively address global animal health issues. Each of the consortium members has established linkages with international institutions in veterinary medicine and the equivalent of the USDA in numerous countries. The vision is that veterinarians with knowledge in international animal health will provide needed expertise within state and federal governments, the corporate animal health industry, and as consultants to US livestock operations with international markets. International externships for veterinary students are being established at universities, research stations, and pharmaceutical companies with offices in other countries.

WSU's International Veterinary Education program (IVE, www.vetmed.wsu.edu/international) was designed to provide students with an opportunity to gain knowledge and understanding of international issues in veterinary medicine, including socioeconomic and cultural systems and the environment. Students can take elective courses (International Veterinary Medicine and International Field Studies), acquire an introductory background in regional animal health issues, and promote an in-depth understanding of specific problems through directed study and international experience. For the field study course, students spend a minimum of one month working in a foreign country, gaining experience in the areas of animal health and well-being, livestock production (including poultry and aquaculture), public health, and trade within the cultural environment of another country.

Other schools provide similar opportunities. For instance, Tufts University has a program focusing on international veterinary medicine. The University of California at Davis has an elective field course in comparative veterinary medicine that provides for an exchange of students between their school and one in Mexico.

Kansas State University (KSU) offers a variety of international activities for its students, including an elective course in Global Veterinary Medicine and study-abroad opportunities. KSU has started a "partner school" relationship with the Sri Venkateswara

Veterinary University (SVV) in southern India. These relationships are sponsored by the Association of American Veterinary Medical Colleges through their Global Initiative in Veterinary Education program (www.aavmc.org/give).

Even without a formal program, students and graduate veterinarians have created their own externships in countries of their choice. They do so by asking that country's veterinary association, or individual veterinarians, about practitioners who are willing to take an extern. Students can also contact professors at their own schools who graduated from veterinary schools in other countries, and ask them for advice about spending a short time in their home country.

For example, a student at the University of Illinois set up an externship with the Kiev Zoo, which included collecting donations of medical supplies in the US and taking them to Ukraine. Another student called US veterinarians with contacts in Spain, and got an externship in Seville simply through "friends of friends." Graduate veterinarians can do the same.

International private practice

It is difficult to get a job in private practice in another country because most countries have stringent licensing requirements that favor their own residents. To find out more about working in a particular country, see the US State Department web site (www.state.gov/travel) and contact the country's consulate (see www.usembassy.gov) and its veterinary association (find via an internet search using the words "association," "veterinary," and the country name).

International Relief Work (Locum Tenens)

There is at least one international relief veterinarian list, called Vetlocums (www.vetlocums.com). This group posts announcements for "relief veterinarian wanted" or "relief position wanted." The web site is arranged in categories: large/small animal practices, wildlife, exotics and international donor projects. They also list a calendar of international veterinary conferences; holidays for veterinarians; and practices for sale. There is a small fee for placing an ad, but none to read the announcements. You can register free at their web site.

Other international relief jobs are found on the variety of "job banks" online. Search for such Internet sites by using the words [veterinarian], [international], and [locum] or [relief].

Teach or learn at other veterinary colleges

Write to veterinary schools in countries of interest, and ask whether there are any courses, internships, or volunteer opportunities. For instance, the University of Pretoria in South Africa offers an opportunity for training in tropical diseases and parasites prevalent in Africa (http://web.up.ac.za > Faculties > Veterinary Science > CE at UP). Short courses (one week to one month long) vary each year; subjects might include veterinary laboratory diagnostics, African epizootic diseases, or wildlife immobilization.

Another idea is to offer to teach basic sciences such as animal anatomy and physiology in a veterinary school or animal science department in a country of interest. For a list of colleges world-wide, go to www.avma.org > education > ECFVG > AVMA listed veterinary colleges.

International consultant

After working for any of the organizations mentioned here, or in government jobs overseas, you may have the knowledge and the contacts to start your own consulting business, or to be hired as a consultant by a development group. (See Chapter 9 for details on setting up a consulting business.)

As an example, Beth Miller, DVM, worked for Heifer Project International (see next section) for 10 years; she now teaches at Pulaski Technical College in Arkansas and also works as an international consultant. She points out the need for a diverse background combined with networking abilities:

> All the veterinarians I have met in international work have broad educations. . . all those years I spent studying French literature before vet school paid off when I started working with the International Goat Association, and the President was from France. I became the Secretary-Treasurer of the Association, which helped me get to know people who hire consultants.

> To build international relationships, try going to international meetings. They are a great place to meet people and learn about opportunities that are not published. Once a friendship is established, keep in touch, and keep it reciprocal; when they visit you, introduce them to everyone in their area of interest, and they'll do the same for you.

> For example, to prepare for a recent consultancy in Pakistan, I contacted a woman I met in 1995 in Beijing, who works with gender economics in southeast Asia, and a Dutch vet working in India. I asked both for advice for outreach to Pakistani women dairy farmers, and their contacts in Pakistan. "Cold calls" without an introduction from a common friend or colleague are not popular in Pakistan (and many developing countries). Who you know can get you the job, *and* more importantly, ensure you can get the job done.

Development Associates, Inc

Development Associates, Inc. (DAI, www.dai.com) is an example of a private, employee-owned development consulting company that contracts with government and service groups. One of DAI's main clients is the US Agency for International Development (USAID). Thus, veterinarians may be employed by DAI but working on USAID projects. (Also see Chapter 16, Government work, USAID.)

DAI provides comprehensive development solutions in several areas that are of interest to veterinarians, including agriculture, agribusiness, and avian influenza control. DAI has a main office in Maryland with all its projects done in other countries.

Veterinarians with a specific area of expertise are hired to work on certain projects for specified time frames. Very short term work of a few weeks may include training groups of people, for example, in responding to an outbreak. Work contracts of one to five years focus on larger projects such as those with USAID.

Qualifications vary with the project. Knowledge of emerging infectious diseases is useful, as is practical field experience. Poultry veterinarians with international experience in developing countries are desired for influenza projects. For example, DAI veterinarians are working in Vietnam to determine whether local free roaming chickens can be grown in semi-confined conditions, which might help during an influenza outbreak. A poultry veterinarian also works out of the main office on the USAID-funded Stamping Out Pandemic and Avian Influenza (STOP AI). A veterinarian having expertise with primates works on the USAID-funded RESPOND project, which seeks to develop capacity in developing countries to identify and control emerging zoonotic diseases.

DAI recruits veterinarians with the necessary expertise on a project by project basis. Occasionally they announce job opportunities in specific trade journals.

Nonprofit international organizations

A wide variety of service and church groups may provide opportunities for short-term international work. When approaching any of these groups, you may be turned away when you ask about positions for veterinarians (once again, the person you are asking may think of veterinarians only as dog doctors). Instead, start by asking about positions related to agriculture, public health, or livestock management. Contact those in your preferred area for more information.

You also can get information about many groups through InterAction, a coalition of more than 150 US-based nonprofits working to promote human dignity and development in 165 countries around the world. Check their web site (www.interaction.org) for a list of the web sites of all 150 groups. In the US, these groups are called "private and voluntary organizations," or PVOs. InterAction coordinates and promotes these activities and helps to ensure that goals are met in an ethical and cost-efficient manner.

Agricultural Cooperative Development International (ACDI)

The name ACDI/VOCA (www.acdivoca.org) dates back to the 1997 merger of Agricultural Cooperative Development International (ACDI) and Volunteers in Overseas Cooperative Assistance (VOCA). This is an economic development organization, funded by the USAID, which fosters broad-based economic growth, raises living standards and creates vibrant communities. Its practice areas are agribusiness, food security, enterprise development, financial services and community development. Most assignments suitable for veterinarians are related to large animals, especially livestock.

ACDI/VOCA assigns veterinarians for 2–12 weeks in volunteer positions worldwide. No wage is paid; however, all costs related to travel (passports, vaccinations, visas, airfare) are paid. Dairy farm management projects could be filled by veterinarians with dairy experience; a recently filled position was for a cattle nutrition specialist. A previous program used veterinarian volunteers to design veterinary programs for Albanian university students interested in ruminants, monogastrics, and poultry. In 2007, veterinarians worked in Georgia on the prevention of the avian influenza outbreak.

Heifer Project International

Heifer Project International (HPI) helps impoverished families worldwide become more self-reliant through the gift of livestock and training in their care (www.heifer.org). To help hungry families feed themselves, HPI provides more than 24 types of food- and income-producing animals, as well as intensive training in community development, animal husbandry, and ecologically sound and sustainable farming. HPI requires recipients to "pass on the gift" of one or more of their animals' offspring to other needy families, which multiplies the benefits of the original gift.

Several veterinarians work at the headquarters in Little Rock, Arkansas. Some are *program officers* for various areas of the world. In addition, 37 program offices in four major geographic areas have a technical staff, each including at least one veterinarian. HPI tries to hire local nationals in other countries, so that veterinarians are hired to work in their own countries. However, some opportunities exist for others to fill paid positions overseas. In the past, veterinarians have been hired in non-clinical areas, such as education, assessment, gender integration, and training. In these cases, while the veterinary education was not essential, it contributed to strategic thinking and won respect from farmers and staff.

In addition to the paid positions, volunteer opportunities are available with HPI. You can volunteer at one of their three Learning and Livestock Centers, one of the five regional offices, or the world headquarters in Little Rock, Arkansas. You might have the opportunity to visit an HPI project in another country as a participant in a work-study or study tour.

This is exciting work that includes helping people around the world who truly need it. Most jobs are not paid, however, and for those that are, the salary never gets very high—although benefits are usually good.

Veterinarians Without Borders

Veterinarians Without Borders was established in 2001 to restore the healthy natural balance among animals, people, and the planet (www.vetswithoutborders.net). It is a volunteer network of veterinarians who travel to countries to provide free veterinary care, and to train communities on responsible animal production, eco-friendly lifestyles, and sustainable human health. Dr. Beth Miller visited Liberia in late 2009 for Veterinarians without Borders-US, and had this to say:

> Liberia had zero vets left after their 14 year civil war, a horrendous feral dog population in the cities, and unknown wildlife population. They desperately needed healthy livestock and an animal health service. The international donors have focused on human health and crops, but there was no one working on the animal side. My friend, Dr. Arlene Gardsbane, got involved through her family, which includes returned

Peace Corps volunteers, who begged her to work on something for Liberia. We organized a small rabies clinic, and vaccinated over 200 dogs in two days. We wrote an assessment report, which VWB-US used to get a grant from USAID to train community animal health workers in animal first aid until professional veterinarians can be trained and placed in the field. A broader proposal for an entire animal health service has been submitted.

Christian Veterinary Mission

The Christian Veterinary Mission (CVM, www.cvusa.org) works to "share the love of Jesus while practicing veterinary medicine" in the US and in countries worldwide. Veterinarians can help CVM with long- or short-term missions.

Short-term missions last weeks to months (2 weeks is average), and are self-funded. On assignment, veterinarians and veterinary students perform basic livestock health, such as vaccination and deworming. Veterinary expertise is shared in a training model such that skills can be left with the visited community.

Long-term positions are often filled by veterinarians who were first involved in the short-term program. Long-term missions are for three years, with two-year renewal options, and are located in Asia, Africa, and Latin America. These projects focus on training local residents to be village animal health workers. Financial support for a long-term position is developed by the veterinarian selected to serve in partnership with the CVM office. Sources include the veterinarian's church, family, and friends, in conjunction with the donor base of CVM and the CVM network throughout the US

A total of 36 full time veterinarians (and many spouses) are currently serving with CVM. Overseas are 17 spouses serving in non-veterinary roles; many are in family support roles, but also almost all are in some form of development work.

Ten veterinarians, including the founder and the current President, work in the CVM Seattle office and in some regional roles. Staff positions include *Program Director; Director of Training; Professional Outreach Director; International Partners Director; Deputation Director; Director of Student Outreach;* and *Region Representative.*

CVM publishes the quarterly *Christian Veterinary Journal*, as well as a monthly e-newsletter with articles, photos, and highlights of the work being done by CVM in the US and abroad.

VETAID

This United Kingdom–based international assistance group (www.vetaid.org) works with agricultural communities in east Africa who depend on animals for their survival. There are approximately 70 employees in offices in Africa (Kenya, Somalia, and Tanzania). They are predominantly staffed in Africa by local people, including veterinarians. Job vacancies are posted on the web site.

Voluntary Service Overseas

Voluntary Service Overseas (VSO, www.vso.org.uk), an independent, international development charity, works through volunteers to fight poverty in developing countries. Search the web site for volunteer opportunities for veterinarians. A recent posting serves as an example.

Sample job announcement

> Urgently recruiting veterinary researcher, Mongolia. You'll work at the State Central Veterinary Laboratory (SVCL), Mongolia's national research and diagnostic centre for veterinary science, medicine and animal disease control. Train staff in the diagnosis of chemical residue in animal origin products through the use of chromatography and mass spectrometer diagnostic methodology; explore ways of coordinating veterinary research with organizations from developed countries; and provide basic English language training for colleagues. Patience, flexibility and a good sense of humor are important qualities in all VSO volunteers, as you'll need to get used to living and working in a new culture with limited resources and facilities.

The Esther Honey Foundation

The Esther Honey Foundation (EHF, www.estherhoney.org) provides compassionate and affordable veterinary services to South Pacific island companion animals in need. EHF works in concert with local government officials, businesses, community members, and others. EHF improves the health conditions and quality of life for these animals by developing partnership programs, raising funds, and recruiting the volunteers necessary to fulfill the Foundation's mission. Volunteers work for a period of two weeks to one year.

Rotary Club International

The Rotary Club International was originally founded on the basis of exchanging information with people in diversified careers, fellowship, and community service (www.rotary.org). It quickly spread into international service. Rotary's Group Study Exchanges are small groups (typically four people) of young professional and business people in their twenties plus an older Rotarian leader. A four- to six-week exchange is arranged with a similar group from another part of the world, with an intensive program of visits involving many talks and presentations. Candidates for these visits are recruited by the district that sponsors them through the local Rotary Club. A rotary member stated that some of their scholarship recipients study veterinary science abroad, and some of the professionals who participate in their exchanges are veterinarians; there have been some grants to developing countries to provide or improve care of livestock. However, most volunteers focus on medical care for people.

People to People Ambassador Program

People to People (www.peopletopeople.com) was founded by President Dwight D. Eisenhower in 1956 and was originally administered by the US State Department. This private, nonprofit organization is dedicated to improving global understanding through international cultural exchange. It develops and administers educational travel programs. Each program arranges for adult professionals to travel abroad together with the purpose of meeting and exchanging ideas with international colleagues who have similar backgrounds, interests, and professions.

Teams of scientists, agricultural producers, crop researchers, agricultural engineers, food processors and packagers, and veterinarians meet with their counterparts, lecture, perform on-site tests and evaluations, discuss recent technical advancements, and assist farmers, breeders, technicians, and researchers in less-developed, traditionally agrarian societies. Delegations also share the latest techniques with their counterparts in developed nations. These exchanges have led to significant research modifications; new technologic applications; and ongoing scientific, technical, and business collaborations. Participants must pay their own expenses.

Government related international groups

Organization of American States student program

The Organization of American States Student Intern Program is designed for junior, senior, and graduate students at the university level to work within their fields of study (www.oas.org). The program, although nonremunerative, is highly competitive. To be selected, students must have at least a 3.0 GPA and a good command of two of the four official languages of the Organization (English, Spanish, French, and Portuguese; preference will be given to the first two official languages).

The United Nations

Many organizations exist under the United Nations (UN) umbrella and some of these offer job opportunities for veterinarians. See http://careers.un.org.

Specialized agencies of the UN such as the following should be contacted directly for job information: Food and Agriculture Organization (FAO, www.fao.org); UN Development Programme (UNDP, www.undp.org); or World Health Organization (WHO, www.who.ch).

Additionally, information on currently vacant positions is available at UN Headquarters, UN Information Centers throughout the world, other offices of the UN family, the foreign ministries of the respective member states, and educational and/or professional institutions such as universities and women's associations.

To be considered for mid-level and higher posts, candidates must possess an advanced university degree (beyond a BS), and have relevant professional experience. Normally, a minimum of six years of professional experience is required. FAO jobs reportedly pay veterinarians $100,000 to $150,000 per year, with excellent benefits.

The UN Peace-keeping Operations agency (www.un.org/en/peacekeeping) seeks professionals with proven track records, an advanced university degree or its equivalent in a relevant discipline, four years of relevant professional experience, and fluency in

English and/or French. Fluency in additional languages, as well as working experience in developing countries, constitute a definite advantage. Applicants must be in excellent health and prepared to work in hardship areas under difficult and sometimes dangerous conditions. They must also be available at short notice. Most missions are classified as "nonfamily" duty stations. The compensation package includes salary and a cost of living allowance.

UN Internships

The UN Headquarters Internship Program is offered to students enrolled in graduate school, with a view to promoting a better understanding of major problems confronting the world and giving them insight into how the UN attempts to find solutions to these problems (www.un.org/en > Resources > Internships). The program consists of three two-month periods throughout the year. There is no pay.

United Nations Volunteers

The United Nations Volunteers (UNV) program, which operates through the Peace Corps, was established in 1971 by the UN General Assembly and is administered by the UN Development Program. The US will send up to 24 US citizens per year to serve as UNVs, in primarily two year assignments. The majority of UNVs serve in Africa, and the Asia Pacific region. Applicants must possess a university degree or technical diploma and preferably have five years of full-time work experience in their field of expertise. Most volunteers have 15–20 years of experience in their respective fields. Application is through the Peace Corps (www.peacecorps.gov).

The Peace Corps

Founded in 1961 by President John F. Kennedy, the Peace Corps is a US government agency that places Americans in foreign countries that have requested Peace Corps volunteers (www.peacecorps.gov). The three goals of the Peace Corps are to promote world peace and friendship; to help promote a better understanding of the American people on the part of the peoples served; and to promote a better understanding of other people on the part of the American people. Peace Corps volunteers work in a variety of fields, including agriculture, community development, education, business, health, nutrition, and natural resources. They fight hunger, disease, illiteracy, poverty, and lack of opportunity around the world. The length of service, including the initial three months of training, is usually around 27 months, and the Peace Corps covers all living, travel, and medical expenses during that time.

To be eligible for Peace Corps service, the applicant must be a US citizen. There is no upper age limit. Married couples may serve in the Peace Corps, but both people must apply and be accepted, and it is usually more difficult for the Peace Corps to place both of them. Those with dependent children are not placed. Most assignments require a bachelor's degree, some require a master's degree, and some require three to five years of work experience instead of, or in addition to, a BA or BS degree. It is recommended that application be made at least six to eight months before the time an applicant is available to depart in order to increase the chances of acceptance.

Applicants must fill out a medical history and undergo physical and dental exams because a health condition easily managed at home can become a serious medical problem in countries that the Peace Corps serves. Host countries do not often have US levels of medical care; sites can be remote, and assignments often are physically and emotionally challenging.

Veterinarians may only be placed for one year rather than the typical two to three years. Pay is low, but the experience is invaluable. For example, many USAID and international development experts from the US served in the Peace Corps.

World Health Organization and Pan American Health Organization

The World Health Organization (WHO; www.who.int/en > employment) and the Pan American Health Organization (PAHO; www.paho.org) are continually seeking the services of highly qualified health professionals. The professional technical staff acts as advisors in public health to member governments. Candidates must possess substantial training and experience in this field before they can be considered for an assignment.

WHO job vacancies are posted online (www.who.int/employment/en). Look at vacancies titled "scientist"; also see the UN web site (www.unsystem.org) for more vacancies. Veterinarians with an interest and background in public health will find many possibilities on the WHO job site. WHO offers internships for students as well.

PAHO operates as the WHO regional office for the Americas, as the specialized agency in health for the Organization of the American States and the United Nations. Within PAHO, the Veterinary Public Health program is under the Division of Disease Prevention and Control. This is a large, unique program with a staff of more than 200 distributed worldwide; 65 percent are at the Pan American Foot-and-Mouth Disease Center in Rio de Janeiro, Brazil.

Most of the PAHO staff are veterinarians with postgraduate degrees in preventive medicine and public health. In addition, most advisor positions require at least seven years of experience at the national level at least two years of participation in technical cooperation programs and activities, and fluency in English and Spanish. Knowledge of Portuguese and French is desirable.

The World Organisation for Animal Health

The need to fight animal diseases at global level led to the creation of the Office International des Epizooties (OIE) through an international agreement in 1924. In 2003, the Office became the World Organisation for Animal Health but kept its historic acronym (www.oie.int). The OIE is the intergovernmental organization responsible for improving animal health worldwide. It is recognized as a reference organization by the World Trade Organization, and as of 2009, it had a total of 174 member countries and territories. The OIE maintains permanent relations with 36 other international and regional organizations and has regional and sub regional offices on every continent.

In addition to its paid staff, the OIE has a number of working groups that consist of veterinary experts (usually with additional degrees) who are volunteers appointed for a number of years. Examples include the Wildlife Working Group and the International Veterinary Biosafety Workgroup.

According to the OIE, it offers an internship for people who wish to

participate in mentored activities of 1–6 months duration at the OIE Headquarters or at the OIE Regional Representations in subjects relevant to their career aspirations and compatible with the objectives of the OIE. Candidates should be advanced veterinary students or recent veterinary or science graduates with special interest and aptitude in the field of epidemiology, microbiology, laboratory technology, information technology, animal welfare or food safety.

The OIE internship does not offer financial assistance. The internships are focused on very specific topics, as shown in the following examples of a web designer and a writer (also see Chapter 10).

Sample OIE internship descriptions: Scientific and technical department

Position 1: **Design of web sites** for OIE Specialist Commissions/ Working Groups. Must be senior veterinary students, veterinary graduates or veterinarians employed by veterinary administrations, with a sound knowledge of terrestrial or aquatic animal diseases, laboratory diagnosis and control of animal diseases, animal disease information systems, and veterinary certifications. Must have good work experience in informatics/web site technology.

Position 2: **Literature review** of the description of major animal diseases. Must be veterinary graduates with a solid background of medicine and/or veterinary epidemiology, experience in literature review of animal diseases, and excellent writing ability. Experience in editing of scientific literature may be an advantage.

Chapter 13 Resources

Groups and web sites

Alliance of Veterinarians for the Environment, www.aveweb.org.

American Academy on Veterinary Disaster Medicine, www.cvmbs.colostate.edu/clinsci/wing/aavdm/aavdm.htm.

American Association of Equine Practitioners Emergency and Disaster Preparedness, www.aaep.org/emergency_prep.htm.

American-Scandinavian Foundation, www.amscan.org.

American Society for Prevention of Cruelty to Animals (ASPCA), www.aspca.org and www.aspcapro.org ; phone: 800-628-0028.

American Veterinary Medical Association, www.avma.org.

Christian Veterinary Mission (CVM), c/o Dr. Kit Flowers, President, 19303 Fremont Ave North, Seattle, WA 98133; www.cvmusa.org; phone: 206-546-7201; fax: 206-546-7458; e-mail: info@cvmusa.org.

Esther Honey Foundation, www.estherhoney.org.

Federation of Asian Veterinary Associations Congress, www.favamember.org

Food and Agriculture Organization (FAO), www.fao.org.

Global Initiatives in Veterinary Medicine, Association of Veterinary Medical Colleges, 1101 Vermont Ave, NW, Suite 710, Washington DC 20005-3521; www.aavmc.org/GIVE.

Heifer Project International, 1 World Avenue, Little Rock, AR 72202; www.heifer.org; phone: 800-422-0474.

Humane Society of the United States (HSUS) Human Resources, 2100 L Street, NW, Washington, DC, 20037; www.hsus. org; HSUS internships: www.hsus.org >about us > employment opportunities.

Humane Society of Veterinary Medical Association (HSVMA), www.hsvma.org.

InterAction, www.interaction.org.

International Veterinary Student Association (IVSA), www.avma.org > Student AVMA > International exchange opportunities.

Latin America Veterinary Conference, www.tlavc-peru.org.

Maddie's Shelter Animal Medicine Program.

Links to programs at veterinary schools, www.maddiesfund.org > Funded Projects > Colleges of Veterinary Medicine. Externship, www.ufsheltermedicine.com > training >Student Externships.

Residency, www.maddiesfund.org > Funded Projects >Colleges of Veterinary Medicine >University of Pennsylvania; www.vet.upenn.edu >Education and Training >Training > Residencies, Internships, and Fellowships >Maddies Residency in Shelter Animal Medicine.

National Alliance of State Animal and Agricultural Emergency Programs, www.nasaaep.org.

National Animal Health Emergency Response Corps (NAHERC), www.aphis.usda.gov/animal_health/emergency_management/naherc.shtml.

National Incident Management Center, www.fema.gov/emergency/nims.

National Veterinary Response Team (NVRT), www.hhs.gov/aspr/opeo/ndms/teams/vmat.html.

Native American Veterinary Services (NAVS), www.pavetfoundation.org; phone: 888-550-7862.

North American Veterinary Conference, www.navc.org.

Office international des epizooties (OIE), 12, rue de Prony, 75017 Paris, France; www.oie.int; oie@oie.int; phone: 33 (0)1 44 15 18 88; fax: 33 (0)1 42 67 09 87.

Organization of American States Student Intern Program, OAS/Public Information, 17th Street and Constitution Avenue, NW, Washington, DC 20006; www.oas.org; phone: 202-458-3754; fax: (202)458-6421.

Pan American Health Organization (PAHO), www.paho.org; e-mail: info@who.int.

Peace Corps, Paul D. Coverdell Peace Corps Headquarters, 1111 20th Street, NW, Washington, DC 20526; www.peacecorps.gov; phone: 800-424-8580.

People to People Ambassador Program, S. 110 Ferrall St, Dwight D. Eisenhower Building, 1956 Ambassador Way, Spokane, WA 99202-4800; www.peopletopeople.com; phone: 509-568-7000; international phone: 866-794-8309, fax: 509-534-5245; e-mail: info@peopletopeople.com.

Rotary International, National Headquarters, One Rotary Center, 1560 Sherman Ave., Evanston, IL 60201; www.rotary. org; phone: 847-866-3000, fax: 847-328-8554.

Rural Area Veterinary Services (RAVS), c/o Eric W. Davis, Director, HSVMA-Field Services, 125 Old Stage Rd., Salinas, CA 93908; www.ruralareavet.org; phone: 831-442-8359; fax: 831-442-8320.

Southern European Veterinary Conference, www.sevc.info.

State Animal Response Teams, www.sartusa.org.

United Nations

UN Employment Information, www.careers.un.org.

UN Internship Program, United Nations, Division for Staff Development and Performance, Policy and Specialist Services, Office of Human Resources Management, Room S-2580, New York, NY 10017; www.un.org/Depts/OHRM/sds/internsh/index.htm www.un.org/en > Resources > Internships.

UN Peacekeeping Operations, UN Personnel Management and Support Service, Field Administration and Logistics Division, Department of Peace-Keeping Operations, S-2280, New York, NY 10017. www.un.org/en/peacekeeping.

UN Personnel Management and Support Service, Field Administration and Logistics Division, Department of Peace-Keeping Operations, S-2280, New York, NY 10017.

UN Staffing Support Section, United Nations, Division for Planning, Recruitment and Operational Services, Office of Human Resources Management, Room S-2555, New York, NY 10017; www.unsystem.org.

University of Florida, www.ufsheltermedicine.com/animalForensicsCrueltyAbuse.html.

University of Pretoria, South Africa, Dept. of Veterinary Tropical Diseases, http://web.up.ac.za/ > Faculties > Veterinary Science > CE at UP or http://scarlacc.up.ac.za/CEatUP/VetSci.aspx; phone: +27 12 529 8000.

US State Department, www.usembassy.gov/ or www.state.gov/travel/.

VETAID, Pentlands Science Park, Bush Loan, Penicuik, Midlothian, EH26 0PL, UK; www.vetaid.org; phone: +44 (0)131 445 6241; fax: +44 (0)131 445 6242; e-mail: mail@vetaid.org.

Veterinarians without Borders, www.vetswithoutborders.net.

Veterinary Forensics, www.veterinaryforensics.com.

Veterinary Medical Assistance Teams, www.vmat.org or www.avma.org/vmat.

Vetlocums, www.vetlocums.com; e-mail: vfeedback@vetlocums.com.

Volunteer Abroad, www.volunteerabroad.com.

Volunteers in Overseas Cooperative Assistance (VOCA), 50 F Street, NW, Suite 1075, Washington DC 20001; www.acdivoca.org; phone: 202-638-4661; fax: 202-783-7204.

World Health Organization (WHO) 20, Avenue Appia, CH-1211 Geneva 27, Switzerland; www.who.int/en; phone: 41-22-791-2111; fax: 41-22-791-2300 or 41-22-791 0746.

WHO job vacancy page, www.who.int/employment/en > vacancies.

WHO Regional Office (US), 525 Twenty-third Street, NW, Washington, DC 20037; www.who.int/en; phone: 202-974-3000; fax: 202-974-3663.

World Small Animal Veterinary Association, www.wsava.org.

World Veterinary Association, www.worldvet.org.

Washington State University (WSU), link to international opportunities, www.vetmed.wsu.edu/international; e-mail: c/o IVE Mushtaq A. Memon, Coordinator, memon@vetmed.wsu.edu.

Books and articles

Axtell, R. E., *Essential Do's and Taboos: The Complete Guide to International Business and Leisure Travel* (Wiley, 2007).

Bimnez, R., et al., *Technical Large Animal Emergency Rescue* (Wiley Blackwell, 2008).

Burns, K, Evolution of Shelter Medicine, *JAVMA News*, November 15, 2006; 229(10): 1543–1545.

Correa, M.T., Employment in International Veterinary Medicine: A Survey of Requirements and Opportunities, *JVME*, Spring 1995; 22: 26 - 27.

Kohls, L. R., et al., *Survival Kit for Overseas Living for Americans Planning on Living and Working Abroad*, 4th ed., (Intercultural Press, 2001).

Kuehn, B. M., Shelter Medicine: A Budding Field that is Helping to Raise the Standard of Care in Animal Shelters, *JAVMA* May 1, 2004; 224(9): 1412–1413.

Larkin M, Veterinarians Leave Their Mark on African Nation. *JAVMA News*, October 15, 2009; 235(8): 911–915.

Martin, J. S., and L.H. Chaney, *Global Business Etiquette: A Guide to International Communication and Customs* (Praeger, 2008).

Merck, M., *Veterinary Forensics: Animal Cruelty Investigations* (Blackwell Publishing, 2007).

National Animal Control Association (NACA), Pros and Cons of Working in the Field of Animal Control, www.nacanet.org/careeropps.html.

Sherman, D. M., *Tending Animals in the Global Village: A Guide to International Veterinary Medicine* (Blackwell Publishing, 2002).

Sinclair, L., et al., *Investigation of Animal Cruelty: A Guide for Veterinary and Law Enforcement Professionals* (Humane Society Press, 2006).

SPCA Opens Largest Nonprofit Hospital in San Francisco. *DVM Newsmagazine*, February 2009: 14; www.sfspca.org.

14 WORKING IN ACADEMIA: TEACHING AND RESEARCH

Veterinarians know a great deal about a variety of scientific subjects. If you enjoy teaching others, you can get a job anywhere from a community college to a veterinary technician school. At a higher level, working at a veterinary teaching hospital includes a mix of teaching and research, and usually has additional education requirements.

For higher education jobs in veterinary medicine, check the Academic Keys web site at http://vetmed.academickeys.com. Also see Chapter 15 for information about extension specialists, who act as educators, and Chapters 16–18 for federal civilian and military jobs (with any agency, you can become a teacher of the skills you learn on the job, teaching other people new to the agency).

College Teaching or Advising Positions

Many teaching jobs can be filled by veterinarians without additional training, and they don't require doing research. For example, veterinarians are qualified to teach a number of college-level science, anatomy, or animal production courses. They also may be hired as advisors for pre-veterinary or veterinary students.

Daily work / Pros and cons

Teaching includes preparing course outlines, materials, and tests; assisting students during and outside class time; giving lectures; and keeping up on the subject taught. A teacher, as part of the faculty, is often required to participate on various committees and give occasional speeches to interest groups.

The advisor's work includes advising students about obtaining the required veterinary experience, and about writing veterinary school applications. The advisor may help with conducting mock interviews and supervising off-campus externships.

It is often rewarding to work with students who are interested in and enthusiastic about science or veterinary medicine. As a faculty member, you are paid to expand your knowledge. Cons may include job uncertainty, the political environment in the university, and at times feeling a bit overshadowed as a veterinarian in a PhD world. Some jobs are part-time and may include no benefits.

At most community colleges, someone with a DVM degree is paid the same as someone with a PhD, since the DVM degree is considered "terminal." Promotion opportunities are in administrative positions, where the DVM degree brings respect and credibility. Contracts are often for 9 months, with summer and winter breaks.

Qualifications / To apply

Some openings are advertised in *JAVMA* or the *Journal of Veterinary Medical Education* (*JVME*), published by the AAVMC (www.aavmc.org). Another source is the *Chronicle of Higher Education*, a weekly tabloid that includes meetings, seminars, workshops, and classified employment advertising for teachers, higher education administrators, and faculty members (www.chronicle.com). Most veterinary schools, universities, and community colleges post job openings on their web sites. Contact veterinary schools and ask about advisory positions. Pay varies widely, from $40,000 to $90,000 per year.

Veterinary Technician Programs

Both part-time and full-time positions are available for veterinarians as teachers in veterinary technician schools; in 2010, there were 160 of these schools in the US. (See avma.org > Education > Accreditation > Veterinary technology programs). A few programs offer distance learning.

Daily work / Pros and cons

Veterinary technician *educators* teach a variety of medical and surgical skills to technicians. Many veterinary technician programs utilize community veterinarians part-time for lectures or for "laboratory" sites where students can get hands-on experience. However, all programs have at least one full-time veterinarian on staff. Teaching time includes lectures, labs, creating and grading class materials, and computer work.

Veterinary technician educators have less hands-on animal contact than do private practitioners, but there is still a significant amount of teaching that involves working with animals (anesthesia, nursing care, and radiology labs). Salaries are often lower than those of veterinarians in industry and government. Rewards include the satisfaction of helping students learn and develop; a good benefits package with scheduled vacation days; no emergency calls; and being able to teach subjects that you learned in veterinary school.

The *Director* of a veterinary technician program is in charge of hiring instructors; coordinating the educational program; developing the curriculum; proposing and managing a budget; and recruiting, interviewing, and counseling students. The director often has teaching duties as well (lectures, laboratories, correcting papers, and so forth), but spends less time at this than do the teachers. Office work, meetings, and telephone time (talking to prospective students and to veterinarians trying to hire a technician) are part of the daily work.

The director has conflicting roles: representing the needs and interests of the program to the administration, and representing the administration's policies and procedures to the faculty and students. Some directors may feel that they have responsibility but limited authority. Pay is moderate, but there are good benefits. The job is challenging and full of opportunities to explore new interests and to meet interesting people. Hours are regular and travel is not usually required.

Qualifications / To apply

A background in mixed practice is helpful, since work with all species is taught in veterinary technician programs. Teachers, and especially directors, have to put up with the bureaucracy and red tape that come with any school or administrative job. Directors need skills in administration, management, and communication.

To find job openings, contact the Association of Veterinary Technician Educators (AVTE; www.avte.net), which holds a three-day AVTE symposium every other year—a good place to go to network. The AVTE produces a quarterly online newsletter that includes job announcements and information about new veterinary technician programs at various colleges. Or write to the veterinary technician schools that are listed in the AVMA Veterinary Career Center web site (www.avma.org > Careers). Another good resource is NAVTA, the National Association of Veterinary Technicians in America (www.navta.org). Pay ranges are not available and are likely to vary widely.

Sample job announcement: Faculty position

> Veterinary Technician School is currently seeking DVM candidates for a faculty position. Requires 3+ years experience. Previous teaching experience is attractive but not required. We offer associate degree programs to aspiring veterinary technicians at several locations. Competitive compensation and benefits as well as stable working hours. Salary commensurate with experience.

Veterinary Teaching Hospital Positions

Dr. John Mattoon reflects on his career in academia:

> I enjoy my interactions with students on a daily basis, and I am rewarded by their successes. I have had the good fortune of interaction with some of the brightest and most enthusiastic veterinarians in the world, not to mention up-and-coming residents and interns, always a source of inspiration and thought-provoking commentary.

> I never had any intention of an academic career. After two years in private practice, I entered a radiology residency program and then was quite eager to re-enter private practice as a specialist. While that was challenging and fun, I was drawn into an academic position at my alma mater, Oregon State University. I soon found myself thoroughly enamored with life as an academician. What I have realized years later is the immense satisfaction of meeting former students and seeing their joy in our profession; it is then that you realize that you have had an impact on their professional lives, sometimes in ways other than rote passage of scientific knowledge.

Living in an academic community has many advantages, including being immersed in a vibrant, continuously invigorating college town atmosphere. While salaries are certainly not on par with our most successful private practitioner colleagues, the university provides unparalleled retirement, health benefits, and vacation time. I have job security (hard-earned, but that's the ladder one climbs in academics), make a very good living, and have the freedom to enjoy a variety of professional opportunities which would be very difficult in the private sector.

An academic career has opened travel opportunities that I thought I could only dream about. To engage with veterinary colleagues throughout the United States and worldwide has been indescribably rewarding professionally and perhaps more importantly culturally.—John Mattoon, DVM, DACVR, Professor of Radiology, Washington State University College of Veterinary Medicine, Pullman WA.

Veterinary teaching hospitals hire veterinarians in a variety of capacities. New graduates are hired as interns; those who have completed an internship are hired as residents. Veterinarians may be hired as clinical instructors or as specialists (see Chapter 4).

Daily work / Pros and cons

Daily work includes creating lesson plans, giving lectures and teaching students in labs. However, only a portion of these jobs involve teaching. Universities usually require that their faculty members also participate in research projects. Clinical hands-on work with animal patients is sometimes but not always part of the job.

The amount of time spent teaching, conducting research, and participating in clinical practice varies greatly, depending upon the appointment. (See Chapter 4 on specialists and Chapter 6 on species variety for details about specialty areas.) Faculty must also publish articles, and participate in committees and university organizations. Time is spent writing notes and papers, attending meetings and conducting research. Occasional travel is necessary to deliver lectures at conventions or meetings.

After the internship and residency, and once board certification is achieved, supervision of interns and/or residents is also part of the job.

The remainder of the work varies with the area of expertise, from canine orthopedic surgery to equine reproduction to wildlife medicine. This work is the same as it would be for any veterinarian working with those species or with that focus.

Universities may have specific cultures, policies, and procedures that are more or less transparent (spoken and unspoken rules), depending on the location. Other attributes of the job are either pros or cons, depending on one's interests. Some love teaching, others love research. Since many different tasks are required, some find the entire situation interesting and others feel pulled down by those aspects less interesting to them. Working with students can be extremely rewarding but also frustrating.

Lack of funding for most colleges has created a tough situation. Veterinary teaching hospitals often have vacant positions, particularly for those specialty areas that are in demand in private practice. Lack of resources can sometimes be frustrating too.

Qualifications / To apply

Veterinarians with "just" a DVM degree may be hired as clinicians. In fact, budget constraints and a lack of sufficient specialists have caused some universities to hire more veterinarians in clinical-track positions, which have less emphasis on research.

Some veterinarians make a career of academia, moving from internship to residency to a university position. Others become board-certified, work in private practice, and then move back to the university setting. Board-certified veterinarians who stay in academia will find they aren't finished yet—they are strongly encouraged to pursue MS and PhD degrees in order to receive tenure, which is the academic method of job security. Many veterinarians choose to pursue a residency and a PhD or MS simultaneously. Advancement often requires moving, on occasion, to positions in different colleges. Although there are exceptions, most academicians do so.

The Pfizer Animal Health / Morris Animal Foundation Veterinary Fellowship for Advanced Study was created as an incentive for veterinarians switching to research. This is a partnership between industry, nonprofit groups, and academia. Applications must be submitted by an institution on behalf of an individual's project. See www.morrisanimal-foundation.org > for grant seekers)

Pay

Pay and benefits are good, although specialists earn somewhat less than those in private practice (see Chapters 2 and 4). See the resource list at the end of this chapter for journal articles related to the need for clinical specialists in academia. Pay and benefits received by veterinarians working in Canada may be found in the Report on Veterinarians in Alternate Career Paths, available from the Ontario Veterinary Medical Association (www.ovma.org).

Research isn't boring

Research is conducted on an astounding array of subjects. One example is Auburn University's Canine Detection Research Institute (CDRI, www.vetmed.auburn.edu/cdri) and its associated Canine Detection Training Center. CDRI has over 20 years of directed research activities encompassing canine detection and the process of canine olfaction. The training center provides problem solving or training solutions, and innovative new ways to use detection dogs.

Washington State University's School for Global Animal Health (http://global-health.wsu.edu) plans a 62,000 square-foot facility that will house over 100 research scientists and graduate students, and state-of-the-art research and diagnostic laboratories.

Also at WSU is the bear research center, the only university facility in the US that houses adult grizzly bears. Researchers are studying the means by which bears can dramatically slow their heart rate and circulation during hibernation without the creation of fatal blood clotting (www.natural-resources.wsu.edu/research/bear-center).

The Aquatic Toxicology Laboratory at the University of California at Davis (www. vetmed.ucdavis.edu > research centers) works to investigate surface water quality and aquatic ecosystem health in watersheds throughout California, and includes both teaching and research.

Colorado State University's Animal Cancer Center (http://csuanimalcancercenter. org/research) has many ongoing projects related to prevention, diagnosis, and treatment of cancer in pets, translating their research and knowledge to also benefit people with cancer.

Researchers at CSU are also studying the impact of climate change on livestock around the globe, particularly in developing countries (www.cvmbs.colostate.edu/aphi).

Kansas State University is working on a proposed US-China Center for Animal Health, a KSU-based training center for the improvement of Chinese animal health education, research, government and industrial work force (www.vet.ksu.edu > development > Newsletters - Lifelines > May 2010).

The Feline Health Center at Cornell University is a veterinary medical specialty center devoted to improving the health and well-being of cats everywhere (www.vet. cornell.edu/fhc).

At Iowa State University, a large number of veterinary researchers are working with swine management issues that range from swine influenza to food borne pathogens in swine and their environment (http://vetmed.iastate.edu > research; and www.ipic. iastate.edu > publications > ISU Swine Researchers).

Ongoing research projects are outlined on every veterinary school's web site, usually with a link titled "research" on the first, main page. Veterinary school links may be found at www.avma.org > education > accreditation > veterinary colleges. Also see the NRC's publication regarding the need for veterinarians in biomedical research. No matter what your interest, you can find a research project!

Chapter 14 Resources

Groups and web sites

Academic keys for veterinary medicine, Higher education jobs in veterinary medicine, http://vetmed.academickeys.com.
Association of American Veterinary Medical Colleges (AAVMC), www.aavmc.org.
Association of Veterinary Technician Educators (AVTE), www.avte.net.
Auburn University Canine Detection Research Institute, www.vetmed.auburn.edu/cdri.
American Veterinary Medical Association, www/avma.org.
  Veterinary Career Center, www.avma.org > Careers.
  Veterinary technician programs list, www.avma.org > education > accreditation > veterinary technology programs.
  Veterinary school links, www.avma.org > education > accreditation > veterinary colleges.
Colorado State University.
  CSU Animal Cancer Center, 970-297-4195; www.animalcancercenter.org.
  CSU Animal Population Health Institute, www.cvmbs.colostate.edu/aphi.
Veterinary Internship and Residency Matching Program (VIRMP), www.virmp.org.
Washington State Univerisity bear research center www.natural-resources.wsu.edu/research/bear-center; WSU School for
  Global Animal Health, http://globalhealth.wsu.edu.

Books and articles

Burns, K, Teaching Hospitals Short on Specialists, *JAVMA News*, August 1, 2006; 229(3): 337–346.
Chronicle of Higher Education, 1255 23rd Street, NW, 7th Floor, Washington, DC, 20037; www.chronicle.com.
Hare, D., Challenges in Clinical Education. *Can Vet J*, February 2007; 48(2): 121–123.
Hubbell, J., et al., Workforce Needs for Clinical Specialists at Colleges and Schools of Veterinary Medicine in North
  America, *JAVMA*, November 15, 2006; 229(10): 1580–1583.
Journal of Veterinary Medical Education (JVME), www.aavmc.org.
National Research Council (NRC), Committee on Increasing Veterinary Involvement in Biomedical Research, *National
  Need and Priorities for Veterinarians in Biomedical Research.* (National Academies Press, 2004); www.nationalacademies.org.
Ontario Veterinary Medical Association, *2010 Report on Veterinarians in Alternate Career Paths*, www.ovma.org.

15 WORKING FOR THE GOVERNMENT

What do the words "working for the government" mean to you? For older generations, they might bring up the image of a military veterinarian (who spent all his time inspecting meat), or a state veterinarian (who spent all his time reading health certificates). For those just coming out of veterinary school, they might bring up a whole new connotation—working for the US Department of Homeland Security, or perhaps doing research on infectious agents at a high-biosecurity facility.

The reality of government work is far more varied than any stereotypic perception. A wide variety of jobs are available that pay well, offer mental stimulation, and can still fill your needs for working with animals, if you so desire. Government jobs are some of the most under appreciated of all careers open to veterinarians. *The vast majority of the government veterinarians interviewed were excited about what they were doing and loved their jobs.*

The titles or "official descriptions" of most government jobs don't tell you a thing. (What does "in charge of disease control" mean?) Take another look, though: these jobs include small animal, equine, and food animal work; hands-on animal work; laboratory and research work; or management and supervisory positions.

The exact job descriptions outlined in this and subsequent chapters may change over time, but the general ideas remain the same. Patience is necessary to wade through each agency's organizational structure.

When considering government jobs, look beyond jobs that require a DVM degree to those that simply ask for someone with a science background or someone with a bachelor's degree that you hold (e.g., microbiology, biology, chemistry). Think of your overall qualifications (e.g., you write well, or have held supervisory positions), not just your degrees.

Pros and cons

Benefits of any government job include good pay and great benefits, guaranteed raises, fairly regular hours, and a clear job description—that is, you know what you're supposed to be doing. Field jobs allow you to continue to work with livestock and with ranchers and farmers without many practice headaches. The type of animals you will work with depends on the location (e.g., pigs in Iowa, cattle in Montana). Jobs can be in rural or urban areas. Sometimes you can travel to interesting places. Once you get over the paperwork and bureaucracy, you can focus on the interesting parts of your job—whether that is pathology, disease management, animal care, or herd health.

All government jobs include plenty of paperwork, policies, procedures, and regulations; veterinarians must be able to write well and be ready to fill out loads of reports. Travel is often required.

Several government workers have described their jobs as requiring a delicate balance between doing a good job, and *not* doing a thorough job. If they are too strict with regulations, they get complaints from the people or groups they are regulating, giving supervisors a headache. Another complaint is that government workers have to spend a certain amount of time *justifying* their own jobs, rather than *doing* them—to make sure that their positions are not eliminated.

Any job descriptions or titles listed in the following chapters may have changed, so consult each agency for up-to-date information. However, these descriptions should give you a good idea of the types of work involved.

State and Local Government Agencies

Approximately 800 veterinarians work for state or local governments. Many cities throughout the US hire veterinarians for positions in public health, animal shelters, or animal care facility inspection.

State positions for veterinarians generally focus on public health, livestock disease, and zoonoses. The main employment opportunities are with the Public Health Department and the Department of Agriculture. State Departments of Public Health are mainly concerned with human health. But, as all veterinarians know, this is directly related to animal health through the food supply and zoonotic disease. State Departments of Agriculture are mainly concerned with animal diseases. Since that can directly affect human health, there can be quite a bit of overlap among job duties in the two state departments.

Some states will put the Department of Health in charge of a certain area, whereas other states put their Department of Agriculture in charge of that very same area. Examples of this potential overlap include a variety of food programs such as milk or egg programs or organic foods certification. Although most job titles with the words "public health" in them are hired in the Public Health Department, there are exceptions. Job titles for veterinarians vary by state.

Animal Shelter Veterinarians

Cities and counties may run their own animal shelter, or more often, may contract with a nonprofit group to carry out animal control and shelter work. See Chapter 13 for more about working with animal shelters and animal rescue operations.

To apply

Every city that has an Animal Control Department should have a veterinarian working part-time, full-time, or on a contractual basis. Call your local department to find out its hiring situation. You may also see job ads in local newspapers, the city's web page, and veterinary journals.

City animal shelter veterinarian

> The City has an immediate part-time opportunity available for a quali-
> fied Veterinarian to provide professional medical care, diagnosis, and
> treatment to animals housed at the City Animal Shelter. Responsibilities
> include staff supervision, medical record keeping, and assisting in the
> development and implementation of goals, policies, and procedure for
> the facility and recommending changes as needed. Starting salary of
> $50.35–$61.18 per hour (2009) plus superb benefits including City-
> contributed retirement plan, cafeteria-style health benefits, and tuition
> reimbursement. Requires DVM + one year of professional veterinary
> medical experience.

County shelter clinic veterinarian

> Bring your compassion for animals to this important role perform-
> ing a broad variety of clinical, laboratory and surgical activities in the
> shelter clinic and mobile unit. Spay, neuter, vaccinate, examine, and treat
> animals; issue certificates containing health status for adopted animals;
> perform emergency treatment and surgery upon injured and diseased
> animals; develop medical protocols and standard operating procedures;
> and write medical reports, processing cruelty cases and presenting cases
> in court. $64,617/yr (2009). County provides an excellent benefits
> package, including medical, dental, and life insurance as well as vacation
> and sick leave, tuition reimbursement, and retirement.

Animal Care Facility Inspector

Daily work / Pros and cons

An inspector's job includes inspecting facilities where animals are raised or cared for,
such as dog breeding kennels, veterinary clinics, and research facilities with laboratory
animals, to ensure animals are properly housed and fed. Most animal care facility inspection is done by federal employees, but some facilities are governed by city regulations
and thus undergo inspection by city veterinarians. See the section on APHIS Animal
Care in Chapter 16 for a complete description of the duties of an animal care facility
inspector.

State law or city ordinance defines which facilities are to be inspected and by whom.
Some inspectors are not veterinarians. In some states and cities, there is no provision for
inspection of veterinary hospitals. In some cities, a shelter veterinarian is also responsible for animal facility inspection. For example, in the state of Pennsylvania, dog law
wardens are charged with inspecting all kennels in the state.

To apply

Contact your local government agencies to find out who is responsible for carrying out those duties where you live. For example, in Colorado, the Pet Animal Care Facilities Act Program is a licensing and inspection program dedicated to protecting the health and well-being of those animals in pet care facilities. (See www.colorado.gov > Divisions > Animal Industry > Pet Animal Care Facilities Program.) In Missouri, the Animal Care Facilities Act regulates individuals and entities that enter dogs or cats into commerce as defined under state statute (http://mda.mo.gov > animals >dogs and cats).

Public Health Veterinarian

The Institute of Medicine defines public health as "what we, as a society, do collectively to assure the conditions in which people can be healthy." States, cities and counties have Public Health Departments that may hire veterinarians.

City or county public health veterinarian

Cities and counties with larger populations may have public health positions that a veterinarian could fill. Contact your city or county Public Health Department for information about specific positions and their titles. Find the department online by first searching for key words [county name] and [.gov], then narrowing that search using key words [public health].

Sample job announcement: County public health veterinarian

> Public Health veterinarian for the County Department of Public Health, Environmental Health Division, Technical Support Section. Requires veterinarian with 1 year of experience preferably in a public health agency or in public health inspection work. Should have a thorough knowledge of infectious diseases common to man and animals and of control measures for such diseases; knowledge of laws relating to animal control and communicable disease control; and knowledge of and skill in performing ante- and postmortem examinations. An MPH is desirable.

State Department of Public Health veterinarian

Veterinarians have many opportunities in various sections of State Departments of Health, which hire a wide variety of scientists. Several states employ a public health veterinarian (PHV).

Veterinarians in environmental health may perform risk assessments of toxic sites or insecticide toxicity studies. State public health veterinarians consult with physicians, emergency rooms, legislators, local officials, schools, health departments, and the general public on preventing exposures to and controlling diseases that humans can get from animals and animal products.

Daily work / Pros and cons

Joni Scheftel, DVM, MPH, DACVPM, enjoys her position as State Public Health Veterinarian in the Minnesota Department of Health, and feels she is making a valuable contribution:

> I love being involved in current infectious diseases issues, which requires keeping up with new information and dealing on a daily basis with relatively stressful situations. I feel that I'm making a difference in the short term through service to the public and other health professionals and in the long term by influencing health policy. I love going to work.

Mira J. Leslie, DVM, MPH, currently a Public Health Veterinarian in the Ministry of Agriculture and Lands, BC, Canada, wrote the following paragraph for the first edition of this book, when she was a State Public Health Veterinarian in Arizona. Although she has moved to other jobs within government, she says it "still describes public health veterinary work in a US state or local health department, though I have "matured" some and would probably have to add the trendy terms like emerging zoonoses, one health, or interdisciplinary."

> I am not a bureaucrat—I really do hands-on active public health work! I deal with Hantavirus, plague, rabies, cat scratch disease, Simian B virus, brucellosis, tick-borne diseases, mosquito-borne diseases, rabies, more rabies, and any other vector borne or zoonotic disease, including reptile-associated Salmonella. I do everything from case investigation and consultation, to field surveillance (collecting rodent blood for hanta, fleas for plague), to writing articles and guidelines, to lecturing and public speaking, to writing and defending legislative issues about rabies and zoonoses, to organizing and collaborating with universities or other organizations on projects that involve zoonotic disease issues. It is very diverse. As you can tell, I love my job, and am always happy to promote PH to veterinarians looking for alternatives.

Qualifications

These state jobs require some knowledge of epidemiology or public health. Thirty-nine PHVs are listed on the web site of the National Association of State Public Health Veterinarians (NASPHV; www.nasphv.org). Of those PHVs, most have a master's or PhD degree. Because Public Health Departments focus on human health, the veterinarian's work will be in zoonotic and food-borne disease, but also may occasionally overlap into human disease issues.

Since the first edition of this book, many veterinary students have been encouraged to focus on public health and to obtain an MPH degree. While that encouragement continues, actual job openings and pay may not be as robust as many would wish. (See Chapter 19 for a discussion on societal needs.)

Dr. Mira Leslie says:

> The evolution of public health vets has ebbed and flowed in the past
> ten years—bioterrorism funds from the late 1990s to 2004 or so
> provided lots of new positions for vets in public health. The dramatic
> cuts recently have cost positions and seriously affected public health
> infrastructure. The good news is that the expertise in population health,
> epidemiology and biomedicine that veterinarians have is increasingly
> influential and integrated into policy making, leadership, and the frame-
> work of public health at all levels (federal, state, and local).

It is possible to get an MPH in one year. You can also acquire new knowledge
without going back to school in the traditional sense. Many accredited universities
offer distance learning, which allows you to take courses online or via correspondence.
EpiVetNet has a list of short- and long-term online courses in epidemiology (www.
vetschools.co.uk/EpiVetNet). You can also join the military to have part or all of your
education paid. See Chapter 18, and the section on going back to school in Chapter 2,
for more information.

States with small budgets and low populations are more likely to hire veterinarians
for jobs with titles such as toxicologist or epidemiologist—even if the applicant doesn't
have a toxicology or epidemiology degree—because these states rarely have the budgets
to hire specialists. For example, Washington State had a veterinarian on staff as an epidemiologist who worked in the area of zoonotic disease. Once you have some experience,
you can move on to a state with a larger budget, with "experience" on your resume. Jobs
may focus on radiation safety, toxicology, epidemiology, and many more areas. DVMs
interested in focusing on the details of one aspect of their training might like this work.
Others may take a job with a narrow focus as a springboard to other jobs.

To apply

Look for job advertisements in each state's personnel division (the easiest way to
find job listings is to look on the state's web site; otherwise, contact the department by
telephone, email, or mail).

As with many government jobs, the best advice is this: take any job with the state
that you can get, then you will find a wealth of other job opportunities that weren't
obvious from the outside. Many management jobs are "exempt" positions—which
means they're appointed or elected, and therefore often are not advertised to the public.
Thus you need to work for the state in order to know about other positions working for
the state.

Also, once you're "in," you can educate others about the qualifications veterinarians
have that make them ideal for jobs for which they might not have been considered in
the past. Apply for any job that involves the subjects you studied in veterinary school. At
least two of the veterinarians interviewed for this section started by taking that approach
in smaller states that were willing to hire veterinarians without advanced degrees. They
have now moved on beyond their initial jobs to those that better serve their needs—but
those first jobs got their feet in the door.

According to one incumbent, turnover in state jobs is slow and is mostly due to retirement. However, a veterinarian in a state without a PHV, for example, could take another Health Department position, and if the environment is supportive, create the PHV position. Openings for State PHVs are typically advertised in *JAVMA* and traditional veterinary-job resources.

Salaries range from approximately $40,000 for an entry-level assistant state public health veterinarian or state public health veterinarian, to more than $100,000 for more senior level positions.

State Departments of Agriculture

Each state has a Department of Agriculture or similar agency with a state-specific name (e.g., Montana's Livestock Board, Louisiana's Livestock Sanitary Board, Nevada's Division of Agriculture). Because each state has a different agricultural emphasis, jobs existing in one state may not exist in another. For instance, North Carolina employs a veterinarian as the state inspector of the National Poultry Improvement Plan, a regulatory program to help ensure healthy poultry from egg to slaughter. In previous years, this has even been a new DVM graduate hired after doing a one-year poultry internship.

The following sections describe positions within specific states' Departments of Agriculture, which may also be typical of other states. See the web site of the National Association of State Departments of Agriculture (NASDA; www.nasda.org), and your state's Personnel Department.

Many management and supervisory jobs for veterinarians exist within each state's Department of Agriculture. The most obvious are the state veterinarian and others who work under that person for "Animal Disease Control." Veterinarians have also worked as directors, assistant directors, and commissioners in state Departments of Agriculture.

Some states hire veterinarians for meat inspection; in other states, meat inspection is done by federal veterinarians (see FSIS in Chapter 16). To find out the case in a particular state, call the state veterinarian's office. See the AVMA web site for contact information in the state, then e-mail or call and ask for job descriptions for all jobs open to veterinarians (www.avma.org > My AVMA > Member Resource Directory > Government agencies).

Animal disease control

Entry-level jobs in animal disease control involve hands-on inspections, investigations, and travel, and they may be based out of more rural locations. Jobs higher up in the hierarchy are supervisory and desk positions, frequently located in more urban settings.

Every state has an "official in charge of animal disease control," but the job title varies. In many states, that official is the state veterinarian. See the AVMA web site for other titles (www.avma.org > Animal health > Disaster preparedness series > State veterinarians). These titles range from "Administrator, Division of Animal Industries" (Idaho) to "Executive director and state veterinarian, Board of Animal Health" (Minnesota), to "Chief, Bureau of Animal Industry" (Iowa).

The *official in charge of animal disease control* generally has several other veterinarians working in the same office. These may include the *assistant state veterinarian, state public health veterinarian, state meat inspector, veterinary medical officer,* and *animal health veterinarian.*

Animal Health Veterinarian (Washington)

The animal health veterinarian (AHV) in Washington State is responsible for public health protection in one of five areas of the state. The AHV performs animal and herd examinations, conducts epidemiologic investigations, establishes and releases quarantines, investigates zoonotic diseases, and investigates animal welfare complaints. The AHV also acts as liaison between the state veterinarian and livestock groups; investigates and prepares cases for fines or prosecution; trains and prepares for animal health emergencies and natural disasters; and investigates meat drug residue findings.

Daily work / Pros and cons

The Washington State animal health veterinarian spends most of the time doing field or epidemiologic investigative work. For example, if a drug residue problem is found, the AHV traces the animal to the farm of origin, contacts the producer, and conducts an on-farm interview to identify the potentials for residue introduction. About one day a week, on average, is spent doing paperwork or working on reports.

The AHVs do all their own office work; because they all work out of home offices, their time is flexible. They file weekly time and project reports and adjust their schedules to a 40-hour week.

The work involves driving and working outdoors, no matter what the weather. In addition, they may be working with ranchers or farmers who are angry about having their premises quarantined or having a disease or drug residue problem.

Qualifications

The AHV must have knowledge of federal and state laws and regulations pertaining to the control and eradication of infectious livestock diseases within the state, as well as investigational procedures for judicial review and legal prosecution. The AHV must be able to work with owners and processors in inspection and control of livestock; plan and direct inspections in the area; work with veterinarians, livestock industry, media, and the public; and write well. The position requires a veterinary degree with at least three years' experience in agricultural veterinary medicine. The salary range in Washington in 2010 for Field Veterinary Medical Officers (non-supervisory) was $61,000 to $80,000.

Veterinarian, Animal Health and Food Safety (California)

California's Division of Animal Health and Food Safety Services in the Department of Food and Agriculture (CDFA, www.cdfa.ca.gov/AHFSS) employs veterinarians that focus on herd health and food safety. These veterinarians are distributed throughout the state

Daily work / Pros and cons

Veterinarians who work for the CDFA are either food safety specialists or animal health veterinarians. Either can advance to supervisory positions.

Meat and poultry food safety specialists work with small poultry processing facilities and custom meat harvest facilities that provide food for urban or rural communities. The veterinarians' work includes conducting inspections and implementing regulatory disease control measures, outreach, and training. Journey level veterinarians may develop training, evaluate legislation, recommend policy and assist with administration of the overall program. For a description of the details of a meat inspection job, see FSIS in Chapter 16.

Animal health veterinarians focus on certain livestock and poultry diseases. Field-level veterinarians implement animal health programs, investigate reports of livestock and poultry diseases, initiate or implement disease control and eradication measures, and provide related outreach and education for their area. Veterinarians with specialized expertise are assigned to state headquarters and are responsible for statewide program areas as well as administration of the overall animal health program.

Qualifications

All applicants for a veterinary position must take a state exam. Top rankings are then considered for open positions. The testing office accepts applications continuously and notifies job applicants as openings arise. (See www.cdfa.ca.gov/Employment.html and www.spb.ca.gov.)

Animal health veterinary jobs require a veterinary degree and state license. The applicant must have detailed knowledge of food animal medicine, and livestock and poultry diseases of severe consequence, be able to speak and write effectively, and be willing to travel.

Meat and poultry food safety veterinarians must have a veterinary degree, but a California veterinary license is not required. The applicant must have knowledge of veterinary pathology, food safety and food safety practices as they relate to meat processing.

For either category, requirements for advancement include experience and knowledge in that area and the ability to plan and direct the work of others. Further advancement requires knowledge of public administration, personnel management, and supervision. Pay varies with the position.

Extension jobs

Susan Kerr, DVM, PhD, Extension Educator, Klickitat County, Washington, appreciates her value as an educator:

> As an extension educator, I help people and don't have to hand them a bill. This is a big change from private practice, where you have to charge for your services to stay in business. I have less direct animal contact than in practice, but I feel I am helping more animals and preventing more problems by educating owners about how to care for their animals properly. It is rewarding to help 4-H youth learn how to be good animal caretakers and gain skills and knowledge they will use their entire life.

Veterinarians may work as *extension agents* (often at the county level) or as *extension specialists* (often associated with a land grant college or university). Several of the veterinarians whose quotes appear in the section on food animal medicine in Chapter 5 are *extension veterinarians*. In addition, veterinarians may also fill extension jobs where only part of their job is directly related to veterinary medicine.

Extension jobs are offered via the government in coordination with teaching institutions. Because most funding comes from the state, and because job applications are made within each state, these jobs are included in this state/local government chapter.

The National Institute of Food and Agriculture (NIFA, www.nifa.usda.gov), formerly the Cooperative State Research, Education and Extension Service (CSREES), is an education network based at 130 of the nation's land-grant colleges of agriculture, plus Tuskegee University, several forestry colleges, 27 colleges of veterinary medicine, and native-serving institutions. Land-grant colleges have a trio of mandates: teaching, research, and service (extension).

Extension personnel are responsible to the taxpayers in the community, so there must be a lot of taxpayers with a particular need to have a specialist for that need (e.g., a dairy extension specialist for dairy farmers). Thus, if you want to work with a particular species such as with horses, then you'll want to apply for an extension job in a county or state such as Kentucky, where the economy depends on that to some extent.

NIFA operates through a model of specialized National Program Leadership (NPL); it currently has 5 people serving as NPLs who are veterinarians. For instance, there are veterinarians serving as NPL for Veterinary Science, NPL for Animal Health, and NPL for Animal Agrosecurity. All the veterinary NPLs hold both DVM and PhD degrees. Working as a team, their jobs involve oversight of NIFA's veterinary and animal health, including research, education and extension.

Daily work

While extension educators work *with* universities, only some work *at* the university campus; others may work in outlying communities. Extension veterinarians at universities often have split appointments such as 50% extension, 25% teaching and 25% research.

Extension educators are basically information brokers with a broad range of duties. They provide educational and technical assistance in livestock and crop production, family life, and community development. They may provide information about subjects as diverse as home economics, raising sheep, caring for horses, planting pastures, or growing oats.

A new extension agent may be asked to do a "community needs survey" to find out what needs exist and what programs are desired. The agent's job is then to deliver the requested information, by looking it up, teaching classes, finding volunteer teachers who are knowledgeable in the subject, or by giving out printed information. Organizing, writing, and distributing educational handouts on a variety of subjects are part of the job. Web sites with this information are available for each county.

Extension educators respond to calls from community members and find materials they need or a person to contact. They also conduct or organize classes on a variety of subjects. They establish collaborative relationships with county commissioners, the 4-H, the state university, schools, organizations, and agencies. The amount of administrative work varies, but is typically 15 percent of the job duties.

A typical winter day in northern states is spent indoors. Summer days may include outdoor work with youth for those who have 4-H responsibilities. Extension agents may coordinate 4-H programs; tell people about the information they offer, and then get it to them by phone, mail, or e-mail; write a newsletter; and organize meetings. They may telephone several people to find someone to write an article about food safety for their upcoming newsletter or to find someone to give an educational talk about dairy herd management. They may conduct tours of crop demonstration plots, coordinate educational workshops for livestock producers and host farm tours.

Most extension agents have assistants, who may include a secretary or 4-H program assistant. They also train local volunteers who train others. Examples include master food safety advisors, master gardeners, weed advisors, livestock advisors, or a subset such as a master goat farmer. The educator must recruit, screen, train, and manage volunteers who help develop and implement these programs.

Veterinarians may fill those volunteer roles as well. Volunteers get something back, too; for example, they may get free classes and materials from the university, for which they give back volunteer hours.

Each county has an extension director who supervises the county's extension educators. This position is from 15 to 100% administrative, depending on the number of extension educators being supervised. County directors are supervised by district directors.

Pros and cons

Extension educators and volunteers can only give advice and information sanctioned by university-based research. Traditionally, this research has focused on conventional farming practices, but is increasingly diversifying into areas of sustainable agriculture, integrated pest management, and organic production.

Extension veterinarians still have contact with animals and animal owners, but without the need to take emergency calls or run a for-profit business. Hours can be long, though, with many educational programs held at night and on the weekend. Extension veterinarians are required to be licensed in their state and participate in continuing education. This is a very people-oriented job, working with people of all ages, including schoolchildren.

Qualifications

An agricultural background is necessary, and a background in education is helpful or required, depending on the position. The extension educator must have effective speaking, writing, and listening skills; experience working with groups and individuals; and the capability to work independently and as a team member.

The area's economic base will determine the amount of time spent using knowledge of livestock or horses versus working in areas such as orchard or pasture management, or gardening. Those with proficiency in many areas are most likely to be hired. Emphasis is placed on people skills, computer and distance education skills, communication skills, and the subject matter directly pertinent to the specific job opening. Teaching and administrative experience and experience working with the news media are desired.

To apply

NIFA operates as a partnership of the federal government through the USDA and state and local governments. About 70 percent of the system's funding originates from state and local sources, with the rest from the federal government. However, extension agents are hired by the state's land grant university.

There is no central repository for extension jobs, which are advertised differently by each state. Potential sources of job announcements include the web site of the state's land grant university (which should have a page devoted to the extension service); the NIFA-USDA web page (www.nifa.usda.gov); advertisements in the classified section of larger cities' newspapers; or the *Chronicle of Higher Education*, a national weekly tabloid of educational jobs and opportunities (www.chronicle.com). The extension director in the state, whose office is usually at the university, may have job notices for other states as well. The American Association of Extension Veterinarians can supply the address of a particular state's organization of extension agents (http://vetmed.illinois.edu/aaev/url.htm). Local extension service offices are listed in the government section of the phone book—under "county," then under "cooperative extension." On the AVMA web site, extension agencies are listed under USDA (www.avma.org > My AVMA > Member Resource Directory > Government agencies). Also see Chapter 14 on working in academia and teaching.

Pay varies widely since each state has varying amounts of local and federal funding. Benefits are usually excellent. Advancement probably requires additional degrees beyond the DVM (e.g., in education or management). Some positions are on the university tenure track, with comparable advancement opportunities.

Interestingly, the NIFA is also the administrator of the VMLRP, which is the Veterinary Medicine Loan Repayment Program implemented in 2010 to encourage veterinarians to work in areas of need. This program is described in Chapter 1. Veterinarians receiving these loans are not extension educators but may work in a variety of job types (www.nifa.usda.gov/vmlrp).

Chapter 15 Resources

Groups and web sites

American Association of Extension Veterinarians, http://vetmed.illinois.edu/aaev/url.htm.

American Association of Public Health Veterinarians, www.acvpm.org; phone: 515-331-4439.

American Humane Association, 63 Inverness Dr East, Englewood CO 80112-5117; www.americanhumane.org; e-mail: info@americanhumane.org.

American Public Health Association, 800 I Street, NW, Washington, DC 20001-3710; www.apha.org; phone: 202-777-2742; fax: 202-777-2533; e-mail: comments@apha.org.

American Society for the Prevention of Cruelty to Animals, www.aspca.org and www.aspcapro.org.

Association of Shelter Veterinarians, www.sheltervet.org.

Cooperative State Research Education and Extension Service (CREES), see NIFA.

EpiVetNet, www.vetschools.co.uk/EpiVetNet.

Humane Society of the United States, 2100 L Street, NW, Washington, DC 20037; www.hsus.org.

National Animal Control Association, PO Box 480851, Kansas City, MO 64148-0851; www.nacanet.org; phone: 800-828-6474; fax: 913-768-0607; e-mail: naca@nacanet.org.

National Association of State Departments of Agriculture, 1156 15th Street, NW, Suite 1020, Washington, DC 20005; www.nasda.org; phone: 202-296-9680; fax: 202-296-9686; email: nsada@nasda.org.

National Association of State Meat and Food Inspector Directors, c/o Mr. Charlie Ingram; e-mail: charlie@nasda.org.

National Association of State Public Health Veterinarians, www.nasphv.org.

National Institute of Food and Agriculture (NIFA), 1400 Independence Avenue, SW., Stop 2201, Washington, DC 20250-2201; www.csrees.usda.gov and www.nifa.usda.gov; phone: 202-720-4423.

Shelter Veterinarian, www.sheltermedicine.com.

University of Florida's Shelter Medicine and Forensics CE, www.ufsheltermedicine.com.

Books and articles

Burns, K, Evolution of Shelter Medicine, *JAVMA*, November 1, 2006; 229(10): 1543–1545.

Chaddock, H.M., Veterinarians: Integral Partners in Public Health. (2007); available at www.aavmc.org/documents/VWEACongressionalPaperPDF.pdf.

Chronicle of Higher Education, www.chronicle.com.

Kuehn, B. M., Shelter Medicine: A Budding Field that is Helping to Raise the Standard of Care in Animal Shelters, *JAVMA* May 1, 2004; 224(9): 1412–1413.

National Animal Control Association (NACA), Pros and Cons of Working in the Field of Animal Control, www.nacanet.org/careeropps.html.

Nolen, R.S., Animal Care faulted for lax oversight of problem dog breeders, *JAVMA News* 237(1), July 1, 2010:8-10.

SPCA Opens Largest Nonprofit Hospital in San Francisco. *DVM Newsmagazine*, February 2009: 14; www.sfspca.org.

Verdon, D, Vet blows whistle on slaughter practices, *DVM Newsmagazine*, Apr 1, 2010. Available at www.dvm360.com.

16 WORKING FOR THE FEDERAL GOVERNMENT

Thanks to Michael Gilsdorf, DVM, MS, Executive Vice President, National Association of Federal Veterinarians, who provided valuable information for this chapter.

Federal jobs can be divided into two broad categories: the uniformed and civil services. Currently, close to 3,000 veterinarians work for the federal government. The vast majority work with the US Department of Agriculture (USDA) or with the US Army (see Chapter 18).

Within the civil services, most government veterinarians—nearly 36 percent—work for the USDA-Food Safety and Inspection Service (FSIS), with another 25 percent working for the USDA-Animal and Plant Health Inspection Service (APHIS). Civilian jobs are scattered throughout the US, with the majority in Maryland, Iowa, Texas, Georgia, and Virginia, and some in Colorado and the Washington, DC, area; many require you to relocate every few years.

Veterinarians can work for a wide variety of government agencies, within a variety of interest areas. An AAVMC article by H. Chaddock (www.aavmc.org) includes an excellent appendix that summarizes the variety of jobs held by veterinarians in the federal government. Reading those summaries can provide some perspective about work with the federal employment. You can also find and talk to federal government veterinarians at the annual meeting of the National Association of Federal Veterinarians (www.nafv.net).

The main US federal agencies that employ veterinarians are listed in Table 16.1. Government agency organization can change any time. However, the basic job descriptions will remain similar.

Because the pay scale and approach to applications is the same for many jobs, this chapter starts with that general information before proceeding to specific government agencies and the positions within them. The first "test" to see if you qualify for a government job is to be able to wade through this chapter. If you can do that, you're ready to read the even more stuffy government literature.

Applying for Federal Employment

Many federal employees will tell you this: The first step to take in investigating any civilian federal job is to apply for one. This does not obligate you in any way, but it will speed up the hiring process once you pursue that. There are several approaches to applying for federal jobs, which are detailed in the sections that follow.

Table 16.1: Main US federal agencies that employ veterinarians

US Dept of Agriculture (USDA)
Animal and Plant Health Inspection Service (APHIS)
Animal Care (Animal welfare) (AC)
Veterinary Services (VS)
Centers for Epidemiology and Animal Health (CEAH)
Center for Veterinary Biologics (CVB)
National Center for Animal Health Emergency Management (NCAHEM)
National Center for Import and Export (NCIE)
National Veterinary Services Laboratories (NVSL)
Food Safety and Inspection Service (FSIS)
Agriculture Research Service (ARS)
Office of Risk Assessment and Cost-Benefit Analysis (ORACBA)
National Institute of Food and Agriculture (NIFA)
US Dept of Health and Human Services (DHHS)
National Institutes of Health (NIH)
Centers for Disease Control and Prevention (CDC)
Food and Drug Administration (FDA)
Center for Veterinary Medicine (CVM)
US Dept of Homeland Security (DHS)
Plum Island Animal Disease Center (PIADC)
US Dept of Commerce
National Marine Mammal Laboratory (NMML)
National Marine Fisheries Service (NMFS)
National Technical Information Service (NTIS)
US Dept of the Interior
Fish and Wildlife Service (FWS)
US Geological Survey (USGS)
US Agency for International Development (USAID)
Veteran's Administration (VA)
Environmental Protection Agency (EPA)
National Science Foundation (NSF)
National Zoo
National Aeronautics and Space Administration (NASA)

The following entry-level opportunities offer a great overview of all government positions.

- The *Veterinary Services Careers Program* hires veterinarians who have little experience or background, and trains them to fill APHIS positions. (See APHIS.)
- APHIS NAHERC offers temporary employment in emergency situations. This is a short term opportunity without long term commitment. (See APHIS.)
- FSIS positions are open to veterinarians with no prior experience. (See FSIS.)
- The *Public Health Service Commissioned Corps* is an all-officer organization that provides a variety of employment opportunities for health professionals and students. Officers are most likely to be assigned to the CDC, EPA, FDA, or NIH. (See Chapter 18.)

The following fellowships usually require more experience than held by a new veterinary graduate, but they are open to veterinarians with a wide variety of backgrounds and experience:

- The *AVMA Congressional Fellowship* offers a year working in Washington, DC—a great way to see what other veterinarians are doing as they work for the government. (See also the section on jobs with the AVMA in Chapter 12.)
- The *AAAS Fellowships* may place you in any agency, working on Capitol Hill (see details in Chapter 2, and USAID in this chapter).

Federal job classification

Each federal job type is given a series number; for example, traditional veterinary medical positions are series 0701. You can search by job series on the usajobs.gov web site. The "0701" key word will show you all the vacant positions within the veterinarian series. However, plenty of other jobs have been classified under other series numbers, but are ideal for veterinarians. It is best to look not only at the 0701 series but to also look for the agency or, better yet, the type of job you want (e.g., technical writer; fish biologist).

Federal jobs are advertised in four categories: 1) only employees of the agency concerned may apply; 2) only employees of the department may apply; 3) all government veterinarians may apply; and 4) any veterinarian may apply. The vast majority of job openings are in categories 1–3; until you are "in," you are seeing only a few of the potential job openings.

If you want a federal job, you should consider accepting the most desirable one available, even though it may not be your first choice. The more announcements you apply for, the better your chances. Most government veterinarians start working with APHIS or with FSIS. They then work their way through various other jobs or agencies according to their interests and to openings that become available.

Note: Many job positions are labeled as veterinary medical officer (VMO). That label applies to a wide variety of jobs that are traditionally for veterinarians. In spite of the "officer" word, these are not military jobs, so it wise to also read beyond the "VMO" for a full job description.

Plan your approach

Submit applications to APHIS and FSIS (www.aphis.usda.gov and www.fsis.usda.gov). Applying through the FSIS means that you're applying for *any* job labeled "veterinary" (i.e., series 701)—it does *not* mean you're applying only for meat inspection jobs. Although this application will be used primarily to fill FSIS positions, other federal agencies, such as the ARS, FDA, and the VA occasionally request names of eligible applicants. Your name will be referred on the basis of how well you meet their qualifications, and that observation depends on how thoroughly you describe your experience and knowledge when you fill out the application form—take your time!

The FSIS application *does not* include many jobs for which you may also be qualified, such as public health official, technical information specialist, fish biologist, and so on. To apply for jobs that don't specifically say "veterinarian," contact the individual agency, as described in the agency sections in this chapter, and search the usajobs.gov web site. However, that general site does not automatically list vacancies from agencies with direct-hire authority, so to be thorough, you should check each agency's job announcements.

When considering a government job, look for jobs that simply ask for someone with a science background or someone with a bachelor's degree that you hold (e.g., microbiology, biology, chemistry). Why get hung up on a title when you could find a job that pays just as well as other "veterinary" jobs, and uses as much of your knowledge? Think of your overall qualifications, not your degrees (you write well, have held supervisory positions, etc.). When filling out your application, don't limit your notes to only medical and technical areas. Include your experience or classes you've taken in management, speaking, writing, and so on.

Once your application is sent in, your eligibility is rated and you are placed on a list of people who are contacted as vacancies occur. You have the option of placing limits on both the location and the number of hours that you will work. Doing so will automatically mean that you are not notified of any jobs that don't meet your strict requirements, so be careful with the limits you set.

The Federal Research Service is an example of a private group specializing in helping people get government jobs (www.fedjobs.com). They provide an extensive, up-to-date listing of job openings and tips about the job application process. In addition, the Federal Information Exchange provides electronic access to federal research opportunities, equipment grants, current events, and minority opportunities (www.fedix.fie.com).

The AVMA lists agencies on their web site (www.avma.org > Member Resource Directory > Government agencies). The National Association of Federal Veterinarians has a helpful information sheet, Sources of Federal Employment Opportunities for Veterinarians (www.nafv.net).

Pay

Government worker pay is primarily rated on the GS scale. There are 15 GS levels and a senior executive service; within each are several steps of advancement. New veterinarian graduates with little experience start at the GS-11 level; most positions for veterinarians are at the GS-12 level and above ($65,000 to $100,000+).

The current GS pay chart is available on the Office of Personnel Management (OPM) web site (www.opm.gov), at www.fedjobs.com, or at any employment office. In addition to the GS scale, other pay systems exist within agencies such as the commission corps, the military, and the National Institutes of Health (NIH). Some jobs with FSIS use a different pay scale system called "pay bands."

In addition to competitive pay, the federal government offers great benefits: paid vacation, sick leave, and holidays; health and life insurance options; and a retirement plan. Don't forget to include these in your calculations when comparing other jobs—benefits are expensive!

The pay received by veterinarians working in various government agencies is shown graphically in a Government Accountability Office (GAO) 2009 report titled Veterinarian Workforce, GAO-09-424T, available at www.gao.gov/htext/d09424t.html. The GAO report outlines some of the issues that can interfere with filling the government need for veterinarians (also see Chapter 15). According to that report:

> USDA agencies compete against one another for veterinarians instead of following a department wide strategy to balance the needs of the agencies. According to FSIS officials, APHIS is attracting veterinarians away from FSIS because the work at APHIS is more appealing, there are more opportunities for advancement, and the salaries are higher. Indeed veterinarians are more concentrated in lower grade levels at FSIS than at APHIS. Moreover, the mean annual salary for veterinarians at FSIS in 2007 was the lowest among the three key USDA agencies…. Salaries for individual veterinarians range from $35,000 for those in the residency program at the National Zoo to $205,000 for the highest paid veterinarian at NIH.

Since then, the FSIS has instituted recruitment bonuses (see FSIS section).

USDA Animal and Plant Health Inspection Service (APHIS)

> I was fortunate to serve in APHIS, for they strongly encouraged continuing education and made many opportunities available. The biggest benefit of all was the fact that I loved my job. It required all my academic training, my continuing education learning and daily striving to learn even more. It gave me opportunities to interact with some of the best and brightest scientists and veterinarians in the USDA, in the federal government, and in the world. What more could one want?—Alwynelle Ahl, PhD, DVM (retired).

Currently, about 670 veterinarians work in the USDA-APHIS (www.aphis.usda.gov). These jobs potentially include small animal, equine, food animal or marine animal work, and management and supervisory positions. Don't let the list of descriptions in this section limit your imagination. If you are interested in any of the divisions or units within APHIS, you may be able to find a job there (or work your way up to a position there).

For students

APHIS is partnering with Mississippi State University to provide outreach to veterinary schools and externships. Linda Detwiler, DVM, from the Department of Pathobiology and Population Medicine, Mississippi State University, currently leads the program. See www.aphis.usda.gov > About APHIS >Programs and Offices > Veterinary Services > Student externships and internships.

APHIS also has a scholarship program that helps veterinary students pay for school, employs them during school breaks, and trains them for APHIS jobs. (See www.aphis.usda.gov > career opportunities > student programs and www.cvm.msstate.edu/usdaextern/index.html)

APHIS Animal Care and Veterinary Services

APHIS veterinarians are most often initially hired as veterinary medical officers (VMOs) in either Veterinary Services or Animal Care (two of the nine APHIS divisions). See www.aphis.usda.gov > about > organizational chart.

Animal Care (AC) determines and promotes standards of humane care and treatment of animals through inspections and educational efforts. Veterinary Services (VS) protects and improves the health, quality, and marketability of animals, animal products, and veterinary biologics.

To advance, you must be willing to move and must sometimes apply for different positions, because you will not necessarily get promoted from your current position.

To apply

To apply for veterinary jobs in USDA-APHIS, information and forms can be found at www.aphis.usda.gov. The easiest method is to apply through APHIS' recruitment program called the Veterinary Services Careers Program (see next section). Another route to a VS or AC job is to first get a job with FSIS and then apply for the VS or AC job while holding the FSIS position.

To advance beyond GS-12, you must move to a position other than VMO. Examples include staff veterinarian, port veterinarian, or area-veterinarian-in-charge, all discussed below. Promotion to the GS-13 and higher levels is competitive but possible with only a veterinary degree.

Temporary work is available with APHIS Emergency response for students and veterinarians (see NAHERC in this chapter).

Sample job announcement: USDA, APHIS, Veterinary Services

Current and anticipated VMO vacancies are located throughout
the US and Puerto Rico. Responsibilities could include assignments

related to epidemiology, import and export, foreign animal diseases, or other regulatory veterinary medicine. The duties may include 1) identifying diseases and recommending treatment or preventive care methods; 2) Certifying the health of livestock, poultry, aquatic species, and by-products for export purposes; 3) Planning and coordinating medical procedures to deal with animals and their by-products offered for importation into the US; 4) Determining the presence of foreign animal disease, infestation, or infectious, contagious, or communicable disease; 5) Conducting licensing inspection and monitoring surveillance systems of establishments involved in handling animals and animal by-products. Salary: GS-701-11/12.

APHIS Careers Program

The APHIS Veterinary Services Careers Program (VSCP) hires veterinarians who have little experience or background, and trains them to fill VS or AC positions. Since the VSCP is a recruitment tool, someone not already working for the government might find a job faster that way. (See www.aphis.usda.gov > about >programs > veterinary services.)

You may apply via the APHIS web site (www.aphis.usda.gov), at the Office of Personnel Management web site (www.opm.gov), or at www.usajobs.gov. Candidates will be hired at the GS-11 or GS-12 salary level, depending upon previous experience. VSCP positions are temporary training positions located at one of several "duty stations" around the country.

APHIS Animal Care

APHIS Animal Care (AC) is responsible for enforcement of the Animal Welfare Act and the Horse Protection Act. Veterinarians concerned about animal welfare might be interested in this type of job.

The Animal Welfare Act protects certain warm-blooded animals raised for commercial sale, used in research, transported commercially, or exhibited to the public, and requires minimum standards of care and treatment. The Animal Welfare Act requires that every research lab have a veterinarian on staff. The Horse Protection Act addresses standards for horses.

Animal Care headquarters, located in Riverdale, Maryland, includes Resource Management Support and Animal Care. Field operations for these are coordinated out of three regional offices, with *Animal Care Veterinary Medical Officers* (AC VMOs) in every state.

Daily work / Pros and cons

AC VMOs inspect animal care facilities, including research laboratories; dog breeding facilities; zoos; horse shows; and amusement parks. Inspection sites vary from circuses to Christmas tree lots where live reindeer are displayed.

The VMOs also inspect horse shows, exhibitions, sales, and auctions, to be sure that there are adequate facilities, proper horse handling, and crowd control. Their work includes performing unannounced compliance inspections; liaison with other agencies and industry groups; and development of regulatory policies. VMOs also present educational seminars to regulated industries and the public.

At research laboratories, VMOs explore the need for each research project in relation to the way the animals are used; ensure that proper anesthetics and analgesics are used; and review water and food, heating and ventilation, sanitation, pest control, animal handling, and record keeping.

VMOs spend time driving around to facilities, then walking through the facility for the inspection and writing a report. If deficiencies are found, the VMOs must educate the facility staff about how to correct the problems.

Many AC VMOs keep offices in their homes. Ongoing training is considered paid work time; attendance at veterinary CE meetings is often paid for as well. A government vehicle is provided. Each VMO may have licensed technicians working under his or her guidance. The work schedule is flexible.

The VMO's job requires tact—particularly with research laboratories, since this is a veterinarian evaluating a veterinarian! The VMO often must deal with facility employees who view the VMO as an adversary; some are hostile. Occasional interactions with angry animal rights groups may arise. One drawback reported by a VMO is that government work often requires being able to balance between regulating facilities according to law and helping facilities to continue operating. If you strictly enforce the laws, perhaps shutting down a facility too quickly, you create complaints (by the facility) and thus a headache for your supervisor (who may take it out on you). At the same time, you can't ignore problems. This issue is described in an article by R. Nolen in *JAVMA*.

The best approach is to figure out how to tactfully educate facility staff such that changes are made without creating antagonism. Change can take a long time, so those eager to correct problems quickly may feel frustrated.

Qualifications

The daily work described above requires skills in writing, speaking, communication, diplomacy, and employee management. Qualifications for AC VMOs include knowledge about a variety of animals, from laboratory mice to marine mammals to zoo animals (their social, behavioral, nutritional, and medical needs); an ability to diagnose lameness in horses; knowledge of the Animal Welfare Act; and knowledge of the operations of research facilities, exhibitors, pet suppliers, and animal transporters.

APHIS Veterinary Services

Veterinary Services (VS) is the animal health section of APHIS. VS is responsible for protecting and improving the health, quality, and marketability of the nation's agricultural animals, animal products, and veterinary biologics. The *Veterinary Service VMO*'s work involves herd health preventive medicine as well as a wide array of other services.

The program staff headquarters of VS is located in Riverdale, Maryland, with regional headquarters in Raleigh, North Carolina, and Fort Collins, Colorado. VS operates on statewide, regional, national, and international levels.

The VS entry level position is casually referred to as the "*field service VMO*." Each state has several field service veterinarians, whose work is often based out of home offices. They are assigned to specific geographic areas and must work with all species. While veterinarians who want to work with one particular species may be able to do so as a species specialist, these positions are rare.

In the past, field service work was the main focus of VS, but today there is more focus on the National Health Monitoring System with more veterinarians working in staff positions doing analysis or surveillance of animal disease.

Daily work / Pros and cons

Field service VMOs go to farms and ranches that have disease problems to evaluate their operations, and to outline procedures to prevent disease transmission and eliminate the disease from the herd or flock. Field work involves physical activity, including physical examination and evaluation of cattle and horses. Driving is part of the job, with one to five nights per month spent away from home. Field VMOs work outdoors most of the time (regardless of the weather) and may be exposed to contagious diseases. Establishing and lifting quarantines are sometimes necessary, which may create anger and pressure tactics from affected ranchers. Inspections of schools and restaurants may also be part of the job (e.g., to evaluate whether they are properly disposing of their garbage and not giving it away to someone to feed to their pigs). Other duties include supervising employees such as animal health technicians, and public speaking to explain disease prevention requirements (e.g., to livestock groups). At times, VMOs may be called to other states for short-term work (of three to four weeks) if, for instance, there is an outbreak of disease that requires additional help.

Qualifications

The VS VMO field position requires a veterinary degree and one year of experience performing similar duties (see VSCP, earlier). Experience with large animals or poultry is necessary, as is knowledge of domestic and foreign animal diseases. The VS VMO must be able to gather and assess data, to resolve conflicts, and to write and speak well.

APHIS Management positions

There is a VS *federal area veterinarian-in-charge* (AVIC) in most, but not all, states. The AVIC is in charge of all federal animal health activities within the state or area they supervise. They coordinate the activities of the VMOs working in the field, as well as those involved with import/export, epidemiology, emergency response, and animal disease eradication and control.

The APHIS *senior staff veterinarian* for each species is a liaison between APHIS and special interest groups (e.g., American Association of Equine Practitioners, for horses; American Association of Bovine Practitioners, for cattle; and so forth). Work includes staff management and administrative duties; scientific reading; meeting with experts about various diseases; providing phone consultation for veterinarians and government agencies; and providing technical support via telephone, written documents (e.g., booklets, letters), e-mail, and other means. About 20 percent of the time is spent traveling.

The senior staff veterinarian must have specific knowledge of the particular species and/or animal disease under his or her jurisdiction. For instance, the senior staff veterinarian for equine diseases was an equine practitioner with many years of experience working with world-class performance horses, and thus had knowledge of equine international travel and import/export requirements, various equine special interest groups, and so on. This person came directly to the supervisory position from private practice rather than from within government.

APHIS VS National Center for Import-Export

The National Center for Import-Export (NCIE) regulates the importation of animals and animal products, including birds and fish, that enter the country through ocean, air, and land ports. It facilitates safe international trade and monitors the health of animals presented at the border.

Daily work / Qualifications
Port veterinarians work at ports that allow international shipments of animals, and at quarantine facilities. This is not an entry-level position; veterinarians must have had prior experience in VS VMO field service.

Quarantine station VMOs supervise loading and unloading of imported and exported animals, take blood samples, and perform physical exams upon arrival and daily during the quarantine period. A wide variety of animals come through the quarantine stations, including Olympic-quality horses, cattle, pigs, ostriches, and vultures.

As an example, the Miami facility employs several veterinarians; some work "in the barn" and others perform more of the office administrative work. Office work includes examining and endorsing health certificates, making sure that both the US and other countries' regulations are being met.

Import-export jobs include overtime work because the VMO must be present when planes arrive or take off. A background in mixed practice is ideal because of the knowledge of large animal diseases, vaccinations, and health certificate procedures.

APHIS *Plant Protection and Quarantine (PPQ) VMOs* are employed by NCIE headquarters in Riverdale, MD, but they work in the field at Customs and Border Protection (CBP) stations. PPQs are the liaison between NCIE and customs/border patrol. PPQs each cover four to six states, spending over half their time travelling between ports. They conduct training and inspections of animals and animal products entering the country, and may have some field service duties in addition to their port duties. PPQ veterinarians must be self starters and have the ability to work without daily direct supervision.

Veterinarians working for NCIE must have had experience as VS field service VMOs. PPQ applicants must be experienced in and knowledgeable about import/export, foreign animal disease diagnostics, and regulatory programs in APHIS. These positions require political savvy and leadership, and to have a security clearance.

APHIS VS Centers for Epidemiology and Animal Health and Center for Veterinary Biologics

The scientific and technical units of VS are the Centers for Epidemiology and Animal Health (CEAH) in Colorado and the Center for Veterinary Biologics (CVB) in Iowa. Veterinarians may work in any of these units, to monitor and regulate vaccines, bacterins, antisera, diagnostic kits, and other products of biological origin used in veterinary medicine. For instance, a veterinarian working in the CVB reviews and licenses veterinary vaccines and diagnostic test kits.

The various centers within CEAH perform work such as information analysis, animal health surveillance, national livestock and poultry health studies, and collaboration on animal health issues and projects both domestically and internationally. One major focus of CEAH is epidemiology.

These positions do not necessarily require an advanced degree in epidemiology, but they do require appropriate experience (often gained in other VS jobs, or by taking courses in epidemiology and statistics); about 30 percent of the work time is spent traveling. See www.aphis.usda.gov > animal health> veterinary biologics and www. aphis.usda.gov > about > programs and offices > Veterinary Services > Centers for Epidemiology and Animal Health.

APHIS VS National Center for Animal Health Emergency Management

VS emergency management works to keep the US free from foreign animal diseases. Within VS, the National Center for Animal Health Emergency Management (known as Emergency Programs) coordinates efforts to prepare for and respond to outbreaks of exotic animal diseases. Emergency Programs manages the National Veterinary Stockpile, which maintains the nation's repository of vaccines and other critical veterinary supplies, equipment, and services.

You can download training videos about emergency response and foreign animal disease online. See www.aphis.usda.gov > Emergency Preparedness and Response > Tools and Training.

Emergency Programs manages the National Animal Health Emergency Response Corps (NAHERC).

APHIS National Animal Health Emergency Response Corps

Temporary work is available with APHIS. The National Animal Health Emergency Response Corps (NAHERC) is a reserve group of veterinarians, students, and animal health technicians who can assist state and federal response efforts during an outbreak. (See www.aphis.usda.gov > emergency response.)

Anyone called becomes a temporary USDA APHIS employee, but has the right to refuse assignments at any time. Most tours last about 21 to 30 days. Previously, NAHERC was activated and responded to the 2001 outbreak of foot-and-mouth disease in the United Kingdom, the 2002 avian influenza outbreak in Virginia, and the 2003 Newcastle disease outbreak in California.

Duties while called up might include caring for companion animals; coordinating boarding, sheltering, and evacuation; conducting surveillance; examining herds or flocks for signs of disease; collecting specimens; vaccinating animals; conducting postmortem examinations; euthanizing animals; supervising the disposal of animal carcasses; collecting epidemiological information; inspecting livestock markets, trucks, and vehicles; and performing exotic, avian, research animal, and zoo care and duties. (See Chapters 6 and 13 for more about disaster and rescue.)

Pay for veterinarians in 2010 was $25/hour with minimal benefits. Travel, lodging, overtime, and workers' compensation are provided.

Other APHIS jobs: Teaching, Foreign Service, and more

Teaching or supervising positions are available within APHIS. One veterinarian who had a teaching background became an "education development specialist" and trained APHIS personnel involved with animals; she also helped to supervise the Veterinary Services Careers Program, which was discussed earlier in this chapter.

Another APHIS job involves supervision of the Risk Analysis Systems Unit, which was organized to develop methods for assessing risks to US agriculture from imported diseases or pests.

There are also a small number of jobs overseas with the Foreign Service, but openings are limited. As with other international jobs, fluency in a language other than English is important. The APHIS international staff helps countries train their own animal health care workers or recommend programs to improve food animal health and productivity.

USDA Food Safety and Inspection Service (FSIS)

In a slaughter plant, you get to see a lot of pathology that you read about in textbooks but you would never see in any other career. I've seen two chickens with melanoma, which is remarkable. The inspectors call them blueberry chickens because they look like a blueberry muffin.

I like working with a group and solving problems. Here I have colleagues that I can easily consult or work with on a project. For example, recently we have been evaluating our training program, interviewing inspectors who have gone through training and then observing them on the job, trying to see how we can better prepare them and get them up to speed.

Many new veterinarians are not aware that FSIS veterinarians supervise inspectors who belong to a union. There are several unions within the federal government. We have a labor management agreement we must abide by. However, I have found that if you are a good supervisor and genuinely interested in the well being of your employees, then union activities are a small consideration of your daily work.

We get excellent benefits, sick leave, vacation, plus time for CE. In general we work 5 days a week, 8 hours a day, although there are night and day shifts. Some veterinarians work at one plant whereas others are "on patrol" for several smaller plants. I did "relief" work during my initial years with FSIS, so I have worked in about 40 plants. At my current assignment, I get to do "temp" work assignments on special projects, like food safety audits.

Of course, this is a bureaucracy; you can't make up the rules as you go. There is quite a bit of structure and a chain of command. Even though there are rules and guidelines, an experienced person can effect change if there is a good reason.—Douglas L. Fulnechek, DVM, USDA FSIS Supervisory Veterinary Medical Officer, Springdale, AR.

People who like pathology may enjoy FSIS jobs. The duties of the Food Safety and Inspection Service (FSIS) are to ensure the wholesomeness of food and assure the safety of red meat, poultry, and egg products sold in interstate commerce. FSIS also makes sure food is properly labeled and packaged. Veterinarians are hired by FSIS as *supervisory public health veterinarians* (SPHVs). Opportunities for fellowships, internships, and externships with FSIS are presented at www.fsis.usda.gov > Careers > Internships and Externships.

Daily work / Pros and cons

An SPHV VMO conducts food safety assessments of slaughter and/or processing establishments to ensure processes, facilities, and equipment are appropriate and clean. FSIS-VMOS, as the "inspectors in charge," supervise several online inspectors and consumer safety inspectors. They direct inspection to detect and diagnose conditions that may render food products unfit for human consumption. They also oversee the humane handling and slaughter of livestock, and perform drug residue checks.

Every decision must be documented with paperwork. Some plants take in more questionable animals than others; at those plants, the VMO inspector has more work to do and ends up spending paid overtime doing the necessary paperwork. This job requires working at least six days a week in physically demanding, noisy, and wet environments.

"Relief" jobs as FSIS VMOs are regular, full-time (sometimes overtime!) positions. The reliever is assigned a duty station in one city but works as a fill-in at plants where there is a vacancy or the regular veterinarian is sick or on vacation. One advantage for them is that they build up their resumes with a variety of experiences—from large plants to small ones, and working with a variety of animals and animal products.

VMOs don't work for the plant itself (they work for the government), but they are working *in* the plant; thus, they may be viewed as the "bad guy." New VMOs may be viewed with suspicion and have their judgment questioned. In contrast, some VMOs have taken heat from the media for being "too friendly" with the plant, resulting in alleged leniency on food safety issues. This issue is described in articles such D. Verdon's in *DVM Newsmagazine*.

Taking a firm and consistent approach to every case is the key to developing respect and accomplishing the mission. Many FSIS veterinarians feel they are making an important contribution in that they perform a critical role in protecting the health of the nation through food safety activities.

Qualifications

The USDA-FSIS hires 50 to 75 new veterinarians annually. These positions are open to new graduates, and do not require an additional degree beyond a DVM. Openings are expected to increase over the next decade.

Advancement to a teaching or management position requires management skills. Duties include recordkeeping, writing and travel. Circuit supervisors keep a home office (even though they are assigned a duty station) and spend much of their time driving to different plants for inspection.

To apply

More than 1,000 veterinarians are employed by FSIS, and continual openings are posted on the USA Jobs web site (www.usajobs.gov). Also see www.fsis.usda.gov and www.foodsafetyjobs.gov; and www.fsis.usda.gov > Careers > Why Join FSIS? > Public Health Human Resources System Demonstration Project.) FSIS veterinarians may belong to the American Association of Food Hygiene Veterinarians, www.AVMA.org/aafhv.

FSIS has the authority to set pay above the minimum rate of pay of the grade for a new appointment or reappointment based on the superior qualifications of the individual or the "special need" of the agency (i.e., the applicant brings knowledge or skill of exceptional value to the agency).

FSIS offers student loan repayments to all newly hired veterinarians. In addition, recruitment bonuses are authorized at 25 percent of base salary each year for four years. Bonuses were available nationwide in 2009; whether this will continue depends on future budgeting priorities.

Other USDA offices

USDA Agricultural Research Service

The Agricultural Research Service (ARS, www.ars.usda.gov) is the USDA's chief scientific research agency. The ARS coordinates over 1,000 research projects within 21 national programs. Most veterinarians working with the ARS have additional degrees.

The ARS does employ several VMOs for clinical work. These veterinarians maintain the health of research animals (dairy and beef cattle, sheep, swine, lab animals, and some cats). They perform experimental surgery, such as installing rumen fistulas or placing catheters in blood vessels. They are responsible for routine health care, such as treatment of mastitis, metritis, and other common disorders seen in practice. They supervise one or more technicians, and attend various committee meetings. On-call duty is expected, but there are few emergencies. Openings are advertised at www.ars.usda.gov > careers, at www.usajobs.gov and in *JAVMA*. Turnover is low.

USDA Office of Risk Assessment and Cost-Benefit Analysis

The role of the Office of Risk Assessment and Cost-Benefit Analysis (www.usda.gov > Office of the Chief Economist > risk assessment) is to ensure that major regulations proposed by the USDA are based on sound scientific and economic analysis. ORACBA provides guidance and technical assistance, including education and training; coordination among agencies; and technical and analytical support to USDA agencies. It coordinates peer reviews of proposed major regulations, and assists in the development of risk assessment information services in the USDA.

USDA National Institute of Food and Agriculture

Although this is a federal agency, jobs with the National Institute of Food and Agriculture (NIFA) are discussed under Chapter 15, because these are extension educators who work on the local level.

Department of Health and Human Services

The Department of Health and Human Services (DHHS) is an agency of the executive branch under the president of the United States. Thus, with every change of administration, regulatory policies can, and often do, change.

To begin your search for DHHS job vacancies, go to www.hhs.gov/careers. Then see the specific information for each agency. The DHHS Office of Public Health and Science (OPHS, www.hhs.gov/ophs) includes the Commissioned Corps, a uniformed service of health professionals who serve at the DHHS and other federal agencies (see Chapter 18). The DHHS agencies of primary interest to veterinarians are the FDA and the CDC. Also see Chapter 13, DHHS National Veterinary Response Team.

DHHS Food and Drug Administration (FDA)

The Food and Drug Administration (FDA) approves and regulates drugs and medical devices and protects consumers from unsafe foods, cosmetics, drugs, and radiological products. They also work on preventing antimicrobial resistance in people resulting from the use of antimicrobial drugs in food animals. They screen for drug residues in both meat and milk and provide ongoing research to support animal drug approvals.

The FDA divisions may hire veterinarians for positions such as veterinary medical officer (VMO), biologist, chemist, consumer safety officer, microbiologist, pharmacologist, toxicologist, or pathologist. Over 100 FDA veterinarians direct science-based programs, or are involved in epidemiology, drug review, risk assessment, food safety, biosecurity, and international trade. Most of those work at the Center for Veterinary Medicine (CVM), where they are involved in scientific research.

FDA Center for Veterinary Medicine

The CVM, which regulates animal drugs and feeds, hires veterinarians to work in any of its four areas: management; premarketing; postmarketing; and research. See the article by S. Sundlof regarding the need for veterinarians working in biomedical research in the FDA and other locations.

Daily work

The *management staff* oversees the day-to-day operation of the CVM, including its goals and direction; they manage personnel and the budget, and disseminate information.

The *research staff* conducts their own research and coordinates outside grants and contracts for research about drugs, additives, and contaminants, such as analyzing the metabolism of those items in animal tissues and food. They also determine the safety and efficacy of diagnostic agents and devices for animal use, and investigate interactions between diet and drugs in food-producing animals.

The *premarketing staff* determines whether a drug should be approved for marketing (these ties in with industry jobs in product development; see Chapter 11). Premarketing reviewers study data submitted by drug sponsors. Veterinarians work in teams focusing on, for example, therapeutic drugs for food animals, companion animals, or wildlife.

The *post marketing staff* monitors marketed animal drugs, food additives, medicated animal feeds, and devices to assure continuing safety and effectiveness. Their work includes ensuring that drug advertisements are in alignment with their approved use, and assessing all reported adverse effects with a drug.

Eric Dubbin, DVM, joined the FDA in 1998 after working for 10 years as a large animal practitioner. He began working as a reviewer for new drugs, working his way up to team leader. He is now the Organization Development Executive Coach at the FDA Center for Veterinary Medicine FDA. Dr. Dubbin describes his career:

> I did not dream of becoming a federal employee as I was considering careers in veterinary medicine. My goal was to be a clinical veterinarian and treat patients and clients, and it was quite gratifying.
>
> To me, veterinary medicine has always placed public service in high regard. All of a sudden, the work I did impacted millions of animals and owners. I dealt with medical issues that were different than I encountered in practice; these issues include study design, policy, group dynamics, leadership, industry, media, and diverse multidisciplinary dialogue, all the while dealing with novel and cutting edge medical advances. Working for the FDA has been quite rewarding.

Qualifications / To apply

Most FDA jobs for veterinarians are with the Center for Veterinary Medicine (CVM) at the Maryland headquarters. However, jobs are also scattered throughout the country, in regional offices, district offices, and resident posts. See these web sites:

- FDA-CVM information, www.fda.gov > About FDA > Centers & Offices > About the Center for Veterinary Medicine.
- FDA-CVM jobs, www.fda.gov > Science & Research > Science Career Opportunities.
- FDA information, www.fda.gov > Animal and Veterinary.
- FDA job vacancies, www.usajobs.gov and www.fda.gov/jobs.

Sample job announcement: FDA-CVM veterinary medical officer

> FDA-CVM VMO, GS-14–15, serving in the Rockville, MD Division of Therapeutic Drugs for Food Animals with responsibility for determining the safety and efficacy of new animal drugs. Reviews and interprets applications and scientific investigations regarding New Animal Drug Applications and Investigational New Animal Drugs, making sure they contain the necessary information and are approvable. Discusses the progress of applications with sponsors and prepares correspondence

describing any deficiencies. Evaluates proposed labeling of new drugs. Integrates conclusions of consulting scientists into a comprehensive review. Requires DVM, 1 year of experience in clinical food animal medicine, writing and speaking skills, and ability to review and evaluate data. GS-12 is required to apply.

FDA Office of International Programs

The FDA has been opening new centers around the world as part of the government's ongoing strategy to ensure the quality and safety of exports to the US. The FDA has identified China, India, the Middle East, Europe, and Latin America as areas in which to establish a permanent in-country presence. While they also have ongoing programs in Africa, there are no on-site offices there.

The current director of the FDA Regional Office in Europe, Linda Tollefson, DVM, MPH, is stationed at the US Mission to the European Union in Brussels, and is responsible for all FDA operations in Europe. She is a Rear Admiral in the Commissioned Corps of the US Public Health Service (see Chapter 18). According to Dr. Tollefson:

> Globalization is no longer unique; it's a fact of life. The human and animal pharmaceutical industry, the food we eat and export or import, the dietary supplements, cosmetics, and toys that we or our families use all come from the global marketplace. Therefore it makes sense to examine the efficacy and the safety of these products on the same basis—globally.

> The US FDA has long been involved in collaborative efforts with its counterpart agencies in most countries of the world. The US-European Union relationship is one of the oldest and strongest in this regard. FDA opened the Europe Office, headquartered in Brussels, to further develop its long-standing cooperation with the European Commission and other European Union agencies.

> Being Director of the FDA Europe Office is tremendously challenging. First, it is necessary to be familiar with the entire spectrum of the FDA, not just veterinary medicine or food issues, but all the regulated products. Second, it is necessary to have at least a basic knowledge of the dynamic scientific issues before the agency. Third, understanding the European Union and its institutions is necessary to comprehend the EU decision-making process. All of this adds up to an incredibly stimulating, but very demanding job, which hopefully will also be rewarding. My primary goal is to enhance FDA's collaboration with the European Union to the point where we can jointly address significant public health concerns.

FDA Fellowship

The FDA Commissioner's Fellowship is a two-year program that provides an opportunity for health professionals to receive training and experience at the FDA. Applicants must have a doctoral-level degree (e.g., DVM). Salary depends on experience, but the range in 2009 was $65,000–$110,000. Fellows undergo their training at an FDA facility of their choosing. See www.fda.gov > About FDA > Working at FDA > Fellowship, Internship, Graduate, & Faculty Programs.

DHHS Centers for Disease Control and Prevention (CDC)

The CDC, with headquarters in Atlanta, Georgia, works in such areas as prevention of infectious and chronic diseases, environmental health, occupational safety and health, international health, epidemiologic and laboratory research, data analysis, and emerging infectious diseases. Titles of jobs for veterinarians include *center director, branch director/chief, epidemiologist, epidemic intelligence service officer,* and *laboratory animal care veterinarian.*

In 2010, the CDC announced that it is creating new divisions: the National Center for Emerging and Zoonotic Infectious Diseases (www.cdc.gov/ncezid) and the Center for Global Health (www.cdc.gov/globalhealth).

Daily work

Jennifer Gordon Wright, DVM, MPH, DACVPM, has worked at the CDC for many years. As a veterinarian, she is employed by the US Public Health Service and currently works for the CDC as an epidemiologist. Dr. Wright could also be assigned to work for the USDA, the FDA, the NIH, or even the EPA. Dr. Wright enjoys the opportunity to impact federal policy that her job affords her:

> As a private practice veterinarian, I very much enjoyed working with clients and animals, but I always felt that I was making a difference only on the "individual level." With a career in public health, I am able to make a difference on a state, national, or even international level. There is nothing more rewarding than seeing months or even years worth of work impact federal policy, whether it be a policy relating to pediatric or adult vaccinations, judicious use of antimicrobials, or on-the-job injury mitigation.

Qualifications / To apply

Most veterinarians working at the CDC have additional degrees beyond their DVMs. However, there are a few entry-level opportunities for veterinarians. Veterinarians who work for the Public Health Service Commissioned Corps (see Chapter 18) may be assigned to work with the CDC. The CDC may also temporarily hire other veterinarians working for different government agencies.

The CDC offers job opportunities in other countries. To qualify for CDC overseas jobs, you must be able to work independently and adapt to new situations and changing environments.

Job openings are posted at www.cdc.gov/employment, www.usajobs.gov, and www.avma.org/vcc.

CDC training and fellowships

The CDC's Epidemic Intelligence Service is a two-year postgraduate program of on-the-job epidemiology and statistics training for health professionals (physicians, dentists, and veterinarians). Veterinarians must also have an MPH degree to be eligible. Many of the veterinarians working with the CDC were hired after going through this program.

A two-year CDC *Public Health Informatics Fellowship* is also available with the CDC (www.cdc.gov/PHIFP). This fellowship requires a master's degree or higher and some experience in public health (which most veterinarians have to some degree upon leaving school), as well as experience (or training) in computers. Fellowship participants will be trained in both informatics and public health. This experience will help to equip fellows to guide the development, evaluation, and implementation a support of public health surveillance and information systems. Fellows who have completed their training within the past three years are preferred. (See Chapter 10.)

DHHS *National Institutes of Health (NIH)*

The National Institutes of Health (NIH) headquartered in Bethesda, Maryland, works to supervise, fund, and conduct research that produces new knowledge about disease and disability in humans. NIH research is oriented toward the prevention, diagnosis, and treatment of disease, and NIH-sponsored research discoveries have led to treatment for afflictions ranging from cancer to schizophrenia.

Some of the NIH branches which may have positions of interest to veterinarians include the National Cancer Institute, the National Institute of Environmental Health Sciences, the Office of Alternative Medicine, the Office of Disease Prevention, and the National Library of Medicine (see Chapter 10).

Daily work / Pros and cons

These are indoor jobs that are often focused on a specific area of interest. Most veterinarians working with the NIH focus on laboratory animal medicine or veterinary pathology. They work in areas of animal care and use, animal welfare, laboratory animal medicine and surgery, epidemiology, toxicology, and veterinary and comparative pathology. Pay and benefits are excellent.

Qualifications / To apply

Veterinarians working with the NIH almost always have additional degrees and qualifications. The NIH web site (www.nih.gov) has a resource guide that lists the contact information for the NIH's component institutes and offices. For series 701 veterinary positions within the NIH, apply through the USDA-FSIS (see this chapter's introductory explanation). Many positions are also filled through the Commissioned Corps (see Chapter 18). For other jobs (science, lab animal research, and epidemiology), go to www.jobs.nih.gov.

The National Cancer Institute has partnered with several veterinary schools to train veterinarians in pathology residencies at one of the veterinary colleges, with dissertation work to be done at an NIH institute.

According to a 2009 GAO report, "Veterinarian Workforce":

> . . . [the NIH] faces challenges recruiting veterinarians that specialize
> in laboratory animal medicine and veterinary pathology, who make up
> the majority of veterinary positions at the agency. Both specialties are
> reporting significant shortages that are not forecast to improve for at
> least 10 years.

Many Agencies, Many Choices

Veterinarians interested in public policy may want to explore the AAAS Fellowships, under which they can work with a variety of different government agencies (see Chapter 2).

Jobs with the National Technical Information Service (NTIS, www.ntis.gov) and the National Agricultural Library (NAL) are discussed in Chapter 10, Information services.

The National Zoo (http://nationalzoo.si.edu > careers and internships), offers volunteer opportunities, internships, and (a few) jobs for veterinarians. Also see Chapter 6.

The National Science Foundation (NSF, www.nsf.gov), hires a variety of scientists for long-term and temporary positions. There are no openings for veterinarians per se, but veterinarians may qualify for positions such as biologist that require an advanced degree that could include the DVM. Current vacancy listings are available at www.nsf.gov > about > careers.

Positions in laboratory animal medicine in the Department of Veterans Affairs (VA) are available for veterinarians. Most require additional degrees or board certification, but experience can be an acceptable substitute. Jobs may include organizing and directing animal research facilities, consulting about laboratory animal research, and training medical personnel and animal technicians. For details about laboratory animal medicine, see Chapters 4, 6, and 11. Some job openings for veterinarians are filled via applications that were submitted through the USDA-FSIS (see earlier discussion). For other VA positions, go to www.va.gov.

Government veterinarians working in many different agencies may elect to work in another country. To do so, you must sign on for worldwide availability (you don't have to take an offer, but you should be open to worldwide offers). You can indicate a preference for a country; if you speak a particular language you will have an edge in the countries where that is spoken. Applicants with foreign travel experience are given priority, but "travel" must be more than an occasional two-week vacation. When you are working for the government, you must represent the government's position, regardless of what you believe. Housing and children's schooling are paid.

Department of Homeland Security, Plum Island Animal Disease Center

The Department of Homeland Security (DHS) has positions open to veterinarians. The Plum Island Animal Disease Center (PIADC) on the northeastern tip of New York's Long Island is under the charge of the DHS (previously it was under the USDA). Scientists and veterinarians with ARS and APHIS carry out USDA activities at PIADC.

There is talk of moving the Animal Disease Center at Plum Island to a new and larger facility, which might be built at Kansas State University. This proposed National Bio and Agro-Defense Facility will be for the study of foreign animal and zoonotic disease. Details may be found at www.dhs.gov/nbaf.

PIADC is charged with helping to protect US livestock from foreign animal diseases. Work is broken into three major categories: diagnosis, research, and education. Scientists and veterinarians study foreign animal diseases using live virus and infected animals. This is a high-security laboratory and is the only one in the US that is allowed to study foot-and-mouth disease. Federal and state veterinarians, along with laboratory diagnostic staff, military veterinarians, and veterinary school faculty attend Foreign Animal Disease Diagnostic School each year. (Biosafety levels are described at www.fas. org/programs/bio/biosafetylevels.html.)

Most positions in the DHS that are currently held by veterinarians do not require a veterinary degree. However, veterinary knowledge provides better overall understanding of the breadth of the animal health activities. When searching for such jobs, do not just look at 701 series jobs (veterinarian), but also 301 series (management).

National Marine Mammal Laboratory and National Marine Fisheries Service

Veterinarians with interest and expertise in marine animals may want to investigate jobs with the National Marine Mammal Laboratory (NMML) or the National Marine Fisheries Service (NMFS). These are both part of the National Oceanic and Atmospheric Association (NOAA) of the US Department of Commerce. (See www. afsc.noaa.gov/nmml and www.nmfs.noaa.gov.)

The NMFS is dedicated to the management, conservation, and protection of living marine resources through science-based conservation and management, and the promotion of healthy ecosystems. Personnel at the headquarters work with six regional offices and science centers, and with scientists and managers throughout the nation.

The NMML conducts research on marine mammals, with particular attention to issues related to marine mammals off the US west coast. Research projects focus on ecology and behavior, population dynamics, life history, and status and trends. Information is provided to various domestic and international organizations to assist in developing rational and appropriate management regimes for marine resources under NOAA's jurisdiction.

All jobs are posted at www.usajobs.com (search for jobs titled "biologist"). Job and internship information are at www.nmfs.noaa.gov/pr/about/jobs.htm. Aquaculture jobs are described in Chapter 6.

Fish and Wildlife Service and US Geological Survey

The Fish and Wildlife Service (FWS; www.fws.gov) and the US Geological Survey (USGS; www.usgs.gov) are bureaus within the Department of the Interior that employ a few wildlife veterinarians. Working with these agencies requires that veterinarians develop respectful relationships with the non-veterinarian biologists who have expertise in working with wildlife.

The Biological Resources Discipline (BRD) of the USGS works with others to provide the scientific understanding and technologies needed to support the sound management and conservation of biological resources. The USGS-BRD includes the Wildlife Health center, which employs veterinarians who work on wildlife disease issues. See http://biology.usgs.gov/wter.

The FWS mission is to conserve, protect, and enhance fish and wildlife and their habitats for the continuing benefit of the American people. Its major responsibilities are migratory birds, endangered species, certain marine mammals, fish, the National Wildlife Refuge System, wetlands, conserving habitat, and environmental contaminants. The FWS veterinarians work in the endangered species division doing classification and conservation; natural resources in conservation planning and policy; migratory bird management in habitat conservation; international affairs; law enforcement; and fish and wildlife management and habitat restoration. For job openings with the FWS, go to www.fws.gov or www.usajobs.gov.

Environmental Protection Agency

The Environmental Protection Agency (EPA, www.epa.gov) implements federal laws designed to protect human health and the environment. It conducts a variety of research, monitoring, standard-setting, and enforcement activities. Currently, the few veterinarians who work for the EPA have been assigned there from the DHHS-PHS, rather than being directly employed by the EPA. (See DHHS in this chapter and the PHS Commissioned Corps in Chapter 18). Areas in which veterinarians have worked include risk assessment and evaluation; policy analysis and development; emergency response for environmental contamination; research into adverse health effects of air, drinking water, and terrestrial pollution; research in animal care; and work on zoonotic disease and associated public health risks (studying such topics as prions), and serving as expert witnesses. Several veterinarians work with the EPA as toxicologists.

The EPA web site provides information about general career tracks within the EPA (www.epa.gov/careers). For job openings, go to www.usajobs.gov and www.epa.gov. For internship and fellowship information, see www.epa.gov > careers > College and Grad School Graduates. Also see the section on environment-related jobs in Chapter 6.

US Agency for International Development

The US Agency for International Development (USAID) is a federal government agency that conducts foreign economic assistance and humanitarian aid missions to advance US economic and political interests overseas. Missions may then hire contractors and interns. Both non–US citizens and US citizens may apply for contract positions, but only US citizens may apply for intern positions.

While veterinarians may qualify for USAID positions, such positions are usually not advertised as "veterinarian wanted." Read the job announcement descriptions to see whether your skills fit with their needs, which fall into either public health or agriculture. Peruse job announcements looking for words like zoonotic disease, public health, animal health, agriculture, or food security.

Positions with USAID are posted on www.usajobs.gov and www.usaid.gov/careers. USAID contract employment opportunities are listed in the *Commerce Business Daily* (http://cbdnet.gpo.gov).

Experience in overseas civil strife is required for domestic and overseas positions (Peace Corps work may provide such experience; see Chapter 13.) The USAID Bureau for Humanitarian Response, Office of US Foreign Disaster Assistance, has positions for US citizens only (www.usaid.gov/careers/applicant.html).

USAID contracts with independent development organizations such as Development Associates Inc (DAI) to carry out certain projects. Veterinarians might be employed by those groups and thus end up working on USAID projects. See Chapter 13, nonprofit work, for details.

The Canadian International Development Agency is Canada's group that functions similarly to USAID. See www.acdi-cida.gc.ca.

USAID Fellowships for Veterinarians

Veterinarians who apply for the American Association for the Advancement of Science (AAAS) fellowships in the area of diplomacy and development could potentially be placed with USAID or the State Department. An example is Kim T. Rock, DVM, MIH, who was granted an AVMA-GRD (AAAS) fellowship to work in the USAID-Africa Bureau, Office of Sustainable Development in Washington, DC. Dr. Rock has a master's in international public health from the University of Uppsala in Sweden. Prior to accepting the fellowship, Dr. Rock was a clinical and shelter veterinarian at the Michigan Humane Society and in private practice.

The fellowship program emphasizes networking among a variety of professionals to solve problems in another country. Current funding tends to focus on biotechnology research, zoo and conservation work, and broad environmental issues.

Daily work includes writing; interacting with other professionals, but also with local people, to help them learn new ways of doing things; and a mix of field work and monitoring the situation once projects have been implemented.

A USAID Fellowship requires some foreign language ability, international experience, the ability to work in teams, to write well (the application includes writing a "memo" or article), to articulate your thoughts clearly, and to take an analytical and scientific approach to problems. A moderate salary is paid ($45,000–$85,000), but the best things about the fellowship are the great contacts, leadership skills, knowledge of international business, and other abilities it offers. Former fellows can use their experience to continue work in the international arena, either as independent consultants or as part of a team (nonprofit agency, governmental agency, etc). (Note that there is little or no opportunity to stay on with USAID.)

See Chapter 2, AAAS Fellowships; Chapter 12, AVMA-GRD Fellowships; http://fellowships.aaas.org > become a fellow; and www.usaid.gov/careers/fellows.

National Aeronautics and Space Administration

The National Aeronautics and Space Administration (NASA, www.nasa.gov >about > careers) has had a few veterinarians on staff. For example, the work of former NASA Chief Veterinary Officer, Joe Bielitzki, DVM, MS, is described on the NASA web site (www.quest.nasa.gov) and is partially excerpted here:

> My responsibilities are to make sure that the NASA animals are always properly taken care of, experience minimal distress, and that everything we do follows the regulations that the government has established for animal care. I provide expert consultation on things like anesthesia, husbandry and nutrition. I am also responsible for the health and well being of animals while they are flying. At NASA the job has to do with being able to identify the risks of space travel for the astronauts. Veterinarians are the first people you look to when you are looking at new treatments or new medicines or new ways to deal with the problems that the astronauts might have, because much of the early work will be done in animal models. One of the positive things that I worked on was establishing bioethical principles for using animals in the research program. We were the first Federal Agency to develop principles like these.

Chapter 16 Resources

Groups and web sites

Agricultural Research Service (ARS), www.ars.usda.gov/Careers.

American Association for the Advancement of Science (AAAS), Fellowships, 1200 New York Avenue, NW, Washington DC, 20005; www.aaas.org; phone: 202 326-6700; fax: 202-289-4950; e-mail: Fellowships@aaas.org.

American Association of Food Hygiene Veterinarians (AAFHV), www.AVMA.org/aafhv.

Animal and Plant Health Inspection Service (APHIS), www.aphis.usda.gov.

    APHIS vacancy announcements, www.aphis.usda.gov/mb/mrphr/vacancy.html; e-mail: Apphelp@aphis.usda.gov.

    APHIS Veterinary Biologics, http://aphisweb.aphis.usda.gov/bbep/vb.

    APHIS Veterinary Services Careers (VSC) Program, www.aphis.usda.gov > about> programs offices > veterinary services.

    APHIS Veterinary Services, www.aphis.usda.gov/vs; e-mail: VS_Content_Management@aphis.usda.gov.

American Veterinary Medical Association (AVMA), list of government agencies, www.avma.org > Member Resource Directory > Government agencies.

Center for Disease Control and Prevention (CDC), www.cdc.gov.

    CDC, Employment Information Service, CDC; Mail Stop K05, 4770 Buford Highway, Atlanta, GA 30341-3724.

    CDC, Epidemic Intelligence Service, 1600 Clifton Rd., NE, Mailstop E-92, Atlanta, GA 30333; www.cdc.gov > EIS; phone: 404-498-6110; fax: 404-498-6135; e-mail: eisepo@cdc.gov.

    CDC, Human Resources Management Office, 4770 Buford Highway, MS K-05, Atlanta, GA 30341-3724; www.cdc.gov/employment; phone: 770-488-1725; e-mail: hrcs@cdc.gov.

    CDC Job Information Center/Announcement Postings: Koger Center-Stanford Building, 2960 Brandywine Road, Atlanta, GA; cdcinfo@cdc.gov; phone: 770-488-1725 or 800-CDC-INFO.

Center for Drug Evaluation and Research, job announcements, www.fda.gov/cder/career.htm.

Center for Veterinary Medicine (CVM), see FDA.

Centers for Epidemiology and Animal Health (CEAH); www.aphis.usda/gov/vs/ceah; e-mail: nahms_web@aphis.usda.gov.

Cooperative State Research Education and Extension Service (CREES), Renamed to the National Institute of Food and Agriculture, see NIFA.

Environmental Protection Agency (EPA), www.epa.gov/epahome.

EPA Human Resources Offices, 1200 Pennsylvania Avenue, NW, Washington, DC 20460; phone: 202-260-3267.

EPA Job Hotline, www.epa,gov; e-mail: EPA-InternProgram@epa.gov.

Federal Information Center, www.usa.gov; phone: 800-688-9889.

Federal Information Exchange (FEDIX), www.fedix.fie.com.

Federal jobs, www.usajobs.gov

Federal Research Service, 7507 Pleasant Way, PO Box 1708, Annandale, VA 22003; info@fedjobs.com; phone: 703-914-JOBS or 800-822-5027; phone: 800-822-5027; fax: 703-281-7639; e-mail: www.fedjobs.com info@fedjobs.com.

Federation of American Scientists, Biosafety Levels, www.fas.org > programs > biosecurity.

FedWorld Information Network, www.fedworld.gov; phone: 703-487-4219.

File Resource Library Federal Job Openings listed by the Office of Personnel Management, http://hi-tec.twc.state.tx.us/fedjobs.htm.

Fish and Wildlife Service (FWS), job information, National Wildlife Health Lab, 6006 Schroeder Rd, Madison, WI 53711; www.fws.gov; phone: 608-271-4640; e-mail: Jobs@fws.gov.

Food and Drug Administration (FDA), 5600 Fishers Lane, Rockville, MD 20857; www.fda.gov or www.hhs.gov/about/regions/fdacer.html.

FDA Center for Veterinary Medicine (CVM), 7500 Standish Place, Rockville, MD 20855; Jobs: www.fda.gov > Science & Research > Science Career Opportunities. Other information, www.fda.gov > Animal and Veterinary and www.fda.gov > About FDA > Centers & Offices > About the Center for Veterinary Medicine.

FDA Commissioner's Fellowship, www.fda.gov/commissionersfellowships/default.htm; www.fda.gov > About FDA > Working at FDA > Fellowship, Internship, Graduate, & Faculty Programs; phone: 888-332-4473; e-mail: fdacommissionersfellows@fda.hhs.gov.

FDA job opportunities, www.fda.gov/jobs/positions08.html.

Food Safety and Inspection Service (FSIS), www.usda.gov/fsis and www.foodsafetyjobs.gov; e-mail fsis.careers@fsis.usda.gov; phone 800-370-3747.

FSIS fellowships, internships, and externships, www.fsis.usda.gov > Careers > Internships and Externships.

FSIS Personnel Operations Branch—Recruitment Examining Section, Butler Square West, 100 N Sixth St, Minneapolis, MN 55403; phone: 800-370-3747 or 612-370-2000; e-mail: fsis.careers@fsis.usda.gov.

National Aeronautics and Space Administration (NASA), www.nasa.gov >about > careers.

National Animal Health Emergency Response Corps (NAHERC), www.aphis.usda.gov > animal health/emergency management > naherc; phone: 301-734–8073; e-mail: NAHERC@aphis.usda.gov.

National Association of Federal Veterinarians (NAFV), 1910 Sunderland Place, NW, Washington, DC 20036-1608; www.nafv.net; phone: 202-223-4878; fax: 202-223-4877.

National Institute of Food and Agriculture (NIFA), www.nifa.usda.gov.

National Institutes of Health (NIH), www.nih.gov and www.aamc.org/research/adhocgp/aboutnih.htm.

NIH Recruitment and Employee Benefits Branch, Bldg 31, Rm B-3, C 15, Bethesda, MD 20892; www.jobs.nih.gov; phone: 301-496-2403; e-mail: odjobsweb@mail.nih.gov.

National Marine Fisheries Service (NMFS), www.nmfs.noaa.gov

National Marine Mammal Laboratory (NMML), 7600 Sand Point Way N.E., F/AKC3, Seattle, WA 98115-6349; www.noaa.gov; www.afsc.noaa.gov/nmml; phone: 206-526-4045; fax: (206) 526-6615; e-mail: nmml.information@noaa.gov.

National Oceanic and Atmospheric Administration (NOAA), 1305 East West Highway, Silver Spring, MD 20910, www.noaa.gov.

National Science Foundation (NSF), 4201 Wilson Blvd., Arlington, VA 22230; www.nsf.gov; phone: 703-306-1234.

NSF current vacancy listings, www.nsf.gov >about >career > vacancies; NSF human resources management, phone: 703 306-1182; NSF publications, www.nsf.gov/publications/ods.

Office of Personnel Management (OPM), 1900 E Street, NW, Washington, DC 20415; www.opm.gov; phone: 202-606-1800; OPM online applications, www.usajobs.opm.gov.

Public Health Service Commissioned Corps, www.usphs.gov.

Public Health Informatics Fellowship, www.cdc.gov/PHIFP; e-mail: phifp@cdc.gov.

US Agency for International Development (USAID), Office of Human Resources, Recruitment Unit; Room 671 SA-36 Washington, DC 20523-3609, or 1550 Wilson Boulevard, Room 658A SA-36, Washington, DC 20523-3607; www.usaid.gov; fax: 703-302-4095.

USAID application, USAID/BHR/ OFDA, Washington, DC 20523-0008; www.usaid.gov/careers/applicant.html; fax: 202-647-5269; USAID positions, www.usaid.gov/careers.

USAID fellowship, http://www.usaid.gov/careers/fellows and www.aaas.org >become a fellow.

US Department of Agriculture (USDA), www.usda.gov.

USDA vacancy announcements, www.usda.gov/da/employ.html.

US Department of Health and Human Resources (DHHS), job vacancies, www.hhs.gov/careers.

US Department of Veterans Affairs (VA), c/o Chief Veterinary Medical Officer, 810 Vermont Avenue, NW, Rm 15E, Washington, DC 20420; www.va.gov; phone: 202-273-8230.

USA Jobs, www.usajobs.gov; phone: 202-606-2525.

Books and articles

Burns, K, Training Program Brings Veterinary Pathologists to NIH. *JAVMA News*, February 1, 2009; 234(3): 306–307.

Chaddock, H. M., Veterinarians: Integral Partners in Public Health. (2007); available at www.aavmc.org/documents/ VWEACongressionalPaperPDF.pdf.

Commerce Business Daily, Subscription phone: 202-512-1800, Government Printing Office Stock Number 703-013-000007, List ID "COBD." http://cbdnet.gpo.gov.

Damp, D. V., *Book of US Government Jobs: Where They Are, What's Available, and How to Get One*, 10th ed (Bookhaven Press, 2008).

GAO, Government Accountability Office, Veterinarian Workforce: Actions Are Needed to Ensure Sufficient Capacity for Protecting Public and Animal Health. February 2009. GAO-09-178, a report to the Chairman, Subcommittee on Oversight of Government Management, the Federal Workforce, and the District of Columbia, Committee on Homeland Security and Governmental Affairs, US Senate.

Jacobs, C, Association Jobs: AVMA-GRD Agriculture Policy Analyst. *JAVMA*, March 15, 1990; 196(6): 858–859.

Rezendes, A., Government Revises Veterinary Medical Officer Standards. Veterinarians in Federal Government Earn More Recognition. *JAVMA News*, July 1, 2006.

Lauber, D., *Government Job Finder: Where the Jobs Are in Local, State, and Federal Government* (Planning Communications, 2009).

Liff, S., *Managing Your Government Career: Success Strategies That Work* (AMACOM Books, 2008).

Meeks, B., Animal Docs Fill Homeland Security Slots: From Farm to Fork, Veterinarians on the Agro-terrorism Frontlines, *MSNBC*, March 18, 2005; available at www.msnbc.msn.com/id/7200413.

Nolen, R.S., Animal Care faulted for lax oversight of problem dog breeders, *JAVMA News* 237(1), July 1,2010:8-10.

Sundlof, S.F., Need for Veterinarians in Biomedical Research, Comments by Stephen F. Sundlof, DVM, PhD., Director, CVM, FDA, for the AAVMC; Aug 2, 2007 Bethesda, Maryland; www.fda.gov > Science & Research > Science and Research Special Topics > Critical Path Initiative and www.fda.gov > Animal & Veterinary > News & Events > *FDA Veterinarian Newsletter* 2007 (XXII:IV).

Verdon, D., Vet blows whistle on slaughter practices. *DVM Newsmagazine*, Apr 1, 2010. Available at http://veterinarynews. dvm360.com.

17 CANADIAN GOVERNMENT JOBS

Provincial Governments

Every Canadian province has a variety of Ministries, which generate public policy. Nearly all the agriculture and public health ministries and agencies in Canada do employ veterinarians. Ministry names, job titles, and roles vary, but veterinary positions generally involve disease surveillance, veterinary expertise, and technology transfer. There may be considerable travel with some of the positions. Advancement within the provincial public service is possible, although it usually involves assuming more managerial and supervisory roles.

Catherine Filejski, DVM, MA, MEPA, PhD [ABD], Ontario Ministry of Health and Long-Term Care, provides insight into the daily work and pros and cons of working for provincial governments in Canada.

> I work for the Ontario Ministry of Health and Long-Term Care as a Veterinary Consultant. My situation is unusual, since I have three graduate degrees in international relations and diplomacy in addition to my DVM degree. In melding my international background with veterinary medicine, I occupy a fairly unique niche in public health policy development. My primary role is to provide specialized veterinary expertise in the development of zoonotic infectious disease prevention and control programs and policies. I work with a wide variety of government partners, ranging from staff in local public health units, to provincial and federal government colleagues, to representatives from the US and Mexico. For example, I just returned from an international conference on rabies, where I chaired the North American Rabies Management Plan meeting between representatives from various government agencies in the US, Mexico, and Canada. That was a lot of fun. Within my Ministry, I have also provided expert advice to the Chief Medical Officer of Health about pH1N1 influenza, which has been a huge issue over the past year.

Most veterinarians working for the provincial government have epidemiology degrees, including many of the staff that work with me, but my specific skill set is stakeholder management and intergovernmental relations, rather than epidemiology.

Working in public health means working in a continually evolving environment, and having the opportunity to make a significant contribution to the "big picture." While this can be a very high pressure environment, particularly in the midst of a major outbreak, it also allows you to broaden your professional horizons into the area of human medical issues, and there is always something new to learn about.

My work is definitely a desk job, which made me exhausted at first, as I came from a very busy, active surgical practice. Currently, I often spend 2 to 3 days a week going to other government offices or public health units, attending meetings and pulling together working groups, but I always do return to my desk.

In Ontario, we have 2 veterinarians in the Ministry of Health; one handles enteric zoonotic diseases and I handle non-enteric zoonotic diseases, like rabies, pH1N1, avian flu, Q Fever, and psittacosis (all the fun stuff!). We also have entomologists within our unit, who consult with us on diseases such as West Nile, Eastern Equine Encephalitis and Malaria.

There are a lot of options for veterinarians in government jobs, especially because of the increasing popularity of the "One Health" concept. In Canada, pay is often better in the entry level public health jobs than in the entry level CFIA Meat Hygiene or Animal Health positions in government. It may take a while to find the right position, but veterinarians who take the time to look will definitely find interesting opportunities with good pay.

Qualifications / To apply
Provincial government jobs require a DVM degree with a license to practice in the province. Postgraduate training or working knowledge in public policy, public health, epidemiology or zoonotic diseases is an asset. In agricultural ministry jobs, experience with food animals is desired.

Applicants for Ontario Public Service jobs do not have to be Canadian residents, however they must at least have a work permit allowing them to be employed in the province. Other provinces may have similar requirements.

Contact information for Canadian Government agencies is found on the AVMA web site (www.avma.org > My AVMA > Member Resource Directory > Government agencies). Also see the Canadian government web site at www.gc.ca. Look up provincial government web sites using a search engine and the words [government], [.ca] and the abbreviation of the provice (e.g., [.on] or [.sk]). Also see the Public Service Commission of Canada jobs website (http://jobs-emplois.gc.ca).

Pay and benefits received by veterinarians working for the Canadian government may be found in the Report on Veterinarians in Alternate Career Paths, available from the Ontario Veterinary Medical Association (www.ovma.org).

Federal Government

Many agencies of the Canadian government employ veterinarians, with jobs that somewhat parallel those in the US. See Chapter 16 for details, then investigate the Canadian agencies described below or look for others that may meet your interests. For example, the Canadian International Development Agency (CIDA, www.acdi-cida.gc.ca) is similar to USAID. Also see the quote from a Canadian livestock consultant in Chapter 5. Three major agencies that employ veterinarians are the Canadian Food Inspection Agency (CFIA), the Public Health Agency of Canada (PHAC), and Health Canada.

Canadian Food Inspection Agency (CFIA)

The Canadian Food Inspection Agency (CFIA; www.inspection.gc.ca) is an agency of Agriculture and Agri-Food Canada. CFIA has jurisdiction over packaging and labeling claims, and over seafood, as well as over public health inspections and all other food-related regulatory activities. Veterinarians are hired for two basic purposes in CFIA: animal health and meat hygiene. Some veterinarians may be "cross-utilized" between the two areas. The CFIA considers applications from all individuals who have legal status to work in Canada and does not give preference to Canadian citizens. Legal status to work in Canada is based on either Canadian citizenship permanent resident status, or possession of a work permit. Some positions require applicants to be bilingual in English and French.

Daily work

Animal health veterinarians go out to farms and investigate suspected diseases of international interest as reported by farmers and practicing veterinarians, and they monitor the paperwork submitted by practicing veterinarians who are certifying animals as fit for export. Their jobs involve traveling (in a government-owned car), taking blood samples, speaking to farmers' groups, examining individual animals and herds, and doing investigative work to trace back sick animals to their original owners. Animal health veterinarians often take blood samples from large numbers of sheep, cattle, pigs, and horses to monitor them for contagious diseases or for export purposes.

Meat hygiene veterinarians monitor the transportation and slaughter of animals destined to become food. Antemortem and postmortem inspections are performed. In Canada, as in the US, the veterinarian is assisted by several non-veterinarian inspectors who monitor every carcass and draw to the attention of the veterinarian any carcasses that are unusual. Animal health veterinarians may travel extensively each day, especially in western Canada, where farms and ranches are far apart.

Meat hygiene veterinarians tend to see some unusual lesions, which provides good experience in animal pathology. They may also see the first signs of any disease trends in farm animal populations. At some plants, the veterinarian may work a four-day week (with longer workdays). They are routinely required to work afternoon and midnight shifts, especially when inspecting poultry.

As in the US government, there is always plenty of paperwork. In both animal health and meat hygiene roles, pay scales are well-defined, and advancement means managing or supervising others. Both positions involve some telephone time with consumers and farmers. Public relations are an important part of the veterinarian's function.

Pros and cons

As with most US government jobs, the pros include good pay and benefits, regular hours, a predictable schedule, access to government library resources, and front-line experience in epidemiology and pathology. Cons include committee meetings, dealing with bureaucrats, the occasional adversarial relationship with industry—including meat plant management—and inadequate communication between headquarters and field.

To apply

New graduates may apply for entry level positions in either Animal Health or Meat Hygiene, often through an "inventory position" job advertisement on the Public Service Commission of Canada jobs website (http://jobs-emplois.gc.ca). The CFIA periodically accesses the applications received, and contacts applicants selected for further assessment. Screening involves security clearance checks and a full medical exam. The inventory process is used to create a pool of successful qualified applications, who are offered specific job positions as these become available.

Public Health Agency of Canada and Health Canada

Veterinarians may work for either of these agencies. The primary goal of PHAC is to strengthen Canada's capacity to protect and improve the health of Canadians and to help reduce pressures on the health care system. Health Canada is the Federal department responsible for helping Canadians maintain and improve their health, while respecting individual choices and circumstances. Health Canada also has a Veterinary Drugs Directorate, which is responsible for evaluating and monitoring veterinary drugs administered to food-producing and companion animals.

Positions in public health often require an additional degree in epidemiology, as described in the previous chapter. See www.phac-aspc.gc.ca. Also see the Ontario VMA report on Canadian veterinarians' incomes.

Chapter 17 Resources

AVMA, www.avma.org > My AVMA > Member Resource Directory > Government agencies.

Canadian Food Inspection Agency (CFIA), www.inspection.gc.ca.

    CFIA Food Production and Inspection Service, Nepean, Ontario, K1A 0Y9; phone: 800-442-2342 or 613-225-2342; Director of Human Resources phone: 613-952-8000, www. inspection.gc.ca.

Canadian Public Service Careers (partial list; other provinces similarly coded).

    British Columbia, http://employment.gov.bc.ca.

    Manitoba, www.gov.mb.ca/csc.

    Ontario, www.gojobs.gov.on.ca/Jobs.aspx.

    Ontario Ministry of Agriculture, www.omafra.gov.on.ca.

    Saskatchewan, www.agriculture.gov.sk.ca/careers; www.careers.gov.sk.ca.

Canadian Veterinary Medical Association, http://canadianveterinarians.net.

Health Canada, www.hc-sc.gc.ca.

Canadian International Development Agency, www.acdi-cida.gc.ca.

Public Service Commission of Canada, http://jobs-emplois.gc.ca.

Public Health Agency of Canada, www.phac-aspc.gc.ca.

Ontario Veterinary Medical Association, 2010 Report on Veterinarians in Alternate Career Paths, www.ovma.org; 1-800-670-1702.

18 THE UNIFORMED SERVICES

About 700 veterinarians work in the US uniformed services, which includes the military and the Public Health Service Commissioned Corps. These jobs can be in any state or overseas, but are concentrated in Maryland, Texas, and US possessions (e.g., Puerto Rico, Guam). To enlist in the armed forces you must be a US citizen or legal resident. To become an officer, you must be US citizen.

This chapter presents descriptions of a variety of US military positions. Since the specifics may change over time, be sure to get current information from your military recruiter. (*Note:* You may have to contact more than one recruiter because, as an example, some Air Force recruiters are unaware that veterinarians are hired as part of the Biomedical Sciences Corps.) Better yet, attend meetings where military veterinarians are present (e.g., the AVMA annual meeting) and ask them about how they like their jobs. Inquire about benefits; although the category of uniformed services has the lowest median income of any veterinary category, those reported statistics do not include benefits such as health insurance and vacation time.

A cautionary note from many people within the Army: "Be very careful of recruiters! They will tell you exactly what you want to hear!" That is somewhat true, in that recruiters can be vague and overly optimistic in describing how much control military veterinarians have over where they are stationed, compared with what military veterinarians actually reported. If you don't mind the lack of control over where you live and how often you move, the uniformed services are a great way to gain experience for future jobs and to get further education paid.

The Navy and Coast Guard don't directly hire veterinary officers. Veterinarians may be assigned to these facilities as part of the PHS Commissioned Corps (described later in this chapter). The US Army provides veterinary services to the Army, Navy, Air Force, and Marines as the Department of Defense (DoD) Executive Agent for Veterinary Services. To enter the US Army Veterinary Corps you must be a graduate of an accredited school of veterinary medicine in the US, or, if a graduate of a foreign veterinary school, have successfully completed certification by the Education Commission for Foreign Veterinary Graduates. You must also be licensed in at least one state in the US, the District of Columbia, or a US territory, such as Puerto Rico. Finally, you must pass a medical fitness examination and background security checks.

Not all military jobs require a full-time commitment. You can serve part-time duty and receive supplemental income of several thousand dollars. Contact information for part-time work with the Army and Air Force Reserves or National Guard is presented in the resources at the end of this chapter. See the GAO report 424 for comparative salary information.

Sample job benefits: Military veterinarian

> *Excerpt:* Benefits include Health Professions Loan Repayment of up to $120,000 over three years, which may be applied toward qualified veterinary school loans; paid continuing education, including master's degree and doctorate programs in public health, tropical medicine, virology, toxicology, pharmacology and physiology; 30 days of paid vacation/yr; no-cost or low-cost medical and dental care for you and your family.

Air Force

Veterinarians may apply to the Air Force as Public Health Officers (PHOs) in the Biomedical Sciences Corps. Their field of work, public health, focuses on disease control. Air Force veterinarians work in the area of human public health; they do not work on animals at all. (Army veterinarians work on any Air Force animals that need veterinary attention.) Air Force public health work can be a good stepping-stone to non-military jobs in public health (Chapters 15–16).

Initial assignments are for three years. The Air Force offers deployment "opportunities" (you're "selected"—you don't choose). PHOs are part of a preventive medicine team that goes into countries ahead of air crew flight lines to set up preventive medical and food safety programs for the troops. These assignments usually last no more than 90 days and can be as short as two to three weeks.

Daily work

Public health officers work on disease surveillance, zoonotic disease control, food inspection, and food facility sanitation. They basically help operate a public health department for their base. That work can involve sexually transmitted diseases, deployment medicine, immunizations, occupational medicine (ergonomics, hearing, and respiratory protection), or vector surveillance and control.

PHOs are in supervisory positions. They work with environmental and disease hazards during disasters and wartime situations. They may collect and analyze data from foreign countries and advise the military of potential health threats. PHOs may work with other health professionals in the areas of preventive medicine and epidemiology.

Communicable disease control includes gathering and analyzing epidemiologic data as well as assisting physicians in determining treatment and disease control. PHOs may gather information on medical factors that may affect the capability of military forces when they deploy, and recommend preventive measures. PHOs inspect dining facilities for proper food service standards.

Pros and cons

When you are recruited for an Air Force position, you can make a specific request to be stationed in one place. You are guaranteed to be placed there, but there's no guarantee you won't be moved at any time. From there, you can go to a variety of locations, based on your application or the needs of the Air Force. In general, you are moved about every three years. Although you can request a change in location, the needs of the Air Force come first. There are at most three PHOs at one facility. You cannot usually get assignments in Alaska, Hawaii, or overseas on your first assignment.

Qualifications / To apply

New graduates can apply. Air Force PHO veterinarians enter active duty as captains (unless they entered veterinary school after three years of undergraduate work, and don't have a BS, in which case they start as first lieutenants). After an initial course at the School of Aerospace Medicine in Texas (12 weeks of training focusing on public health; 4 weeks of basic military training), they are sent to their assignments.

After their first three years in the Air Force (first appointment), PHOs are strongly encouraged to get an MPH or another degree. The Air Force offers two ways to do so: either continue in the job and pursue the degree part-time (the Air Force pays 75 percent of tuition costs), or attend school full-time on a full Air Force scholarship, with some flexibility in choice of school. (They say you can apply anywhere you want, but they "assist" with that selection and have final say.) With either route is an obligation to "repay" your schooling with several years of work in the Air Force.

With your additional education, you may go into teaching, research, or a commander position in a hospital or clinic. See www.airforce.com > opportunities > healthcare > careers > biomedical sciences > allied health > public health officer.

Pay

Starting salary for a captain averages around $60,000 (2009) and varies based on experience and location (cost of living). There are additional stipends for housing and food (which are nontaxable), and full benefits such as medical and dental coverage and a retirement plan.

Army

The US Army Veterinary Corps (VC) hires veterinarians to provide veterinary public health capabilities through veterinary medical and surgical care, food and water safety, disease control, biomedical research and development, epidemiology, and management. The VC provides military veterinary expertise in response to natural disasters and other emergencies. They also provide services for pets of military personnel. All veterinarians enter the VC with at least the rank of captain. To qualify, you must be under 42 years old. If you are up to age 44, see the section on Public Health Service Commissioned Corps later in this chapter.

The Army Veterinary Corps conducts and oversees all Department of Defense veterinary missions in more than 40 countries. Most personnel in the US are located in Alaska, Hawaii, or Puerto Rico. Overseas, the majority of VC personnel are stationed in Germany, Italy, Spain, the UK, Turkey, Bahrain, Saudi Arabia, Sinai, Japan, Korea, Thailand, and Guam. They serve in three areas: research and development, food safety and defense, and animal medicine. Veterinarians played a large role in the Iraq war and continue to be posted there as well as in Afghanistan.

Army Public Health Command

The Army is combining some veterinary and human health operations. The Army Veterinary Command and the Army Center for Health Promotion and Preventive Medicine will merge to form the US Army Public Health Command as part of a larger reorganization of the Army's medical services. Some animal care, food safety, and food defense missions will be assigned to medical treatment facilities with preventive human medicine services. The command will implement a one-health approach to some of the Army's public health missions, and is scheduled to be operational in 2011. However, the Army states they anticipate neither significant additions nor reductions in staff, veterinary or otherwise. Veterinarians will continue to support their missions (i.e., do the same jobs)—clinical veterinary care, food safety and quality assurance, and animal disease prevention and control.

Daily work

New members of the VC must first spend 12 weeks at the Officer Basic Leadership Course. After military orientation and food inspection/public health courses (each lasting several months), Army veterinarians are assigned to work at a military base. First assignments generally include care of military working dogs and privately owned animals of military personnel at a veterinary treatment facility. Army veterinarians also give medical and surgical care to government-owned animals, including laboratory animals, marine mammals, or ceremonial horses. The Army is responsible for providing care to all working dogs and other animals for all the Departments of Defense—the Air Force, Navy, Marines, and Army. Only preventive medicine is done. They are also responsible for inspection of all meat that comes into the commissaries (military grocery stores). Human disease cases suspected to be of animal origin may require quarantines and epidemiologic investigations. The amount of time spent working in the base veterinary clinic versus doing meat inspection will vary with the needs of the location.

The Army veterinarian's duties may include public health education programs, stray animal control, and liaison with local disease control authorities or monitoring programs that identify the existence of zoonotic disease in wild animals. Veterinarians may also initiate and supervise pet-facilitated therapy programs. These programs include small animal screening for hospital visitation and therapeutic horsemanship.

The Army's mission requires operation in a field environment. In the event of a national emergency, the veterinarian helps protect the livestock industry, providing foreign countries with assistance in animal disease control, and providing emergency medical support in veterinary-related areas.

The Veterinary Corps also trains officers to provide support in areas of low-intensity conflict. In the past, special emphasis has been placed on training for deployment to areas of Central and South America and Asia. As conflict develops around the world, this emphasis can change.

Long-term overseas positions are also available. A year's assignment in the US is required before being sent overseas. On assignment in other countries, duties can include inspection of foods and commercial food establishments, public health support, herd health, and food animal medicine.

Higher-ranking officers or those who have completed further training may become instructors or supervisors of these programs. For example, one position would involve traveling around Europe as an inspector of dairy processing plants that sell dairy products to the military.

Another example position is an officer in charge of a veterinary services squad, responsible for preparing soldiers (technicians and food inspectors) to deploy anywhere in the world in support of US forces. Soldiers are prepared to move into the field and to establish and operate a food inspection and animal medicine program within 72 hours. Their primary mission is food inspection, with a secondary mission as first-line care for military working dogs.

Army veterinarians develop vaccines and antidotes to protect troops from the possible effects of biological and chemical warfare. Almost a third of all veterinary officers are engaged in biomedical and subsistence R&D for the military. Before entering biomedical research, or following initial assignments, veterinarians are offered an advanced training residency in laboratory animal medicine or pathology at one of several Army institutes. Approximately a third of veterinary officers have attained board certification.

Pros and cons

Army veterinarians have access to continuing education, including the pursuit of additional degrees. (However, training opportunities are limited to those that the military needs at that time.) There are long-term civilian training opportunities in public health, lab animal medicine, pathology, and a few clinical specialty slots with full pay and benefits. Army veterinarians can compete for specialized education in civilian institutions leading to graduate degrees in public health, laboratory animal medicine, veterinary microbiology, pathology, physiology, toxicology, pharmacology, and food technology, for example. Army preceptorship programs are also available in veterinary pathology and laboratory animal medicine.

Being in the Army means being flexible about moving to different areas of the country or the world. You can have fun with this, learning about and enjoying different cultures and interests. But you can also suffer, being placed in an area you don't enjoy, or moving more often than you'd like. According to one source, relocation is expected every 24–36 months. When moving to new assignments, payment of travel expenses and shipping charges for families and personal goods is provided.

You can request assignment to a certain country, but you aren't guaranteed placement there. Daily travel depends on your duty position; with that comes a per diem payment. Those veterinarians with a nonmilitary spouse may encounter marital stress due to the frequent moves and sometimes the travel requirements (daily or weekly travel).

The clinical medicine you will practice is basic preventive medicine; if you want to see a variety of cases, you most likely won't find that in the Army. In most cases, there are no emergency calls. You'll have limited animal work, endless paperwork, and potential for long-term deployments.

Qualifications / To apply

To apply, contact any regional Army medical recruiter, or go to www.goarmy.com or http://vetopportunities.amedd.army.mil.

All Army officers must complete a series of educational courses in their branch as well as in the management and command structures of the military as a whole. All medical branches (veterinarians, physicians, and dentists) spend several weeks in Fort Sam Houston, Texas. After that, all Veterinary Corps officers take a three-month course in Chicago (mainly learning food inspection).

To qualify for positions and promotions, VC officers take courses such as the Officers Advanced Course for AMEDS (Army Medical) officers. To be promoted to lieutenant colonel, they take the Command and General Staff Course. If they join a Civil Affairs Unit, they take additional courses in civil affairs. They can also take a number of courses on subjects of personal interest, such as marine navigation and ship handling. The Army encourages board certification for continued promotion.

Pay

Salaries and benefits are good and parallel those of the Air Force. Advancement in rank is competitive and based on a time scale. Pay increases are based on a published schedule. Retirement is available after 20 years with 50 percent of base pay and a 2.5 percent increase each year after 20 years, capped at 75 percent after 30 years. Board-certified specialists are paid extra.

Benefits include a 30-day paid annual vacation; all federal holidays off; regular hours (most of the time); convenient post exchanges and commissaries; medical benefits for you and your dependents; tax-free housing allowance or government housing provided in some military communities; tax-free food allowance; and more. Women report that health care during pregnancy and child-care quality are excellent. Access to officers' clubs, tennis courts, golf courses, swimming pools, libraries, theaters, hobby and craft shops, and other services may also be included.

Through the Active Duty Health Professions Loan Repayment Program, payments over three years may help repay veterinary school loans.

US Public Health Service Commissioned Corps

The Department of Health and Human Services (DHHS) Office of Public Health and Science (OPHS, www.hhs.gov/ophs and www.usphs.gov) includes the Commissioned Corps, a uniformed service of health professionals who serve at the DHHS and other federal agencies.

The Commissioned Corps is an all-officer organization that provides employment opportunities for health professionals and students. As part of the DHHS, the Commissioned Corps has officers assigned to all of the Public Health Services agencies and program offices. (See Chapter 16 and www.hhs.gov > about us > Organization chart.)

USPHS officers are most likely to be assigned to the CDC, EPA, FDA, or NIH. In addition, commissioned officers are also assigned to certain agencies outside the PHS, to help meet their health professional staffing needs. At the professional level, each agency that uses officers determines those positions best suited for a commissioned officer and seeks the most qualified candidates.

Individuals are commissioned in the corps for a career with the PHS rather than for a position in a particular program area. The initial assignment should provide experience and/or training that will prepare the officer for possible future assignments. Most positions that would be open to a veterinarian are in biomedical animal research or epidemiology. Typical positions include laboratory animal veterinarian, veterinary pathologist, epidemiologist, and regulatory veterinarian.

Veterinarians working in the Corps work on animal and human disease outbreaks; management of disease prevention and control programs; medical and biological research; drug regulation; and monitoring of vaccine development.

See the profiles in Chapter 16, under FDA and CDC, of veterinarians whose government careers have developed through the Commissioned Corps.

Daily work / Pros and cons

Regulatory veterinarians review and evaluate applications of new animal drugs, devices, food, food additives, and other chemicals intended for use in animals. They consider adequate labeling, the effects of various agents on animal systems, and questions of drug safety or effectiveness. They determine the need for revised labeling or withdrawal of a drug from the market, inform application sponsors of any deficiencies in their applications, and help to plan and implement various disease studies. Regulatory veterinarians can advance to supervisory positions that include more authority and autonomy, including serving as expert federal consultants to industry on drug approval policy.

The Corps is a great way to get an overview of potential government jobs. You can use this experience to move into a civilian federal job, or you can remain in the Corps for a long-term career. Many of the jobs you could get via the Corps are the same as those you could get as a civilian, so it's important to weigh the pros and cons of being a uniformed versus a civilian government employee (see government jobs, PHS in Chapter 16). The Corps may offer a higher or a lower salary, and different benefits, for the same type of work. View the informative "Comparison of Civil Service and Commissioned Corps," which is oddly positioned on the web site of the Indian Health Service of the DHHS (www.ihs.gov/jobscareerdevelop/navajojobs > Compare).

Two publications that address possibilities in veterinary public health care are a *JAVMA* article by Wohl and Nusbaum, and the WHO report, *Future Trends in Veterinary Public Health.*

Qualifications / To apply

Lower-level jobs require only a DVM; promotion requires more experience, and advancement to the highest level may require board certification or another advanced degree.

Staff epidemiologist or pathologist positions require an additional degree or residency. Note, however, that you must have completed only the coursework for an additional degree—you needn't have been awarded the degree itself. While having an additional degree will make you a more competitive applicant, nondegree applicants are considered on a case-by-case basis.

To be appointed, you must be under 44 years old, pass a physical examination, and be willing to be assigned wherever needed—although you are encouraged to get involved in the search for an appropriate position. All initial appointments are made to the Reserve Corps, and reserve officers serve a three-year probationary period.

Pay

The Commissioned Corps offers a base salary and benefits similar to those provided to officers in the other uniformed services: medical and dental coverage; low-cost life insurance; 30 days paid vacation each year; a noncontributory retirement plan; and travel, housing, and subsistence allowances.

Chapter 18 Resources

Groups and web sites

Air Force, Chief, Military Public Health, HQ USAF SGPA, Bolling AFB, DC 20332-5113; www.airforce.com; phone: 202-767-1838 or 800-423-USAF.

Air Force Reserve, http://afreserve.com; phone: 800-257-1212.

Air National Guard; NGB/DPR; Andrews AFB, MD 20331; www.ang.af.mil; phone: 301-981-8569.

Army, www.goarmy.com

National Guard Readiness Center, Attn: NGB-ARP-HN; 111 S George Mason Dr, Arlington, VA 22204- 1382; www.ng.mil; phone: 703-607-7145.

Army recruiter, USA PERSCOM, TAPC-OPH-VC, 200 Stovall St, Alexandria, VA 22332-0417; www.goarmy.com; phone: 703-325-2360 or 800-USA-ARMY.

Army Veterinary Corps; Chief, US Army Veterinary Corps, Attn: MCVS; 2050 Worth Rd, Ft Sam Houston, TX 78234-6000; http://vetopportunities.amedd.army.mil/index.html; phone: 210-221-8149 or 210-221-6564; e-mail: VSOpportunities@LN.amedd.army.mil.

US Department of Health and Human Services (DHHS), Office of Public Health and Science, www.hhs.gov/ophs.

US Public Health Service Commissioned Corps Recruitment, 1101 Wooton Parkway, Plaza Level, Rockville, MD 20852; www.usphs.gov; phone: 877-463-6327 or 800-279-1695.

USPHS Job announcements, http://dcp.psc.gov > jobs.

US Army Reserve, Attn: ARPC-OPS-MC Cdr, ARPERCEN 9700 Page Blvd, St Louis, MO 63132-5200; www.usar.army.mil phone: 314-538-2121 or 800-325- 4973.

Books and articles

Comparison of Civil Service and Commissioned Corps, www.ihs.gov/jobscareerdevelop/navajojobs > Compare.

Future Trends in Veterinary Public Health Report of a WHO Study Group. Technical report series No. 907 (World Health Organization, 2002). Available at http://libdoc.who.int/trs > WHO TRS 907.

GAO, Veterinarian Workforce: The Federal Government Lacks a Comprehensive Understanding of Its Capacity to Protect Animal and Public Health. Statement of Lisa Shames, Director Natural Resources and Environment. February 26, 2009. Testimony before the Subcommittee on Oversight of Government Management, the Federal Workforce, and the District of Columbia, Committee on Homeland Security and Governmental Affairs, US Senate, GAO-09-424T. Available at www.gao.gov/htext/d09424t.html.

Wohl, J. S, and K. E. Nusbaum, Public Health Roles for Small Animal Practitioners. *JAVMA*, February 15, 2007; 230(4): 494–500.

19 LONG-RANGE OUTLOOK AND FUTURE GOALS

> Veterinary medicine is integral to the well-being of any future society. This is a pivotal moment for the veterinary profession and for veterinary medical education. Leadership, collaboration, and a shared vision will determine the destiny of the profession.—N. Willis et al., The Final Report of the Foresight Project.

Veterinary medicine was named as one of the fastest growing fields by *Money* magazine (2009) and one of the 50 best careers by *US News* (2010). According to the AVMA Food Supply Veterinarian Medicine Coalition Report, the increase in national demand for veterinarians will increase 12 to 13 percent by 2016, with the shortage remaining at 4 to 5 percent annually thereafter. This is partly attributed to the restricted number of openings in veterinary colleges, with a total graduating class size of 2,700 new veterinarians in the US each year, as well as to the difficulty of non-US graduates to enter the US labor market. Retirement of the baby boomers is also predicted to create a void. However, this rosy outlook is countered by negative economic data. Opinions vary about whether such forecasts for demand are realistic.

Major issues facing the veterinary profession today include scope of practice, changes in the role of companion animals, veterinary student debt, income challenges, and diversity. Questions about supply and demand, particularly in food animal medicine, are topics of much debate. This chapter addresses those diverse challenges.

Scope of Practice

One medicine, one health

> Animal health is truly at a crossroads. Its convergence with human and ecosystem health dictates that the "one world, one health, one medicine" concept must be embraced. We need our colleagues in human medicine, public health, and the environmental health sciences. Together, we can accomplish more in improving global health than we can alone, and we have the responsibility to do so.—Roger Mahr, DVM, AVMA past president, in *JAVMA* (article by R.S. Nolen).

Veterinary medicine is no longer a world of the small animal and large animal veterinarian. Although veterinarians are uniquely capable of aiding in public health issues, they are not yet looked to as a primary source to fill these roles.

> One of the things I find shocking is when I go to these human public health conferences, I'm always asked, "What are veterinarians doing here?"—Charles M. Hendrix, DVM, PhD, AVMA past vice president, in *JAVMA* (article by R.S. Nolen).

The One Health Initiative is a movement to forge co-equal, all inclusive collaborations among physicians, veterinarians, and other scientific health-related disciplines. It has been endorsed by many major medical organizations and health agencies, including the AVMA, the American Medical Association, and the Centers for Disease Control and Prevention, among others. For details, see www.avma.org >Public health > One health; www.onehealthinitiative.com; and the related but separate www.oneworldonehealth.org.

As this idea gains momentum, veterinarians may find increasing opportunities in such fields as public health, biomedical research, and government service; international policy is also taking on a larger role. However, the number of job openings appears to be small (see Chapters 15-18).

The "one health" idea carries some potential conflicts of interest for veterinarians. Are we concerned about food animal producers (who may want to use growth-promoting daily antibiotics), or are we concerned about public health (and potential antibiotic resistance)? Food animal veterinarians may be at odds with veterinarians working with the FDA and CDC on some "one health" issues. Additionally, potential conflicts exist among MDs and DVMs defining "their" territory, with, so far, MDs winning out (holding more public health jobs, for example).

Doctor and technician roles

Scope of practice also includes the work that is done by veterinarians and veterinary technicians. The AVMA Biennial economic survey (2010) said:

> Employing technicians with greater skill sets would allow technicians to do work that otherwise might be performed by veterinarians, freeing veterinarians to perform work requiring a different degree of expertise or skill. The more work technicians are qualified to do, the more veterinarians can leverage their time within the practice, generating additional revenue. The normalized results indicated the average veterinarian's gross revenue would increase by $93,311 for each additional credentialed veterinary technician per veterinarian.

A strong partnership between veterinarians and technicians can allow doctors to focus on their skill set (diagnosing, prescribing and performing surgery). Also, as more veterinarians become specialists, so too the number of technician specialties and specialists is increasing (see Chapter 4). Chapter 5 includes a description of the potential increased role of technicians in food animal practice.

Technicians empowered to do the jobs they are trained for are more satisfied with their career choice. That, plus improved pay, may be the solution to a perceived shortage of veterinary technicians (which may be related to high numbers exiting the technician profession, rather than to inadequate numbers of technicians or technician schools).

Debate about who "owns" particular tasks varies with the economy; when veterinarians are busy doing work that requires a doctor, then the skills of a technician (nurse) become easier to discern. The difficult conversation involves defending territory versus a realistic evaluation of the training that is required to perform certain tasks. As with other debates, this one may be ultimately settled by the public and the economy, and not by veterinarians themselves.

A look at the literature in human medicine reveals a parallel debate as nurses with varying credentials have been awarded greater responsibility over the years. The trend in human health care for diverse roles of paraprofessionals may serve as a model, for both desired and undesired outcomes, should the veterinary profession be so bold as to lead this change rather than react to it. A newspaper article by D. Yetter stated

> Registered nurse practitioners say they are able to increase access to health care and make it more affordable... advocates for nurse practitioners say it is these primary care nurses who will make up for the shortage of primary care physicians and at the same time keep the costs down.

The article quoted a registered nurse practitioner:

> None of us are trying to play doctor. If we had wanted to be doctors, we'd have gone to medical school.

A likely future scenario is that, like nurses, veterinary technicians may fill a wider variety of roles, with many states modifying their practice acts and continually redefining the roles and responsibilities of credentialed technicians. For example, the New Hampshire VMA is considering having a category of licensed food animal technicians, as outlined in a 2010 *JAVMA* article by G. Cima:

> The state veterinary practice act requires that veterinarians arrange to provide emergency coverage for clients... fellow veterinarians realize they would be on call continuously if they open mixed animal practices in these areas.

Different stances are taken by different states regarding who can perform dentistry, chiropractic and massage therapy in large and small animals (Chapters 3-5). These debates and discussion of other potential roles for veterinary technicians are outlined in the book, *Career Choices for Veterinary Technicians*, by Rose and Smith. (For legal details, refer to each state's Veterinary Practice Act.)

Human Medicine as a Harbinger of the Veterinary Future

Observing trends in human medicine can provide a wake-up call to veterinarians for the future. One such trend is the use of insurance to cover health care costs. The number of companies offering pet health insurance is growing continually, as is the debate about the pros and cons of such coverage.

Another trend is that pet food and pharmaceutical companies have increasing influence in the veterinary schools and at veterinary continuing education meetings, both of which receive significant funding from such companies. As government funding for research at academic institutions dwindles, and large companies are relied upon to provide research and scientific papers, the perception of the public is that the profession will lose objectivity in evaluating new diagnostic and treatment regimens. Conflict of interest is greatly underestimated by many in the veterinary profession, who assume that good intentions and honesty will solve the problem.

> Physicians and industry have a shared interest in advancing medical knowledge. Nonetheless, the primary ethic of the physician is to promote the patient's best interests, while the primary ethic of industry is to promote profitability. Although partnerships between physicians and industry can result in impressive medical advances, they also create opportunities for bias and can result in unfavorable public perceptions. Many physicians and physicians-in-training think they are impervious to commercial influence. However, recent studies show that accepting industry hospitality and gifts, even drug samples, can compromise judgment about medical information and subsequent decisions about patient care.—S. Coyle, Ann Intern Med 2002.

Acknowledging conflict of interest, rather than denying its existence, provides the clearest path toward reducing its impacts. The profession will gain by being proactive rather than waiting to react to increasing pressure by the public. One example of the latter is the passage of the 2010 Physican Payment Sunshine Act, which requires annual reporting of any gifts (money, food, travel, or any item) over a cumulative value of $100 made to physicians or physicans groups by any company. (See www.prescriptionproject. org, and Weintraub, Kaiser News.)

Editors of some of the world's top medical journals have recently agreed to standardize their requirements for authors to disclose conflicts of interest to include financial and nonfinancial relationships and affiliations.

Of course, good work and research is done by many companies. Many argue that it is impossible to turn down opportunities to learn from and partner with industry, especially when there truly is a breakthrough that can move veterinary medicine forward. Full disclosure is not the same as forbidding partnerships; at the same time, disclosure alone is not always sufficient.

One example of the fine lines among these issues is the recent creation of medical guidelines for management of various diseases (e.g., by the AVMA, AAHA and the AAFP). Although funding is provided by various companies, the associations choose independent experts to write the documents without allowing any company to actively participate. For such guidelines to be well-respected by both veterinarians and pet owners, the process of their creation must be as "clean" as possible, and guided by medical evidence published in peer-reviewed journals. Useful resources include the Evidence-based Veterinary Medicine Association (www.ebvma.org) and the US Preventive Services Task Force (www.ahrq.gov > Clinical Information > Prevention and Care Management > US Preventive Services Task Force).

Publication of such guidelines has highlighted the dearth of evidence regarding disease incidence and treatment outcomes in veterinary medicine. The small size of most veterinary practices, combined with a lack of a consistent medical record keeping system among them, has made comparison among practices nearly impossible. Unfortunately, although such information has been compiled by some corporate veterinary practices, it remains proprietary and is not available for general reading. The recent adoption of a shared nomenclature is the first step towards gathering useful information (see Chapters 9 and 10).

The Changing Role of Pets

The veterinary profession in the US and Canada remains one dominated by companion animal practice (Table 19.1, at end of chapter). Of particular significance to the long-range outlook for private practice is the changing perception of the role of pets in family life (see Helms article in *JAVMA*). Over the last 50 years, the dog has moved from the backyard, to the house, to the bedroom. Where it was once a challenge to get pet owners to vaccinate their pets regularly, people are now having brain surgery performed on their beloved "family members."

New issues arise as the definition of a pet is challenged. Will society continue to define a pet as property, giving sole custody to the owner? Or will the relationship between animal and human be redefined as one of "guardian"? What will animals' rights be in the future?

The law in the US and Canada recognizes animals as property dependent on people for basic care, and thus "damages" to animals are generally limited to their value as property. If that legal definition changes, veterinarians will find themselves increasingly exposed to liability, including being scrutinized for their treatment of animals or for failing to report animal abuse. This may bring about more lawsuits and increased liability insurance costs. The profession must be proactive in facing these issues. The public, as much or more than the veterinary profession, will ultimately make these decisions.

Diversity Issues

Although gender certainly falls under the category of "diversity," the gender shift (toward increasing numbers of female veterinarians) has overshadowed a more troubling fact: The veterinary profession does not reflect the diversity of society today. Efforts to increase discussion and action about diversity have increased recently, although discussion seems to be more prevalent than action. The Association of American Veterinary Medical Colleges (www.aavmc.org) has a committee on diversity; the Association of

Women Veterinarians Foundation is a diversity partner with AAVMC. There is a Lesbian and Gay Veterinary Medical Association, and an Association of Medical Professionals with Hearing Losses which includes veterinarian members, but no associations of Latino, Asian American, or African American veterinarians (although a Facebook™ group for the latter was created in 2009).

Colleges of veterinary medicine have begun to address diversity. For example, in 2005, the AAVMC launched *DiVersity Matters*—an initiative to increase diversity among students, faculty, and leadership of the US Colleges of Veterinary Medicine (see www. aavmc.org/DVM). A few veterinary internships have been set aside for minority or "underrepresented" groups. Four such internship slots were found during a search of the VIRMP web site (www.virmp.org, accessed 4/7/2010).

As with other hot topics, it is critical to not make assumptions about the causes of this lack of diversity; doing so can waste enormous time and resources "fixing" problems before a real diagnosis is made. A great deal of social science research addresses the origins of and influences on individual career choice among young people of different backgrounds. Examining such work can help guide the course of future action.

Economic Challenges

One of the greatest challenges facing the profession is whether graduating students are able to earn the salaries they need to pay off student loans (see Table 19.2 at chapter end). Rapidly increasing tuition costs are one cause that is not limited to veterinary schools. However, for veterinarians the average debt upon graduation is about double the average starting salary (see Chapters 1 and 2). When adjusted for inflation, student debt load has increased more than three times faster than starting salaries over the last 21 years. (See *JVME* article by N. Kieves.) Mean educational debt among those with debt was $133,873 in 2010. Excluding salaries for graduates pursuing advanced study, mean full-time starting salary was $67,359 (AVMA).

Still, the return on investment (ROI) for a veterinary degree is not the same as the starting salary. Debt may be viewed as an investment, and the DVM degree arguably has a good long-term rate of return. Nonetheless, debt constitutes a real expense for new graduates.

The increase in numbers of students entering internships provides a further negative influence on both short-term and long term income, with data to date showing the lost income during that internship year not being recouped by higher earnings (See L. Choca's article in *Trends*, AVMA data in *JAVMA*, and Chapter 2). If the internship becomes a standard for all new graduates, that has a profound effect on the economics of the profession overall.

Economics of companion animal practice

It is easy to recognize the increasing importance of pets in family life, but the number of pets per family and the growth of the pet population in relation to the growth of the graduating veterinary pool are worthy of inspection.

According to the American Pet Products Association (APPA, www.americanpet-products.org) biennial survey of pet owners, the percentage of the US population who owned a pet rose from around 52 percent in 1988 to 62 percent in the year 2000; since then it has ranged up and down from 61 percent to 63 percent of households—staying steady, but not growing further.

The fact that pet care is not free—pet owners must pay directly for animal health care—is another factor that drives change. As veterinary care becomes viewed as a "right" and a "necessary expense," alternatives such as insurance and creative credit options are being explored and debated. The NCVEI and AAHA have published guides to pet health insurance.

So-called "compliance studies" by AAHA and AVEPA (Spain) have shown that pet owners are increasingly willing to spend money on their pets whenever the veterinarian offers a clear and honest recommendation for each pet. Nonetheless, during the economic downturn of 2008–2010, many practices had stagnant growth, and job offers for new graduates decreased. In 2008, of the graduates who reported the number of job offers received, 57.8% received 2 or more job offers; in 2010, that had dropped to under 40% (AVMA data).

One topic of debate is whether companion animal medicine is saturated with veterinarians. The recession revived discussion of mergers and other cooperative business models. Despite reports of practices becoming larger, the average practice still consists of two veterinarians. The situation of redundant hospital resources that has existed (and been decried) for decades still exists. For example, radiographic equipment sits unused for the majority of the day in practices all over the country, but competing practices refuse to pool resources. Few practices are busy enough to have to turn away new clients. Many do not utilize veterinary technicians to their fullest (which might reveal decreased need for doctor time, i.e., decreased demand). Nonetheless, well-managed practices do exist and are quite successful.

Another question is whether the increasing percentage of minority-group households in the US may affect veterinary income, since certain minority groups appear to spend less on veterinary care. (See Wolf et al, in *JAVMA*).

A final topic of concern is whether there is a decreased interest in practice ownership, and if that is the case, what are its causes? As with other debates, this one is confounded by a lack of good data. Surveys of people's intentions are commonly cited but are not an accurate reflection of their actions. Practice brokers report that sales of good practices (those that have value in a business sense) continue to do well. Young veterinarians are learning that practice ownership results in higher incomes, and with increasing concern about debt, many of these doctors may decide to become owners.

Increasing business knowledge

One action to diminish economic challenges is educating students on business and life skills through programs such as the Business Certificate Programs at the University of Pennsylvania and the University of Minnesota. Many students are taking their future into their own hands, as is shown by the student-created Veterinary Business Management Association, which is active in many schools (www.vbma.biz).

It is not just students who need to appreciate the business side of veterinary medicine. Private practitioners must also begin to run their clinics as a business if they are going to survive and prosper. At the same time, they must be aware of client perceptions of whether the emphasis is on medical care or on profit only. Good medical care does result in a good income, so ethical veterinarians can be good at business while focusing on good medical care and client communication.

Some veterinarians and students are pursuing MBAs to supplement their DVM degrees. While the MBA might provide additional knowledge, it is not clear that it provides a significant advantage to those in private practice.

Gender and economics

The veterinary profession has seen a profound shift from being primarily a male profession to one that is primarily female. Discussions of economics often drift into gender issues, with some stating that perceived "shortages" in rural or food supply medicine would be solved if only veterinary schools could attract more students who are male and/or from rural backgrounds. There is no clear evidence to show that lack of such students is the cause of this "shortage," nor any evidence that attracting such students would abate such expressed need. Where there is no feasibility of economic survival, neither men nor women will provide services. One study, by A. Villarroel et al in *JAVMA*, actually showed few differences between men and women on reasons for getting into or for leaving rural practice.

There is a gender income gap in veterinary medicine, though, as in other professions. Because the profession is becoming dominated by women, it becomes more difficult to compare income by gender. Instead, the issue returns to the economics of the entire profession, compared with professions that require similar education. Historically, men have dominated higher-paying professions among those that require equivalent education. (See articles by C. Smith.)

The veterinary profession has responded to these issues by creating ongoing discussions and forums for sharing information. One example is the National Commission on Veterinary Economic Issues web site (www.ncvei.org,), where veterinarians can view and share financial data from their practices. The AVMA and AAHA publish regular financial data that includes gender comparisons.

Loan forgiveness programs

The federal government and many states are sponsoring economic aid and loan forgiveness programs. The approval of such programs and their funding are separate steps; the question of funding is usually revisited each year. Most if not all of these programs are targeted towards the small percentage of students who have an interest in food animal medicine or public health, or who agree to work in underserved areas.

The FSIS has instituted loan repayment programs and recruitment bonuses of significant value for those who agree to work in government food safety jobs (see Chapter 16).

The Veterinary Medicine Loan Repayment Program (VMLRP) provides student debt relief to veterinarians who agree to practice in designated veterinary shortage situations (food animal and/or rural areas; see Chapter 2). The Veterinary Public Health Education and Workforce Act proposed a competitive grant program to veterinary schools to be used for facility expansion, curriculum development, or faculty. It also would create a fellowship program with the DHHS and would create a new Division of Veterinary Medicine and Public Health at the Health Resources and Services Administration.

The Veterinary Services Investment Act would provide grants to relocate or recruit veterinarians and veterinary technicians into shortage areas, and support veterinary students seeking training in food-supply veterinary medicine (www.avma.org >press releases).

Food Supply, Rural, and Large Animal Medicine

Food animal welfare

The issues that arise regarding food animal welfare were highlighted with the release of a 2008 report from the Pew Charitable Foundation: *Putting Meat on the Table: Industrial Farm Animal Production in America*. The Pew report acknowledged that current production methods decrease costs and increase the consistency and amount of food produced. Yet, according to the report, "one of the most serious unintended consequences of industrial food animal production is the growing public health threat of these types of facilities." The report went on to discuss animal welfare with regard to confined food animals.

The response to this report highlighted the potential conflicts of interest among "veterinarian as an advocate for the farmer," "veterinarian as a public health advocate," and "veterinarian as a leader in animal welfare." The AVMA responded to the Pew report with outraged indignation, describing it as

> a prolonged narrative designed to romanticize the small, independent farmer. . . . While we believe there is value in some of the recommendations offered by the Pew Commission . . . the Pew report contains significant flaws and major deviations from both science and reality.

The AVMA and the Pew Foundation are both reputable groups that have good scientists and veterinarians working with them. In whatever manner one might debate individual points from either side, it is clear that the AVMA (and thus the veterinary profession) may lose ground in its desired position as a respected voice in public health and animal welfare, if it is not able to bridge these differences.

Supply and demand: Shortage?

According to the Foresight Report cited at the beginning of this chapter,

> The current number of veterinarians is inadequate to address the present and future needs of society. To remain relevant, academic veterinary medicine must prepare veterinarians for what may come in the future.

Data and opinions vary, however, about whether such forecasts for demand are realistic. The veterinary literature abounds with discussions of a veterinarian shortage in fields such as food supply and rural practice, and of the need for veterinarians to work in public health. Although the total number of veterinarians in these fields is fairly small, their importance to disease control and global health is quite high.

Chapter 5 presented the definitions of rural, mixed animal, large animal, and food animal veterinarians. These definitions and the distinctions among them are important because of the dramatic differences in supply, demand, and income for each. For example, mixed animal practitioners have some of the lowest incomes in the profession, whereas 100 percent food animal veterinarians earn some of the highest incomes (see Table 3.2 in Chapter 3).

The discussion over interconnected issues such as economics, public health, and food supply veterinarians are confounded by the use of vague terms, such as "demand" and "need," that are poorly understood.

Supply: The quantity of a good or service available for sale.

Demand: The desire for a good or service supported by the possession of the necessary means of exchange to effect ownership.—*Economist Dictionary of Economics.*

Need: A necessary duty; a lack of something desirable or useful.

Shortage: A lack or deficit.—*Merriam Webster's Online Dictionary*

Actual demand requires that there is a "buyer with the necessary means of exchange," that is, a large number of actual job openings for which a veterinary degree is required and which provide professional-level pay. For example, although there is agreement in the profession that more veterinarians are needed to fulfill the concept of "One Health" (e.g., in public health), the number of job openings to fill that need is uncertain. Additionally, many of these positions require additional training beyond the DVM degree, yet the pay may not be sufficient to attract many to that career path.

Likewise, although many rural areas "need" a veterinarian, there are often not significant numbers of job openings or waiting clients to be able to support a veterinarian. Some areas of the country with large numbers of livestock are not served by any veterinarian at all. Livestock owners in those areas may individually feel the need for a veterinarian, but sufficient work may not be available to support a veterinarian in the area.

Shifts in global agriculture have profoundly impacted the veterinary profession. Current data suggest a decrease in demand for food animal veterinary services. For example, the numbers of cattle, hogs, breeding sheep, and turkeys in the US have all declined (see Chapter 5). In 2008, US cattle feeders lost more money on average for each animal sold than at any other time in history. Low milk prices are contributing to a decrease in the number of dairies, while research continues to increase milk production per cow.

Veterinary herd health is replacing individual animal care. As veterinarians become consultants to industry, their role widens to include issues such as animal welfare, risk management, and environmental impacts of food animal waste. However, agribusiness has consolidated to the point that very few veterinarians are needed to serve a large number of animals. Lay personnel perform basic tasks such as pregnancy diagnosis on larger production facilities. Arguably, much of the need for health care services could be supplied by veterinary technicians.

Recent reports from new graduates point to a dearth in openings in food animal or mixed practices. Several letters to *DVM Newsmagazine* during 2009 were from recent graduates who were confused about the talk of a shortage when they could not find jobs. More recent anecdotal reports from the 2010 graduating class also state that new grads were not able to find desired positions in food or mixed animal practice. There is discussion of many rural practices that are for sale with no buyer, and others that have advertised for associate veterinarians without finding someone to fill that position. However, it is less clear whether a perceived lack of buyers is due to an actual buyer shortage, to tightening of credit, or to practice valuations that are not appealing to the buyers who are shopping. (See www.vetpartners.org for the No-Lo™ Practice Valuation Worksheet.)

A search on the AVMA Veterinary Career Center (VCC) web site (www.avma.org/jobs/default.asp, on 10/24/09) with the criteria "veterinarian," "food supply," "any species," and "any location" yielded only one job announcement, for a mixed animal practice in North Dakota. Using instead the criteria of "any/all cattle, swine, and/or poultry," the search revealed 16 ads, 14 for mixed practice and only two for food-animal only. This was in contrast to 15 "association" positions, most of which reflected openings at animal shelters; 17 ads for academia; and more than 250 openings in private practice (40 of those with a single large corporate practice). (It is currently not possible to search for "public health" jobs on the VCC site.)

Food animal veterinarians counter that company or industry jobs are often posted with specific interest groups rather than on general sites such as that of the AVMA. Might those who desperately need veterinarians broaden the places they place their ads? APHIS, but not FSIS, places ads on the VCC site. The AVMA and AABP are members of a group called the Veterinary Career Network, which shares job databases. A search on the AABP web site (www.aabp.org) revealed a list of 20 job openings, of which only 2 were 100 percent bovine and the rest were mixed animal practices. Likewise, the ARV web site jobs (www.ruralvets.com) are nearly all for mixed animal practices (see also Chapter 5).

Government positions may be advertised only on government web sites. The FSIS welcomes applicants at any time. In 2008, the USDA-FSIS reported 100 open positions for veterinarians, with "no change foreseen in the near future." However, most of those positions were filled when the FSIS began to offer more recruitment bonuses.

Responding to "need"

Responses to any shortage or need via the knee-jerk reaction of attracting more students to public health or food animal practice will not be effective if those students end up in small animal practice due to economic necessity.

Focusing on students (supply) rather than on the demand side could divert unnecessary energy that might otherwise be better used. From an economic perspective, there is little evidence that one can create demand by increasing supply.

Furthermore, it is questionable whether it is cost effective to design entire programs at veterinary schools to address food supply or public health veterinary shortages when the total number of those jobs is tiny (in the hundreds) in proportion to about 90,000 total veterinarians in the US.

This is a book about jobs. Thus, when we describe a "need," we are speaking of an economic need where specific job openings are waiting. Unless they receive government support, positions for food supply veterinarians require a sufficient client base to pay a living wage, not just people and animals that, as individuals, do not have ready access to a veterinarian. Public health, biosecurity, and zoonotic concerns, while real, require government funding to create specific positions that veterinarians can actually fill.

The problem is not lack of interest

Some decry the "lack of student interest" in public health or food supply medicine, yet there is no evidence that this is a cause of the low number of veterinarians in those positions.

What's more, many of those showing initial interest in those paths will change focus during school or shortly after graduation. One study, by M. Jalinski in the *Canadian Veterinary Journal,* compared veterinarians' career interests over time from pre-veterinary through graduation, postgraduation, and the present; the interest in small animal practice doubled over that time, with corresponding decreases in interest about food animal and mixed animal practices.

Many students change their minds about their career paths while still in school; the most important reasons cited were "exposure to other choices," "anticipated on-call demands," and "could not efficiently pay off debt" (Osborne). Students who are initially enthusiastic about entering rural and/or mixed practice often change their goals when they graduate and must pay their bills as well as their loans. For many, the combination of work hours and pay don't add up.

In a study published in *JAVMA* by A. Villarroel et al., the main reasons cited for leaving rural practice were "practice atmosphere" and "practice location." D. Osborne's study in *Focus* showed that 50 percent of those who entered large animal practice had left it after five years. The 2010 Report on Veterinarians in Alternate Career Paths, from the Ontario Veterinary Medical Association (www.ovma.org), found that almost half of those who left mixed animal practice did so because they wanted fewer work hours; 37% left due to stress.

Is the nation at risk?

The outcome of the discrepancy between need and realistic job openings is summed up in one article that addresses the shrinking number of veterinarians in rural areas:

> A shortage of those frontline veterinarians who discover and control livestock diseases could mean economic disaster for producers and the industries that carry the product to the end user.—C. Dumas.

In another article addressing public health needs:

> The impact of veterinary medicine on national security, the national economy, and international trade is also far-reaching. For example, all [the greatest] threat agents are zoonotic. These challenges, combined with the fact that veterinarians are the only health professionals trained in multispecies medicine, present an unparalleled opportunity to provide a bridge between agriculture and human medicine.—H. Chaddock.

Finally, in a Government Accountability Office report:

> "The federal government lacks a comprehensive understanding of the sufficiency of its veterinarian workforce. Four agencies . . . have identified current or future concerns: APHIS, FSIS, ARS, and the Army. Current and future shortages, as well as noncompetitive salaries, were among the concerns identified by these agencies. . . there is no government-wide effort to search for shared solutions, even though 16 of the 24 federal entities that employ veterinarians raised concerns about the sufficiency of this workforce.—GAO 09-424.

Future Goals

Economics

Since the first edition of this book was written, the US economy has undergone significant changes—from the recovery from the recession of the 1980s to the tech-stock bubble of the late 1990s, to the huge economic gains, increasing personal debt, and housing bubble of the early 2000s, to the economic crisis beginning in 2008. Two key studies performed near the turn of the century lend perspective to historical thinking: The NCVEI Current and Future Market for Veterinarians outlined the future forecast as of 1999; the 2005 AVMA-Pfizer Business Practices Study, by J. Volk et al., raised questions about veterinarians' business acumen.

Private practice veterinarians are taking on the challenge of learning business principles, and they must temper that with continual attention to client service and quality medical care. Pet owners have access to more information than ever before, and will resist any perception they have of being "sold to" rather than "informed about" medical care for their pets. Veterinarians must do more than just raise their fees to increase their incomes—instead, attention to good business practices and basing medical recommendations on evidence-based medicine will help ensure continued trust from their clients.

Underserved areas

In order to recruit, maintain, and actively engage new graduates in underserved or critical areas, government support may be required. If the goals of maintaining public health and keeping the food supply safe require veterinary expertise (versus veterinary technician expertise), then such funding must be targeted towards creating sufficiently-paid jobs for which a veterinary degree is required.

A broader perspective is helpful about the need for *any* kind of services in rural areas, from human medical facilities to ministries, which have trouble recruiting professionals. (See articles in *Time* magazine by D. VanBiema, in the *Journal of Rural Health* by G. Barley, and in the *Journal of the American Board of Family Practitioners* by K. Ellsbury.) According to L. Clark in a *Washington State Magazine* article:

> Over the last 20 years, the number of health care students in the US choosing primary care careers in rural areas has dropped precipitously due to a number of factors: lower compensation, professional isolation, limited time off, and lack of respect and prestige among peers.

With regard to the need for veterinarians in rural areas, as has happened in human medicine, perhaps communities may begin to work together to create incentives to attract their own veterinarians. However, we could find no examples of that occurring.

An additional approach is to assist and encourage non-US veterinary schools to pursue accreditation, which might provide for additional qualified veterinarians to work in the US. However, reactions to immigration since 2001 have made it more difficult to enter the country for work. Furthermore, there has been a paradoxical negative reaction by some parties regarding the University of Mexico's veterinary school working towards US accreditation—this in spite of the fact that the US accreditation body has considered schools outside the US for 60 years. (See the *JAVMA* articles by M. Larkin.)

Finally, a novel approach might be to reconsider the "need," as described by John Albers, DVM, in a 2009 article in *Trends magazine*:

> I firmly believe that, in order to meet today's challenges, we need to get away from the idea that meeting society's needs automatically means producing more veterinarians.

Veterinary schools

During 2009, AAVMC organized and launched the North American Veterinary Educational Consortium (NAVMEC; www.navmec.org). This consortium is holding national discussions on several important questions in planning the future of veterinary medical education. What is meant by meeting societal needs, and what knowledge, skills, and competencies should all new graduates of veterinary medical colleges possess at graduation to ensure societal needs are met? What are different educational models that will prepare all new graduates to meet societal needs?

One problem is that schools must prepare future veterinarians for passing the National Board Examination. The North American Veterinary Licensing Examination (NAVLE), in turn, is meant to protect the public from harm, and thus focuses on traditional veterinary practice. With this criterion as a main focus of our teaching hospitals, veterinary students may find it difficult to discover and prepare for options beyond private practice.

What additional skills and knowledge will give students an edge? While employers emphasize nontechnical skills such as business management and communication, veterinary school faculty aren't strong supporters of teaching such skills. A 2010 *JAVMA* article by I. Lane found that

> The disconnect between faculty perspectives and employer or alumni needs regarding business and leadership skills is striking. . . In regard to fostering business acumen, teaching faculty also may be losing touch with veterinary student needs. . . Weak support was also apparent for coaching and leadership skills in veterinary graduates. . . Despite the importance of economic issues facing livestock owners and large animal veterinarians, there was low support for development of business skills by (faculty) large animal veterinarians as well.

New models for veterinary teaching hospitals include partnerships with private practice, as is exemplified by the veterinary teaching hospitals in Southern California and in Mexico City. While many universities experience shortages of certain specialists, many are also not ready to accept this paradigm as a new approach to teaching. (See M. Larkin's articles in *JAVMA*, and www.westernu.edu > colleges > veterinary medicine). Other teaching models discussed by NAVMEC are outlined by M. Larkin in *JAVMA*.

Action steps

Actions our associations might take

- Take the "high road" with any debates, and particularly with conflict of interest areas. Focus on evidence, even when that means shifting the association stance on issues.
- Become proactive leaders in creating expanded and defined roles, responsibilities, and expertise requirements for veterinary technicians and other skilled paraprofessionals to help fill the needs of society.
- Honestly evaluate the influences that cause the high attention paid to a need for food production veterinarians. Who benefits from the emphasis on having veterinarians fill this need? Acknowledge and address the fact that many veterinary schools and governmental agencies rely on this "need" for their continued funding. How can they survive under a different paradigm?

Actions employers might take

- Establish externships for students and for veterinarians to learn about different careers. The sooner students are exposed to new career paths, the sooner they can become passionate about them and embrace them fully. They can also gain invaluable hands-on experience that will help them get jobs in the more obscure sectors.
- Re-examine job descriptions and considering the wide array of positions that veterinarians may fill. Veterinarians have a wide variety of skill sets, many of which are frequently overlooked.
- Lobby more strongly for funded programs to provide veterinarians in areas of need.

Actions veterinary teaching hospitals might take

- Align pre-veterinary requirements with general knowledge needed for all career paths in veterinary medicine. These areas might include business, sociology, communications, and psychology, as well as the basic sciences. (The argument that students "won't take" these courses doesn't fly; they will take what is required to apply to veterinary school.)
- When working to attract students who might show interest in underserved areas, balance the numbers of such students and the amount of the curriculum to the actual job demand.
- Use caution when considering any attempt select the "right" individuals based on aptitude, personality or behavioral traits. Rely on recent, peer-reviewed and statistically-valid studies to evaluate the effectiveness, or lack thereof, regarding predictive tests for performance and behavior.
- Offer certain "tracks" at only some schools (also called Centers of Emphasis); this is most effective if students opting for these are not required to pay out-of-state tuition. (See www.avma.org > Advocacy > Congressional activities > Current agenda > 110th agenda > Issue brief > Centers of Emphasis in Food Systems Veterinary Medicine, and also M. Larkin in *JAVMA*.)
- If using such tracks, create a plan to evaluate the outcome—will this give the desired results of filling those niche areas, or will it only limit the future choices for those graduates? One of the key recommendations of the 1989 Pew Report, Future Directions for Veterinary Medicine, was for "multiple re-entry points" at the colleges, to allow those who had tracked in one area to return to the CVM for additional training if they wanted to now focus on another species or area.
- Acknowledge the conflict of interest that exists between their sources of funding, the types of jobs for which they train their students, and the actual job market. For example, if school funding is agriculture based, then schools will feel obligated to educate students along those lines, regardless of potential jobs that await them.
- Expose students to their choices through experiential examples as early as possible.

- Help students understand balancing the human-animal bond with performing health care in a for-profit business environment, and how to manage the inherent conflict of interest that ensues.

Need for more information

More information will help to guide future actions. Some of the items mentioned in the first edition of this book have only now begun to be evaluated. For example, instead of asking practice owners why they can't seem to hire an associate, a more useful approach would be to find out why job-seekers don't find those jobs appealing. Instead of lamenting the apparent disinterest of young people in practice ownership, a more useful approach might be to explore their assumptions and stereotypes about what that involves, and to help practice owners create a business worth buying. Instead of trying to "fix" students by changing their career paths, a more useful approach might be to find out what attracts them or deters them from certain career paths.

The number of graduates who drop out of the profession entirely is unknown. See Table 19.1; over 15% of veterinarians' career paths are not known. Are they dropouts? Furthermore, "drop out" must be defined, since this book shows that is a fuzzy line.

Acknowledgement of the economic forces driving choice is essential. Trying to change student attitudes or student composition may not be an effective approach to changing market forces. Arguably, market forces themselves act to change student attributes and/or composition, not the other way around.

Our challenge as a profession is in protecting the public while still preparing for the future of veterinary medicine. All veterinarians must ask themselves what they can do to effect change. What should the future look like, and what can you contribute to make that happen? Ultimately, our profession must come back to the oath we, as veterinarians, all took upon graduation:

> Being admitted to the profession of veterinary medicine, I solemnly swear to use my scientific knowledge and skills for the benefit of society through the protection of animal health, the relief of animal suffering, the conservation of animal resources, the promotion of public health, and the advancement of medical knowledge.
>
> I will practice my profession conscientiously, with dignity, and in keeping with the principles of veterinary medical ethics.
>
> I accept as a lifelong obligation the continual improvement of my professional knowledge and competence.

Table 19.1: Employment of US veterinarians by job category

	Number	Percent of total (rounded)		
Companion animal exclusive private practice	41,117	44%		
Companion animal predominant private practice	6,001	6%	50%	
Mixed animal private practice	4,328	5%		
Food animal predominant private practice	3,937	4%	10%	65%
Food animal exclusive private practice	1,103	1%		
Equine private practice	3,699	4%		
Other private practice	710	1%		
Employment unknown	15,092	16%		16%
College or university	6,356	7%		
Industry	3,235	3%	12%	
Other Public and Corporate	2,029	2%		
Federal government	1,753	2%		
State or local government	1,118	1%	4%	
Uniformed services	688	1%		
Other not listed	1,881	2%		2%
Total	93,047			

AVMA data, 2009; www.avma.org > reference > marketstats > US Veterinarians

Table 19.2: Mean starting salary by job category

Companion animal exclusive private practice	$71,000
Companion animal predominant private practice	69,000
Mixed animal private practice	62,000
Food animal predominant private practice	62,000
Food animal exclusive private practice	69,000
Equine private practice	38,000
Uniformed services	65,000
Advanced education (mainly internships)	29,000

AVMA, 2010. Starting salary unavailable for some job catetories. Values rounded.

Chapter 19 Resources

Groups and web sites

Association of Medical Professionals with Hearing Losses, www.amphl.org.

American Veterinary Medical Association (AVMA), www.avma.org

AVMA Veterinary Career Center (VCC), 1931 N Meacham Rd Schaumburg IL 60173-4360; 800 248 2862; vetcareers@avma.org www.AVMA.org/vcc.

AVMA, Centers of Emphasis in Food Systems Veterinary Medicine, www.avma.org > Advocacy > Congressional activities > Current agenda > 110th agenda > Issue brief.

AVMA Biennial Economic Survey, See current results at www.avma.org > products >resources.

Lesbian and Gay Veterinary Medical Association, www.lgvma.org.

National Commission on Veterinary Economic Issues (NCVEI), www.ncvei.org > Resource library. (Note: The NCVEI recently announced the potential formation of a partnership with Kansas State University to create a Center for Veterinary Economics.)

North American Veterinary Medical Education Consortium (NAVMEC), www.navmec.org.

One Health Initiative (One Medicine, One Health), www.onehealthinitiative.com.

One World–One Health, www.OneWorldOneHealth.org.

Veterinary Career Center (VCC), AVMA, 1931 N Meacham Rd Schaumburg IL 60173-4360; 800 248 2862; vetcareers@avma.org; www.AVMA.org/vcc.

Veterinary Medicine Loan Repayment Program (VMLRP) www.nifa.usda.gov/vmlrp; www.avma.org > Advocacy > State legislative resources > Issues > Veterinary loan repayment; Email: vmlrp@nifa.usda.gov.

Books and articles

Albers, J., From the Executive Director: Thoughts on veterinary medicine, companion animal practice, and AAHA. *Trends magazine*, Nov/Dec 2009:13-15.

American Animal Hospital Association (AAHA), www.aahanet.org

AAHA, *Compliance: taking quality care to the next level*. Lakewood, Colo: AAHA Press, 2009.

AAHA, *The Path to High-Quality Care: Practical Tips for Improving Compliance*. Lakewood, Colo: AAHA Press, 2003.

American Veterinary Medical Association (AVMA), www.avma.org

Biennial Economic survey of US veterinarians *JAVMA*, (236) 8, April 15, 2010.

Response to the Final Report of the Pew Commission on Industrial Farm Animal Production. 2009; available at www.avma.org.

AVMA Communications Division, Shepherd A., Employment, Starting Salaries, and Educational Indebtedness of Year 2009 Graduates of US Veterinary Medical Colleges. *JAVMA*, September 1, 2009; 235(5): 523–526.

AVMA Communications Division, Shepherd A., Employment of Female & Male Graduates of US Veterinary Medical Colleges, 2009, *JAVMA*, October 1, 2009; 235(7): 830–832 (similar report published periodically).

AVMA Communications Division, Shepherd A., Employment, starting salaries, and educational indebtedness of year-2010 graduates of US veterinary medical colleges. *JAVMA*, October 1, 2010; 237(7): 795-798

AVEPA, Asociación de Veterinarios Españoles Especialistas en Pequeños Animales, Instituto Veterinario De Estudios Económicos, Hill's Pet Nutrition; *Healthy Pets Mean Healthy Business: How Increased Compliance Makes Good Sense in Building a Modern, Caring Veterinary Practice*; Barcelona, Spain, 2007.

Andru, D., et al., Job Satisfaction, Changes in Occupational Area, and Commitment to a Career in Food Supply Veterinary Medicine, *JAVMA*, June 15, 2006; 228(12): 1884–1893.

Bannock, G., et al., *The Economist Dictionary of Economics*, 4th ed, (Bloomberg Press, 2003).

Barley G.E., Reeves C.B., et al., Characteristics of and issues faced by rural female family physicians. *J Rural Health*. 2001 Summer; 17(3):251-8.

Brown, J. P., and J. D. Silverman, Study of the Current and Future Market for Veterinarians and Veterinary Services in the United States. Executive Summary, *JAVMA*, 1999; 215(2):161–183; Study is available in abridged version: C. Smith, editor, National Commission on Veterinary Economic Issues, Schaumburg IL (2000).

Carter, C.N., *One Man, One Medicine, One Health—the James H. Steele Story* (BookSurge Publishing, 2009).

Chaddock, H.M., Veterinarians: Integral Partners in Public Health. (2007); available at www.aavmc.org/documents/VWEACongressionalPaperPDF.pdf.

Cima, G., NH considering licensing nonveterinarian livestock care, *JAVMA News*, Mar 15, 2010, 236(6):612-613.

Clark, L., Recruiting Rural Health Care Providers. *Washington State Magazine*, Fall 2010; 10-11.

Coyle SL; Ethics and Human Rights Committee, American College of Physicians-American Society of Internal Medicine. Physician-industry relations. Part 1: individual physicians, *Ann Intern Med*. 2002 Mar 5;136(5):396-402

Cron, W., et al., Executive Summary of the Brakke Management and Behavior Study, *JAVMA*, 2000; 217: 332–338.

Dininny, S., Dearth of Rural Veterinarians Raises Food-Safety Concerns, *Associated Press,* March 16, 2008.

Dumas, C., Veterinarian Shortage Threatens Producers, Public Health, *Farm & Ranch Guide*, January 31, 2009.

Ellsbury, K.E., Baldwin L.M., et al. Gender-related factors in the recruitment of physicians to the rural Northwest. *J Am Board Fam Pract.*, 2002 Sep-Oct; 15(5):391-400.

Food Supply Veterinary Medicine Coalition Report, available at www.avma.org/fsvm.

GAO, Veterinarian Workforce: Actions Are Needed to Ensure Sufficient Capacity for Protecting Public and Animal Health. February 2009. GAO-09-178, a report to the Chairman, Subcommittee on Oversight of Government Management, the Federal Workforce, and the District of Columbia, Committee on Homeland Security and Governmental Affairs, US Senate. Available at www.gao.gov.

GAO. Veterinarian Workforce: The Federal Government Lacks a Comprehensive Understanding of Its Capacity to Protect Animal and Public Health. Statement of Lisa Shames, Director Natural Resources and Environment. February 26, 2009. Testimony before the Subcommittee on Oversight of Government Management, the Federal Workforce, and the District of Columbia, Committee on Homeland Security and Governmental Affairs, US Senate, GAO-09-424T. Available at www.gao.gov/htext/d09424t.html.

Gwinner, K., et al., Attracting Students into Careers in Food Supply Veterinary Medicine, *JAVMA*, June 1, 2006; 228(11): 1693–1704.

Harmon R, AAHA Pet Insurance Buyer's Guide, *Trends magazine* Nov/Dec 2009.

Helms, T. D., and M. J. Bain, Evaluation of Owner Attachment to Dogs on the Basis of Whether Owners Are Legally Considered Guardians of Their Pets, *JAVMA*, April 1, 2009; 234(7): 896-900.

Herbold, J. R., et al., Vet Med Today: Public Veterinary Medicine, *JAVMA*, December 15, 2000, 217(12): 1812–1836.

Hoblet, K. N., A. Maccabe, and L. E. Heider, Special Report: Veterinarians in Population Health and Public Practice: Meeting Critical National Needs, JVME, 2003; 30: 287–294; available at. www.aavmc.org/JVME_hoblet.htm.

Jelinski, M., et al., Factors Associated with Veterinarians' Career Path Choices in the Early Postgraduate Period, *Can Vet J*, September 2009; 50: 943–948.

Larkin, M., Veterinary schools have their pluses, minuses. *JAVMA*, Sept 1, 2010, 237(5):478-480.

Ontario Veterinary Medical Association, *2010 Report on Veterinarians in Alternate Career Paths*, www.ovma.org; 1-800-670-1702.

Weintraub, A.,*Kaiser Health News*, New Health Law Will Require Industry To Disclose Payments To Physicians; www.kaiserhealthnews.org/Stories/2010/April/26/physician-payment-disclosures.aspx.

Kieves, N., Roark, A., Sparks, T., Business Education in Veterinary Schools: The Potential Role of the Veterinary Business Management Association; *JVME* 34(5): 678-682.

Lane, I., and Gobue, E.G., Perspectives in professional education: Faculty perspectives regarding the importance and lace of nontechnical competencies in veterinary medical education at five North American colleges of veterinary medicine. *JAVMA* 237(1), July 1, 2010: 53-64.

Larkin M., Veterinary education receives a workup: Academic leaders ponder teaching models, *JAVMA News* 236(12), June 15, 2010:1270-1275.

Larkin M., Speaking Different Languages, *JAVMA News*, May 15, 2010; also see *JAVMA* Letters to the Editor, July 15, 2010, (237) 2, p 150-152.

Larkin M., Board Weighs In On Foreign Accreditation, *JAVMA News*, July 15, 2010.

Lloyd, J. W., Current Economic Trends Affecting the Veterinary Medical Profession, *Vet Clin Small Anim*, 2006; 36: 267–279.

Macejko, C., Choice Veterinary Jobs Hard to Find in Tough Economy, *DVM Newsmagazine*, June 2009:1.

Macejko, C., Public-Health DVM Shortage Called "Critical," *DVM360*, April 1, 2009; www.dvm360.com.

Merriam Webster's Online Dictionary, www.merriam-webster.com.

Money magazine, Best Jobs in America, 2009, http://money.cnn.com/magazines/moneymag/bestjobs > job growth.

National Commission on Veterinary Economic Issues (NCVEI). (Note: The NCVEI may be forming a partnership with Kansas State University to form a Center for Veterinary Economics.)

NCVEI, A Veterinarian's Guide to Pet Health Insurance, www.ncvei.org/resources.aspx.

NCVEI, *Current and Future Market for Veterinarians and Veterinary Medical Services in the United States. KPMG LLP Study Report, Abridged version*. National Commission on Veterinary Economic Issues, 2000.

Nolen, R.S., One-Health Wonders, *JAVMA*, December 15, 2008; 223(12): 1828–1829.

Nolen, R.S., Mahr calls for "one health' initiative, *JAVMA News*, September 1, 2006.

Nolen R.S., Promoting One Medicine Among Veterinary Students, *JAVMA News*, February 1, 2007.

Osborne, D., Predicting the Future of Large Animal Practice, *Focus*, September/October 2007; 26(5): 14–16.

Pew Commission on Industrial Farm Production, *Putting Meat on the Table: Industrial Farm Animal Production in America*, final report available at www.ncifap.org or www.pewtrusts.org. Also see Letters to the Editor, *JAVMA*, October 15, 2008; 233(8): 1227–1228.

Pew National Veterinary Education Program, Future directions for veterinary medicine: The Pew report; *Can Vet J*, 1989 June; 30(6): 472–476. Copies available by request; e-mail info@pewtrusts.org.

Prince, J. B., et al., Future Demand, Probable Shortages, and Strategies for Creating a Better Future in Food Supply Veterinary Medicine, *JAVMA*, July 1, 2006; 229(1): 57–69.

Public Health Reality Check. *DVM Newsmagazine*, Opinion/Letters, June 2009; 32.

Remsburg, D., et al., A Proposed Novel Food Animal Health Care Delivery System, *JAVMA*, September 15, 2007; 231: 6.

Rezendes, A., One World, One Health, One Medicine, *JAVMA News*, September 15, 2007.

Rose, R, and C Smith. *Career Choices for Veterinary Technicians: Opportunities for Animal Lovers.* AAHA Press, 2009.

Sacks J.J., Sinclair L., et al., Breeds of dogs involved in fatal human attacks in the United States between 1979 and 1998. *JAVMA* 2000; 217:836-840.

Schoenfeld-Tacher, R., et al, Comparison of strength of the human-animal bond between Hispanic and non-Hispanic owners of pet dogs and cats, *JAVMA* 2010; 236:529–534.

Smith, C., Gender and Work: What Veterinarians Can Learn from Research about Men, Women, and Work, *JAVMA*, May 1, 2003; 220(9): 1304–1311.

Smith, C., Gender Shift in Veterinary Medicine: Cause and Effect, *Veterinary Clinics of North America: Practice Management Issue* (Elsevier Publishing, 2006), chapter 4.

Tremayne, J. Kansas Program to Increase Rural DVMs, *DVM Newsmagazine*, July 2006; 62.

VanBiema, D, Rural Churches Grapple with a Pastor Exodus, *Time magazine*, Thurs Jan. 29, 2009. Available online at www.time.com/time/magazine.

A Veterinarian's Guide to Pet Health Insurance, NCVEI; available at www.ncvei.org/resources.aspx.

Veterinary Hospital Managers Association Salary Survey, www.vhma.org.

VetPartners, No-Lo™ Practice Valuation Worksheet, available at www.vetpartners.org.

Volk, J., et al., Executive Summary of the AVMA-Pfizer Business Practices Study, *JAVMA*; 2005; 226: 212–218.

Willis, N., et al., Envisioning the Future of Veterinary Medical Education: The Association of American Veterinary Medical Colleges Foresight Project, Final Report, *JVME*, 2007; 34(1): 1–41.

Wolf, C., Lloyd, J., Black, J., An examination of US consumer pet-related and veterinary service expenditures, 1980–2005; *JAVMA* 233(3), August 1, 2008, 404-413.

Wood, F., Is Purchasing Power Shrinking? Vet Econ, August 2007; 36.

Yetter, D., and Halladay, J., Nurses Covering More Health Care: KY is among states looking to fill gaps by expanding roles of other caregivers. *USA Today*, March 12, 2010:3A.

ABOUT THE AUTHOR

Carin A. Smith, DVM, President of Smith Veterinary Consulting, works to help veterinarians and their teams create successful lives and careers. She is a consultant, speaker, trainer, and author who gained experience in both large and small animal practice before devoting her time to consulting. Dr. Smith conducts workshops and gives presentations worldwide. She is a Certified Mediator and a Certified English Language Instructor.

Dr. Smith is a member of the Association for Conflict Resolution, the American Society of Training and Development, and the Society for Human Resource Management. She is a member and has served on the board of directors of the American Veterinary Medical Law Association and of VetPartners, a veterinary consultants' association. She is also as a member of the National Academies of Practice, an organization of distinguished practitioners representing 10 different health care professions which works to advise governmental bodies on our health care system. Dr. Smith was honored with the 2010 Distinguished Service Award from the Association for Women Veterinarians Foundation. This award recognizes special effort and contributions of that individual to advance and improve the status of women in veterinary medicine.

Dr. Smith is a nationally-recognized, award-winning author of hundreds of articles and many books, including:

- *Client Satisfaction Pays: Quality Service for Practice Success*
- *Team Satisfaction Pays: Organizational Development for Practice Success*
- *Career Choices for Veterinarian Technicians (with Rebecca Rose, CVT)*

Please see Dr. Smith's web site (www.smithvet.com), which presents complete details about Smith Veterinary Consulting.

Contributing Author

Nina Kieves, DVM, graduated from the University of Minnesota College of Veterinary Medicine in 2009. She then completed a one-year small animal rotating internship at her alma mater and continued with a surgical internship in Maryland. Dr. Kieves worked in marketing for several years prior to attending veterinary school.

Dr. Kieves helped advance veterinary business education by serving on the National Veterinary Business Management Association executive board while in school. Dr. Kieves has attended the AVMA Veterinary Leadership Experience as both a participant and as a mentor. She also completed the Penn Executive Veterinary Leadership: Making an Impact as a Health Leader Program conducted at the Wharton School of Business, University of Pennsylvania.

APPENDIX A: CAREER PREP

For information about pre-veterinary requirements, applying to veterinary school, and state and federal licensing requirements go to the web sites of the American Veterinary Medical Association (AVMA; www.avma.org) and the Association of American Veterinary Medical Colleges (AAVMC; www.aavmc.org).

The AVMA information includes a downloadable brochure with a brief overview of careers in veterinary medicine (www.avma.org > Animal Health > AVMA brochures > Veterinarians). The AAVMC web site has links to all the veterinary colleges, information about applying to veterinary schools, and more.

High school and college students may also be interested in the book, *Career Choices for Veterinary Technicians*, by R. Rose and C. Smith.

In addition to the veterinary medical degree, most veterinary positions require federal and state licensing.

Veterinary exams and licensure

The new graduate with a veterinary degree in hand must take and pass national and state exams in order to work in private practice in the US. The AVMA Model Veterinary Practice Act lists common exceptions to the requirement for state licensure. For more specific information, go to www.avma.org > Issues > Policy > Model Veterinary Practice Act.

Graduates of US-Accredited schools

The National Board of Veterinary Medical Examiners (NBVME, www.nbvme.org) provides standardized examinations for use by state and provincial licensing boards as part of their licensure procedure for veterinarians. The North American Veterinary Licensing Examination (NAVLE) by the NBVME is a multiple-choice exam that can be taken by senior veterinary students and graduates of any US-accredited veterinary school.

Veterinarians who have graduated from a non-US school that has been AVMA-accredited have the same testing requirements as those from accredited schools in the US. For a list of currently-accredited colleges, go to www.avma.org > education > accreditation > veterinary colleges. The debate about US-accreditation of other schools is described in a *JAVMA* article by M. Larkin.

Graduates of other veterinary schools

Graduates of nonaccredited schools must pass additional exams. The NBVME web page has an overview of requirements that must be filled by graduates of nonaccredited veterinary colleges who want to practice in the US. See www.nbvme.org > NBVME examinations > Foreign trained veterinarians and www.aavsb.org > PAVE.

The Educational Commission for Foreign Veterinary Graduates may provide help with the transition to working and living in the US. See www.avma.org > education > ECFVG.

State exams and licensing

Most states require that practicing veterinarians have passed a state veterinary exam in addition to the national tests. Each state sets its own requirements for licensure, which may include an oral or practical exam in addition to a traditional multiple choice written test.

Some states offer the new graduate a temporary license before the test is taken. Others require the new veterinarian to work under supervision for six to 12 months.

There is a trend for states to offer a license by endorsement or reciprocity, which means that if the veterinarian is licensed in another state, has passed the NAVLE, and has practiced for a specified period of time (e.g., three to five years) without disciplinary action, then the board can issue a license by endorsement, requiring at most only a simple test covering state rules and regulations. More than half the states have some type of license by endorsement or reciprocity now, and more are adopting it each year.

Because it becomes more difficult to pass tests after being out of school for many years, the best advice for a recent graduate is to take tests in all the states in which you think you may want to practice, pay the fees for several years until you feel settled, then drop those licenses you are fairly sure you won't ever use.

Other licenses and accreditation

Certain jobs have additional requirements. A Drug Enforcement Administration (DEA) license is required in order to prescribe controlled substances and thus is necessary for private practice, as well as work in animal shelters and some other jobs. State accreditation in order to fill out health certificates is also required for private practitioners and some other positions. You can inquire about these (or will be informed about them) when you apply for or accept certain jobs.

Jobs that don't require licensure

Veterinarians who have not passed the NAVLE, or those who have not taken or passed the state exam in a particular state, may still be eligible for certain nonpractice jobs. Jobs that don't require passing the NAVLE may be found in government, industry, and academia.

Each state has its own definition of "practice"; that definition tells you which jobs require that the veterinarian has passed that state's exam. In general, veterinarians must be licensed if they are serving the public for a fee. Exceptions may include some positions in industry, consulting or research. Jobs that may require *a* state license, but not necessarily one in the state where the veterinarian is working, include many government and military positions and some university positions.

APPENDIX B: ACRONYMS

AAALAC	Association for Assessment and Accreditation of Laboratory Animal Care (International)
AAAS	American Association for the Advancement of Science
AABP	American Association of Bovine Practitioners
AACPPV	American Association of Corporate and Public Practice Veterinarians
AAEP	American Association of Equine Practitioners
AAFHV	American Association of Food Hygiene Veterinarians
AAFP	American Association of Feline Practitioners
AAHA	American Animal Hospital Association
AAHV	American Association of Housecall Veterinarians
AALAS	American Association for Laboratory Animal Science
AASRP	American Association of Small Ruminant Practitioners
AASV	American Association of Swine Veterinarians
AAV	Association of Avian Veterinarians
AAVMC	Association of American Veterinary Medical Colleges
AAVSB	American Association of Veterinary State Boards
AAZV	American Association of Zoo Veterinarians
ABD	All but dissertation (PhD [ABD])
ABVP	American Board of Veterinary Practitioners
ABVT	American Board of Veterinary Toxicology
AC	Animal Care (USDA-APHIS)
ACCC	Animal Chiropractic Certification Commission
ACDI	Agricultural Cooperative Development International
ACDI	Canadian International Development Agency)
ACLAM	American College of Laboratory Animal Medicine
ACPV	American College of Poultry Veterinarians
ACT	American College of Theriogenologists
ACVA	American College of Veterinary Anesthesiologists
ACVB	American College of Veterinary Behaviorists
ACVCP	American College of Veterinary Clinical Pharmacology
ACVD	American College of Veterinary Dermatology
ACVECC	American College of Veterinary Emergency and Critical Care
ACVIM	American College of Veterinary Internal Medicine
ACVM	American College of Veterinary Microbiologists
ACVN	American College of Veterinary Nutrition
ACVO	American College of Veterinary Ophthalmologists
ACVP	American College of Veterinary Pathologists
ACVP	Association Canadienne des Vétérinaires Porcins (see CASV)
ACVPM	American College of Veterinary Preventive Medicine
ACVR	American College of Veterinary Radiology
ACVS	American College of Veterinary Surgeons
ACVSMR	American College of Veterinary Sports Medicine and Rehabilitation
ACZM	American College of Zoological Medicine
ADSA	American Dairy Science Association
ASVMAE	American Society of Veterinary Medical Association Executives
AEMV	Association of Exotic Mammal Veterinarians
AGRICOLA	Agricultural Online Access
AHVMA	American Holistic Veterinary Medical Association
AJVR	American Journal of Veterinary Research
AKC	American Kennel Club
AMA	American Marketing Association
AMA	American Medical Association
AMA	American Management Association

AMIA	American Medical Informatics Association
AMVEC	Asociación Mexicana de Veterinarios Especialistas en Cerdos
AMWA	American Medical Writer's Association
APCRO	African Predator Conservation Research Organization
APHIS	Animal and Plant Health Inspection Service (USDA)
APPA	American Pet Products Association
APVS	Asia Pig Veterinary Society
ARAV	Association of Reptilian and Amphibian Veterinarians
ARS	Agricultural Research Service (USDA)
ARV	Academy of Rural Veterinarians
ASJA	American Society of Journalists and Authors
ASLAP	American Society of Laboratory Animal Practitioners
ASPCA	American Society for Prevention of Cruelty to Animals
ASTD	American Society for Training and Development
AVCA	American Veterinary Chiropractic Association
AVDC	American Veterinary Dental College
AVE	Alliance of Veterinarians for the Environment
AVEPA	Asociación de Veterinarios Españoles Especialistas en Pequeños Animales
AVHIMA	American Veterinary Health Information Management Association
AVI	Association for Veterinary Informatics
AVMA	American Veterinary Medical Association
AVMF	American Veterinary Medical Foundation
AVMLA	American Veterinary Medical Law Association
AVTE	Association of Veterinary Technician Educators
AZA	Association of Zoos and Aquariums
BA	bachelor of arts
BHR	Bureau for Humanitarian Response (USAID)
BS	bachelor of science
CADIA	Center for Animal Disease Information and Analysis
CAHI	Canadian Animal Health Institute
CAHIA	Center for Animal Health Information and Analysis (USDA-APHIS CEAH)
CASV	Canadian Association of Swine Veterinarians (see ACVP)
CBE	Council of Biology Editors, Inc.
CBP	Customs and Border Protection (US)
CD	compact disk
CDC	Centers for Disease Control and Prevention (FDC)
CE	continuing education
CEAH	Centers for Epidemiology and Animal Health
CEO	chief executive officer
CFIA	Canadian Food Inspection Agency
CFP	Certified Financial Planner
CMA	Certified management accountant
CMAR	Certified Manager, Animal Resources
CPCVM	Center for Public and Corporate Veterinary Medicine
CPIA	Certified Professional IACUC Administrator
CREES	Cooperative State Research, Education and Extension Service (now NIFA)
CSREES	See CREES
CSU	Colorado State University
CV	curriculum vitae
CVB	Center for Veterinary Biologics
CVC	Central Veterinary Conference
CVM	Center for Veterinary Medicine (FDA)
CVM	Christian Veterinary Mission
CVMA	Canadian Veterinary Medical Associatoin
CVMA	California Veterinary Medical Association
CVPM	Certified Veterinary Practice Manager
D+	Diplomate (see Chapter 4)
DABVP	Diplomate, American Board of Veterinary Practitioners
DABVP-SHM	Diplomate, American Board of Veterinary Practitioners, Swine Health Management
DABVT	Diplomate, American Board of Veterinary Toxicology

DACLAM	Diplomate, American College of Laboratory Animal Medicine
DACPV	Diplomate, American College of Poultry Veterinarians
DACT	Diplomate, American College of Theriogenologists
DACVA	Diplomate, American College of Veterinary Anesthesiologists
DACVB	Diplomate, American College of Veterinary Behaviorists
DACVCP	Diplomate, American College of Veterinary Clinical Pharmacology
DACVD	Diplomate, American College of Veterinary Dermatology
DACVECC	Diplomate, American College of Veterinary Emergency and Critical Care
DACVIM	Diplomate, American College of Veterinary Internal Medicine
DACVM	Diplomate, American College of Veterinary Microbiologists
DACVN	Diplomate, American College of Veterinary Nutrition
DACVO	Diplomate, American College of Veterinary Ophthalmologists
DACVP	Diplomate, American College of Veterinary Pathologists
DACVPM	Diplomate, American College of Veterinary Preventive Medicine
DACVR	Diplomate, American College of Veterinary Radiology
DACVS	Diplomate, American College of Veterinary Surgeons
DACVSMR	Diplomate, American College of Veterinary Sports Medicine and Rehabilitation
DACZM	Diplomate, American College of Zoological Medicine
DAI	Development Associates, Inc
DEA	Drug Enforcement Agency (US)
DHHS	Department of Health and Human Services (US)
DHS	Department of Homeland Security (US)
DIA	Drug Information Association
DoD	Department of Defense (US)
DVM	Doctor of Veterinary Medicine (Veterinarian); see also VMD
EBVMA	Evidence-based Veterinary Medicine Association
ECFVG	Educational Commission for Foreign Veterinary Graduates
EHF	Esther Honey Foundation
ELF	Edward Lowe Foundation
EMR	electronic medical record
FAVRRP	Food Animal Veterinarian Recruitment and Retention Program
FDA	Food and Drug Administration (US)
FEDIX	Federal Information Exchange
EPA	Environmental Protection Agency (US)
ER	emergency room
FAD	foreign animal disease
FAO	Food and Agriculture Organization (UN)
FDA	Food and Drug Administration (US)
FSBPT	Federation of State Boards of Physical Therapy
FSIS	Food Safety and Inspection Service (USDA)
FWS	Fish and Wildlife Service (US)
GAO	Government Accountability Office (US)
GIS	geographic information system
GIVE	Global Initiative in Veterinary Education
GPVEC	Great Plains Veterinary Educational Center (University of Nebraska)
GRD	Governmental Relations Division (AVMA)
GTB	global tuberculosis
HACCP	Hazard Analysis and Critical Control Point
HPI	Heifer Project International
HSS	Department of Health and Human Services (US)
HSUS	Humane Society of the United States
HSVMA	Humane Society of the Veterinary Medical Association
IAAHPC	International Association for Animal Hospice and Palliative Care
IABC	International Association of Business Communicators
IACUC	Institutional Animal Care and Use Committee
IAED	International Association of Equine Dentistry
IAVRPT	International Association of Veterinary Rehabilitation and Physical Therapy
IBPA	Independent Book Publishers Association
ICMJE	International Committee of Medical Journal Editors
IHTSDO	International Health Terminology Standards Development Organization

IPVS	International Pig Veterinary Society
IRS	Internal Revenue Service (US)
ISFM	International Society of Feline Medicine
ITAA	Information Technology Association of America
IVAS	International Veterinary Acupuncture Society
IVE	International Veterinary Education (WSU program)
IVSA	International Veterinary Student Association
IWRC	International Wildlife Rehabilitation Council
JVME	Journal of Veterinary Medical Education
JAVMA	Journal of the American Veterinary Medical Association
KSU	Kansas State University
MA	Master of Arts
MBA	master of business administration
MEPA	Master of European Politics and Administration (European Union's College of Europe)
MGVP	Mountain Gorilla Veterinary Project
MIH	Master of International Health
MOU	memorandum of understanding
MPA	Master of Public Administration
MPH	Master of Public Health
MPVM	Master of Preventive Veterinary Medicine
MS	Master of Science
NAAJ	National Association of Agricultural Journalists
NACA	National Animal Control Association
NAFV	National Association of Federal Veterinarians
NAHERC	National Animal Health Emergency Response Corps
NAHMS	National Animal Health Monitoring System
NAL	National Agricultural Library
NASDA	National Association of State Departments of Agriculture
NASPHV	National Association of State Public Health Veterinarians
NAVC	North American Veterinary Conference
NAVLE	North American Veterinary Licensing Examination
NAVMEC	North American Veterinary Educational Consortium
NAVS	Native American Veterinary Services
NAVTA	National Association of Veterinary Technicians in America
NBAF	National Bio and Agro-Defense Facility
NBCAAM	National Board of Certification for Animal Acupressure & Massage
NBVME	National Board of Veterinary Medical Examiners
NCAHP	National Center for Animal Health Programs
NCBTMB	National Certification Board for Therapeutic Massage and Bodywork
NCIE	National Center for Import and Export
NCVEI	National Commission on Veterinary Economic Issues
NFAIS	National Federation of Abstracting and Information Services
NGO	nongovernment organization
NIFA	National Institute of Food and Agriculture
NIH	National Institutes of Health
NLM	National Library of Medicine
NMFS	National Marine Fisheries Service
NMML	National Marine Mammal Laboratory
NOAA	National Oceanic and Atmospheric Administration
NOAH	Network of Animal Health
NSF	National Science Foundation
NSU	National Surveillance Unit (CEAH)
NTIS	National Technical Information Service
NVRT	National Veterinary Response Team
NVS	National Veterinary Stockpile
NVSL	National Veterinary Services Laboratories
NWRA	National Wildlife Rehabilitation Association
NWU	National Writers Union
OFA	Orthopedic Foundation for Animals
OFDA	Office of US Foreign Disaster Assistance

OICC	Office for International Collaboration and Coordination
OIE	Office International des Epizooties; now the World Organisation for Animal Health
OPHS	Office of Public Health and Science
OPM	Office of Personnel Management (Federal)
ORACBA	Office of Risk Assessment and Cost-Benefit Analysis (USDA)
OSHA	Occupational Safety & Health Administration (US)
PAHO	Pan American Health Organization
PAVE	Program for the Assessment of Veterinary Education Equivalence
PD	product development
PDS	Professional Development Staff (USDA-APHIS VS)
PHAC	Public Health Agency of Canada
PhD	Doctor of Philosophy
PhD [ABD]	Doctor of Philosophy, all but dissertation
PHO	public health officer
PHS	Public Health Service (US)
PHV	public health veterinarian
PIADC	Plum Island Animal Disease Center
PIC	Primate Information Center
PIN	Primate Info Net
PPQ	Plant Protection and Quarantine (USDA-APHIS)
PRRS	Primate Resource Referral Service
PVO	private and voluntary organization
PVPCP	Public Veterinary Practice Career Program (APHIS)
R&D	research and development
ROI	return on investment
RPRC	Regional Primate Research Center (University of Washington)
RVP	rural veterinary practice
SBA	Small Business Administration
SCAVMA	Student Chapters of the American Veterinary Medical Association
SCORE	Service Corp of Retired Executives
SHM	Swine health management
SHRM	Society for Human Resource Management
SIAA	Software & Information Industry Association
SNOMED	Systematized Nomenclature of Medicine
SOP	standard operating procedure
SPCA	Society for Prevention of Cruelty to Animals
SPHV	supervisory public health veterinarian
STC	Society for Technical Communication
SVV	Sri Venkateswara Veterinary (University)
TSR	technical service representative
UN	United Nations
UNDP	United Nations Development Programme
UNV	United Nations Volunteers
URL	Uniform Resource Locator (web address)
USAID	United States Agency for International Development (Department of State)
USDA	United States Department of Agriculture
USPHS	See PHS
UVIS	Universal Veterinary information System
VA	Department of Veteran Affairs (US); Veterans Administration (US)
VBMA	Veterinary Business Management Association
VC	Veterinary Corps (US Army)
VCC	Veterinary Career Center (AVMA)
VCSA	Veterinary Clinical Skills Assessment
VESPA	Veterinary Emergency and Specialty Practice Association
VHMA	Veterinary Hospital Managers Association
VIN	Veterinary Information Network
VIRMP	Veterinary Internship and Residency Matching Program
VIVA	Volunteers in International Veterinary Assistance
VMLRP	Veterinary Medicine Loan Repayment Program
VLS	Veterinary Learning Systems

VMAT	Veterinary Medical Assistance Teams
VMD	Veterinary Medical Doctor (University of Pennsylvania)
VMLRP	Veterinary Medicine Loan Repayment Program
VOCA	Volunteers in Overseas Cooperative Assistance
VS	Veterinary Services (USDA-APHIS)
VSCP	Veterinary Services Careers Program (USDA-APHIS)
VSIPP	Veterinary Specialists in Private Practice
VWEA	Veterinary Workforce Expansion Act
WAVMA	World Aquatic Veterinary Medical Association
WCS	Wildlife Conservation Society
WHO	World Health Organization (UN)
WNPRC	Wisconsin National Primate Research Center
WSAVA	World Small Animal Veterinary Association
WSU	Washington State University
WTO	World Trade Organization
WVA	World Veterinary Association
WVC	Western Veterinary Conference
WWW	World Wide Web

APPENDIX C: RESOURCES

Groups and Web Sites

Please see notes in the introduction about how to access or obtain these resources.

Academic keys for veterinary medicine, higher education jobs in veterinary medicine, http://vetmed.academickeys.com.

Academy of Rural Veterinarians, www.ruralvets.com.

Academy of Surgical Research at www.surgicalresearch.org.

Academy of Veterinary Consultants, www.avc-beef.org.

Academy of Veterinary Homeopathy, PO Box 9280, Wilmington, DE 19809; www.theavh.org; phone: 866-652-1590.

Advanstar, Calendar of veterinary events www.dvm360.com > events > calendar.

Advanstar communications, Advanstarvhc.com and www.DVM360.com.

African Predator Conservation Research Organization, www.apcro.org.

Agricultural Research Service (ARS), www.ars.usda.gov/Careers.

Air Force, www.airforce.com

Careers, www.airforce.com > opportunities > healthcare > careers > biomedical sciences > allied health > public health officer; Chief, Military Public Health, HQ USAF SGPA, Bolling AFB, DC 20332-5113; phone: 202-767-1838; 800-423-USAF

Air Force Reserve, http://afreserve.com; phone: 800-257-1212.

Air National Guard; NGB/DPR; Andrews AFB, MD 20331; www.ang.af.mil; phone: 301-981-8569.

Alliance of Veterinarians for the Environment, P.O. Box 50046, Nashville, TN 37205; 615-353-0272; gwengriffith@gmail.com; www.AVEweb.org.

AltVetMed, www.altvetmed.org.

American Academy on Veterinary Disaster Medicine, www.cvmbs.colostate.edu/clinsci/wing/aavdm/aavdm.htm.

American Agricultural Editors Association, c/o Den Gardner, Executive Director, PO Box 156. New Prague, MN 56071; www.ageditors.com; phone: 952-758-6502; fax: 952-758-5813; e-mail: Ageditors@aol.com.

American Animal Hospital Association (AAHA), 12575 West Bayaud Ave, PO Box 150899, Denver, CO 80215-0899; www.aahanet.org; phone: 303-986-2800; 800-883-6301.

AAHA management seminars, www.aahanet.org > education.

AAHA guidelines, www.aahanet.org > resources.

American Association for Laboratory Animal Science (AALAS), www.aalas.org.

American Association for the Advancement of Science (AAAS), fellowships, 1200 New York Avenue, NW, Washington DC, 20005; www.aaas.org >become a fellow; phone: 202 326-6700; fax: 202-289-4950; e-mail: Fellowships@aaas.org.

American Association of Avian Pathologists, www.aaap.info/mc/page.do.

American Association of Bovine Practitioners, www.aabp.org.

American Association of Corporate and Public Practice Veterinarians (AACPPV), 6060 Sunrise Vista Drive, Suite 1300, Citrus Heights, CA 95610-7098; www.aacppv.org; phone: 916-726-1560; e-mail: info@aacppv.org.

American Association of Equine Practitioners, www.aaep.org > career center.

AAEP Emergency and Disaster Preparedness, www.aaep.org/emergency_prep.htm.

American Association of Extension Veterinarians, http://vetmed.illinois.edu/aaev/url.htm.

American Association of Feline Practitioners, www.catvets.com.

American Association of Food Hygiene Veterinarians, www.avma.org/aafhv.

American Association of Housecall Veterinarians, www.housecallvets.org; www.homevets.org.

American Association of Mobile Veterinary Practitioners www.aamvp.org.

American Association of Public Health Veterinarians, www.acvpm.org; phone: 515-331-4439.

American Association of Rehabilitation Veterinarians, www.rehabvets.evetsites.net.

American Association of Small Ruminant Practitioners, www.aasrp.org.

American Association of Swine Veterinarians, www.aasv.org.

American Association of Veterinary Laboratory Diagnosticians, www.aavld.org.

American Association of Veterinary Medical Colleges, 1101 Vermont Avenue, NW, Suite 301, Washington, DC 20005; www.aavmc.org.

American Association of Veterinary State Boards, 4106 Central St., Kansas City, MO, 64111; www.aavsb.org; phone: 877-698-8482; fax: 816-931- 1604; e-mail: aavsb@aavsb.org.

American Association of Zoo Veterinarians, www.aazv.org.
American Board of Veterinary Practitioners, www.abvp.com.
American Board of Veterinary Toxicology, www.abvt.org.
American College of Laboratory Animal Medicine, www.aclam.org.
American College of Poultry Veterinarians, www.acpv.info.
American College of Theriogenologists, www.theriogenology.org.
American College of Veterinary Anesthesiologists, www.acva.org.
American College of Veterinary Behaviorists, www.dacvb.org.
American College of Veterinary Clinical Pharmacology, www.acvcp.org.
American College of Veterinary Dermatology, www.acvd.org.
American College of Veterinary Emergency and Critical Care, http://acvecc.org.
American College of Veterinary Internal Medicine, www.acvim.org.
American College of Veterinary Microbiologists, www.acvm.us.
American College of Veterinary Nutrition, www.acvn.org.
American College of Veterinary Ophthalmologists, www.acvo.org.
American College of Veterinary Pathologists, www.acvp.org.
American College of Veterinary Preventive Medicine, www.acvpm.org.
American College of Veterinary Radiology, www.acvr.org.
American College of Veterinary Sports Medicine and Rehabilitation, www.vsmr.org.
American College of Veterinary Surgeons, www.acvs.org.
American College of Zoological Medicine, www.aczm.org.
American Veterinary Dental College, avdc.org.
American Dairy Science Association, www.adsa.org.
American Fisheries Society, Fish Health Section, www.fisheries.org/fhs.
American Goldfish Association, www.americangoldfish.org.
American Holistic Veterinary Medical Association, www.ahvma.org; phone: 410-569-0795; e-mail: office@ahvma.org.
American Humane Association, 63 Inverness Dr East, Englewood CO 80112-5117; www.americanhumane.org; e-mail: info@americanhumane.org.
American Kennel Club, www.akc.org.
American Management Association, www.amanet.org.
American Marketing Association, www.ama.org.
American Medical Association, www.ama-assn.org.
American Massage Therapy Association, www.amtamassage.org; phone: 877-905-2700.
American Medical Informatics Association, 4915 St Elmo Ave., Suite 302, Bethesda, MD 20814; www.amia.org/; phone: 301-657-1291; fax: 301-657-1296.
American Medical Writer's Association, 40 West Gude Drive, Suite 101, Rockville, MD 20850-1192; www.amwa.org; phone: 301-294-5303; e-mail: amwa@amwa.org.
American Pet Products Association, www.americanpetproducts.org; phone: 203-532-0000.
American Public Health Association, 800 I Street, NW, Washington, DC 20001-3710; www.apha.org; phone: 202-777-2742; fax: 202-777-2533; e-mail: comments@apha.org.
American Sheep and Goat Center, phone: 800-951-1373; 202-350-9065; www.sheepandgoatsusa.org.
American Society for Training and Development, www.astd.org.
American Society of Association Executives, 1575 I St NW, Washington, DC 20005-1168; www.asaenet.org; phone: 202-626-ASAE; fax: 371-8825; e-mail: asae@asae.asaenet.org.
American Society of Journalists and Authors, 1501 Broadway Suite 302, New York, NY 10036; www.asja.com; phone: 212-997-0947; fax: 212-937-2315.
American Society of Laboratory Animal Practitioners, www.aslap.org.
American Society for the Prevention of Cruelty to Animals, www.aspca.org and www.aspcapro.org; phone: 800-628-0028.
American Society of Veterinary Medical Association Executives, PO Box 280425, Lakewood, CO 80228, www.vmaexecs.org.
American Veterinary Chiropractic Association, 442154 E. 140 Rd., Bluejacket, OK 74333; www.animalchiropractic.org; phone: 918-784-2231, fax: 918-784-2675.
American Veterinary Health Information Management Association, www.avhima.org; phone: 662-325-1166.
American Veterinary Medical Association (AVMA), 1931 N Meacham Rd, Suite 100, Schaumburg, IL 60173-4360; www.avma.org; phone: 800-248-2862, e-mail: avmainfo@avma.org.
AVMA Biennial Economic Survey, www.avma.org > products > resources.
AVMA career information, www.avma.org > Public resources.
AVMA, Centers of Emphasis In Food Systems Veterinary Medicine, www.avma.org > Advocacy > Congressional activities > Current agenda > 110th agenda > Issue brief.

AVMA Governmental Relations Division (GRD), 1101 Vermont Ave NW, Suite 710, Washington, DC 20005-3521; www.avma.org > advocacy > federal > legislative activities; externs, www.externsonthehill.com; phone: 202-789-0007; 800-321-1473.

AVMA list of government agencies, www.avma.org > Member Resource Directory > Government agencies; phone: 847-925-8070.

AVMA list of veterinary medical associations, www. avma.org > Advocacy > State legislative resources > Allied veterinary medical associations.

AVMA list of veterinary technician programs, avma.org > Education > Accreditation > Veterinary technology programs.

AVMA Model Veterinary Practice Act, www.avma.org > Issues > Policy > Model Veterinary Practice Act.

AVMA position announcements online, www.avma.org/jobs/default.asp.

AVMA Professional Liability Insurance Trust, www.avmaplit.com.

AVMA Veterinary Career Center, www.AVMA.org/vcc; www.avma.org > Careers; phone: 800 248 2862; e-mail: vetcareers@avma.org.

American Veterinary Medical Foundation, www.avmf.org.

American Veterinary Medical Law Association, www.avmla.org; phone: 312-233-2760.

American Veterinary Society of Animal Behavior. www.avsabonline.org.

American-Scandinavian Foundation, www.amscan.org

Animal and Plant Health Inspection Service (APHIS-VS), USDA, www.aphis.usda.gov.

APHIS Animal Care, www.aphis.usda.gov > animal welfare.

APHIS Center for Epidemiology and Animal Heath, www.aphis.usda.gov > about > programs and offices > Veterinary Services > Centers for Epidemiology and Animal Health.

APHIS Center for Veterinary Biologics, www.aphis.usda.gov > animal health> veterinary biologics.

APHIS externships and internships, www.aphis.usda.gov > About APHIS >Programs and Offices > Veterinary Services > Student externships and internships.

APHIS job vacancy announcements, www.aphis.usda.gov/mb/mrphr/vacancy.html; e-mail: Apphelp@aphis.usda.gov.

APHIS National Animal Health Emergency Response Corps, www.aphis.usda.gov > emergency response.

APHIS student scholarships, www.aphis.usda.gov > career opportunities > student programs.

APHIS Veterinary Services, www.aphis.usda.gov > animal health.

Animal health jobs, www.AnimalHealthJobs.com.

Animal Hospice Compassionate Crossings, www.animalhospice.org.

Aquaculture Network Information Center, http://aquanic.org.

Aquatic Veterinary Medicine Links, http://cvmstudent.cvm.msu.edu/ac/aquarium.htm.

Aquavet, www.aquavet.info.

Army (US)

Army National Guard Readiness Center, Attn: NGB-ARP-HN; 111 S George Mason Dr, Arlington, VA 22204- 1382; www.ng.mil; phone: 703-607-7145.

Army recruiter, USA PERSCOM, TAPC-OPH-VC, 200 Stovall St, Alexandria, VA 22332-0417; www.goarmy.com; phone: 703-325-2360; 800-USA-ARMY.

Army Reserve, Attn: ARPC-OPS-MC Cdr, ARPERCEN 9700 Page Blvd, St Louis, MO 63132-5200; www.usar.army.mil phone: 314-538-2121; 800-325- 4973.

Army Veterinary Corps; Chief, US Army Veterinary Corps, Attn: MCVS; 2050 Worth Rd, Ft Sam Houston, TX 78234-6000; http://vetopportunities.amedd.army.mil; phone: 210-221-8149; 210-221-6564; e-mail: VSOpportunities@ LN.amedd.army.mil.

Asociación Mexicana de Veterinarios Especialistas en Cerdos (AMVEC,; Mexican Association of Veterinarians Specializing in Swine), www.amvec.org.

Associated Koi Clubs of America, www.akca.org.

Association for Assessment and Accreditation of Laboratory Animal Care, www.aaalac.org.

Association for Veterinary Informatics, http://avinformatics.org/avinform; phone: 425-455-0727.

Association for Conflict Resolution, www.acrnet.org.

Association of American Publishers, Inc., 50 F Street, NW 4th Floor, Washington, DC 20001; www.publishers.org; phone: 202-347-3375. New York Office: 71 Fifth Ave, New York, NY 10003; phone: 212-255-0200.

Association of American Veterinary Medical Colleges (AAVMC), www.aavmc.org.

Association of Avian Veterinarians, www.aav.org.

Association of Exotic Mammal Veterinarians, www.aemv.org.

Association of Medical Professionals with Hearing Losses, www.amphl.org.

Association of Primate Veterinarians, www.primatevets.org; phone: 215-774-9603; email info@primatevets.org.

Association of Reptilian and Amphibian Veterinarians, www.arav.org.

Association of Shelter Veterinarians, www.sheltervet.org.

Association of Veterinary Technician Educators (AVTE), www.avte.net.

Association of Zoos and Aquariums, www.aza.org; phone: 1-301-562-0777.

Auburn University Canine Detection Research Institute, www.vetmed.auburn.edu/cdri.

Australian College of Veterinary Scientists, acvsc.org.au.

Bankrate.com.

BNet business tools, www.bnet.com.

British Veterinary Camelid Society www.camelidvets.org.

Business forms and copyright information, www.copyright.gov and www.legalzoom.com.

Cafevet.com.

Canadian Animal Health Institute, www.cahi-icsa.ca.

Canadian Association of Swine Veterinarians, www.casv-acvp.ca.

Canadian Food Inspection Agency (CFIA), www.inspection.gc.ca.
  CFIA Food Production and Inspection Service, Nepean, Ontario, K1A 0Y9; phone: 800-442-2342; 613-225-2342; Director of Human Resources phone: 613-952-8000.

Canadian International Development Agency, www.acdi-cida.gc.ca.

Canadian Public Service Careers (partial list; other provinces similarly coded).
  Ontario, www.gojobs.gov.on.ca/Jobs.aspx.
  British Columbia, http://employment.gov.bc.ca.
  Saskatchewan, www.careers.gov.sk.ca.

Canadian Veterinary Medical Association, http://canadianveterinarians.net.

Careerbuilder.com.

Careers.com.

Careersniff.com.

Cat Writer's Association, www.catwriters.org; e-mail: comments@catwriters.org.

CATalyst Council, www.catalystcouncil.org.

Center for Disease Control and Prevention (CDC), www.cdc.gov.
  CDC, Center for Global Health, www.cdc.gov/globalhealth.
  CDC, Employment Information Service, CDC; Mail Stop K05, 4770 Buford Highway, Atlanta, GA 30341-3724.
  CDC, Epidemic Intelligence Service, 1600 Clifton Rd., NE, Mailstop E-92, Atlanta, GA 30333; www.cdc.gov > EIS; phone: 404-498-6110; fax: 404-498-6135; e-mail: eisepo@cdc.gov.
  CDC, Human Resources Management Office, 4770 Buford Highway, MS K-05, Atlanta, GA 30341-3724; www.cdc.gov/employment; phone: 770-488-1725; e-mail: hrcs@cdc.gov.
  CDC, Job Information Center, Koger Center-Stanford Building, 2960 Brandywine Road, Atlanta, GA; cdcinfo@cdc.gov; phone: 770-488-1725; 800-CDC-INFO.
  CDC, National Center for Emerging and Zoonotic Infectious Diseases, www.cdc.gov/ncezid.
  CDC, Public Health Informatics Fellowship, www.cdc.gov/PHIFP.

Center for Public and Corporate Veterinary Medicine, www.vetmed.vt.edu/org/md/cpcvm.

Center for Veterinary Economics, see NCVEI

Center for Veterinary Medicine (CVM), see FDA.

Central Veterinary Conference, www.thecvc.com.

Certified Association Executives, www.asae.org; phone: 269-429-0300.

Certified Meeting Professionals, www.conventionindustry.org; phone: 517-527-3116.

Christian Veterinary Mission (CVM), c/o Dr. Kit Flowers, President, 19303 Fremont Ave North, Seattle, WA 98133; www.cvmusa.org; phone: 206-546-7201; fax: 206-546-7458; e-mail: info@cvmusa.org.

Chronicle of Higher Education, 1255 23rd Street, NW, 7th Floor, Washington, DC, 20037, www.chronicle.com; phone: 202-466-1000; fax: 202-452-1030.

Colorado State University (CSU).

CSU Animal Cancer Center, 970-297-4195; www.animalcancercenter.org.

CSU Veterinary Medical Massage course, www.colovma.org; phone: 303-318-0447.
  CSU Animal Population Health Institute, www.cvmbs.colostate.edu/aphi.

Cooperative State Research Education and Extension Service, see National Institute of Food and Agriculture (NIFA).

Cost of Living Calculator, www.bankrate.com/brm/movecalc.asp.

Council of Biology Editors, Inc., www.councilscienceeditors.org; phone: 703-437-4377, fax: 703-435-4390; e-mail: CSE@CouncilScienceEditors.org.

Craigslist.org.

Delta Society, 425-679-5500; www.deltasociety.org.

Dodgen, www.dodgenmobiletech.com/products.php.

Dog Writer's Association, c/o Secretary Pat Santi, 173 Union Rd, Coatesville, PA 19320, www.dwaa.org; e-mail: pat@dwaa.org.

Drug Information Association (DIA), www.diahome.org.

Eastern Cougar Foundation, www.easterncougar.org.

Educational Commission for Foreign Veterinary Graduates (ECFVG), www.avma.org/education/ecfvg.

Edward Lowe Foundation, 58220 Decatur Road, P.O. Box 8, Cassopolis, MI 49031-0008; www.edwardlowe.org; phone: 800-232-LOWE (5693); fax: 269-445-2648; e-mail: info@lowe.org.

Entrepreneur Media Inc., 2445 McCabe Way, Ste. 400, Irvine, CA 92614; www.entrepreneur.com; phone: 949-261-2325 (customer service); 800-274-6229 (subscriptions).

Environmental Careers Organization, www.eco.org; 810-960-5857.

Environmental Protection Agency (EPA), www.epa.gov/epahome.

EPA Human Resources Offices, 1200 Pennsylvania Avenue, NW, Washington, DC 20460; phone: 202-260-3267.

EPA Job Hotline, www.epa,gov; e-mail: EPA-InternProgram@epa.gov.

Envirovet, http://vetmed.illinois.edu/envirovet.

EpiVetNet, www.vetschools.co.uk/EpiVetNet.

Equissage, www.equissage.com; phone: 1-800-272-2044.

Esther Honey Foundation, www.estherhoney.org.

European Board of Veterinary Specialisation, ebvs.org.

Evidence-based Veterinary Medicine Association, www.ebvma.org.

Federal Career Opportunities, Federal Research Service, www.fedjobs.com; phone: 800-822-5027.

Federal Information Center, www.usa.gov; phone: 800-688-9889.

Federal Information Exchange, www.fedix.fie.com.

Federal pay scale, www.fedjobs.com.

Federal Research Service, 7507 Pleasant Way, PO Box 1708, Annandale, VA 22003; info@fedjobs.com; phone: 703-914-JOBS; 800-822-5027; fax: 703-281-7639; e-mail: www.fedjobs.com info@fedjobs.com.

Federation of American Scientists, Biosafety Levels, www.fas.org > programs > biosecurity.

Federation of Asian Veterinary Associations Congress, www.favamember.org

Federation of State Boards of Physical Therapy, Physical Therapy State Practice Acts, www.fsbpt.org; phone: 703-299-3100.

FedWorld Information Network, www.fedworld.gov; phone: 703-487-4219.

Feline Advisory Bureau, www.fabcats.org.

Feline Health Center at Cornell University, www.vet.cornell.edu/fhc.

File Resource Library Federal Job Openings listed by the Office of Personnel Management, http://hi-tec.twc.state.tx.us/fedjobs.htm.

Fish Health Medicine Certificate Program, www.vetmedce.vetmed.wisc.edu/fhm.

Fish and Wildlife Service (FWS), www.fws.gov.

FWS job information: National Wildlife Health Lab, 6006 Schroeder Rd, Madison, WI 53711; www.fws.gov; phone: 608-271-4640; e-mail: Jobs@fws.gov.

Food and Agriculture Organization, www.fao.org.

Food and Drug Administration, 5600 Fishers Lane, Rockville, MD 20857; www.fda.gov; www.hhs.gov >about.

FDA information, www.fda.gov > Animal and Veterinary.

FDA job vacancies, www.usajobs.gov; www.fda.gov/jobs.

FDA Center for Veterinary Medicine (CVM), 7500 Standish Place, Rockville, MD 20855;

FDA-CVM Jobs: www.fda.gov > Science & Research > Science Career Opportunities.

FDA-CVM information, www.fda.gov > Animal and Veterinary; www.fda.gov > About FDA > Centers & Offices > About the Center for Veterinary Medicine.

FDA-CVM information, www.fda.gov > About FDA > Centers & Offices > About the Center for Veterinary Medicine.

FDA Commissioner's Fellowship, www.fda.gov > About FDA > Working at FDA > Fellowship, Internship, Graduate, & Faculty Programs.; phone: 888-332-4473; e-mail: fdacommissionersfellows@fda.hhs.gov.

Food Animal Veterinarian Recruitment and Retention Program www.avma.org > AVMA journals > *JAVMA News* > March 15, 2010 ; www.avmf.org/FAVRRP.

Food Safety and Inspection Service (FSIS), www.usda.gov/fsis.

FSIS fellowships, internships, and externships, www.fsis.usda.gov > Careers > Internships and Externships.

FSIS Personnel Operations Branch—Recruitment Examining Section, Butler Square West, 100 N Sixth St, Minneapolis, MN 55403; phone: 800-370-3747; 612-370-2000; e-mail: fsis.careers@fsis.usda.gov.

Global Initiatives in Veterinary Medicine, Association of Veterinary Medical Colleges, 1101 Vermont Ave, NW, Suite 710, Washington DC 20005-3521; www.aavmc.org/GIVE.

Harvard Business School Executive Education Office, www.exed.hbs.edu/programs/agb; phone: 800-HBS-5577 (outside the US, dial 617-495-6555); fax: 617-495-6999, e-mail: executive_education@hbs.edu.

Health Canada, www.hc-sc.gc.ca.

Heifer Project International, 1 World Avenue, Little Rock, AR 72202; www.heifer.org; phone: 800-422-0474.

Humane Society of the United States (HSUS) Human Resources, 2100 L Street, NW, Washington, DC, 20037; www.hsus.org.

HSUS internships: www.hsus.org >about us > employment opportunities.

HSUS Field Services, www.hsvma.org/field_services.

Humane Society Veterinary Medical Association (HSVMA), www.hsvma.org.

Independent Book Publishers Association, 627 Aviation Way, Manhattan Beach, CA 90266; www.ibpa-online.org; phone: 310-372-2732; fax: 310-374-3342; e-mail: info@IBPA-online.org.

Information Technology Association of America, 1401 Wilson Boulevard, Suite 1100, Arlington, VA 22209; www.itaa.org; phone: 703-522-5055; fax: 703-525-2279; Western Region Office, San Mateo, CA; phone: 650-357-7728.

Institutional Animal Care and Use Committee, www.iacuc.org.

InterAction, www.interaction.org.

International Association for Aquatic Animal Medicine, www.iaaam.org.

International Association of Business Communicators, One Hallidie Plaza, Suite 600, San Francisco, CA 94102; www.iabc.com; phone: 415-544-4700; 800-776-4222; fax: 415-544-4747.

International Association of Equine Dentistry, www.iaedonline.com.

International Association for Hospice and Palliative Care, www.iaahpc.org.

International Association of Veterinary Rehabilitation and Physical Therapy, www.iavrpt.org.

International Committee of Medical Journal Editors, www.icmje.org.

International Coach Federation, www.coachfederation.org

International Health Terminology Standards Development Organization, www.ihtsdo.org.

International Institute For Animal Law, www.animallawintl.org.

International Pig Veterinary Society, www.ipvs.de.

International Society of Feline Medicine, www.isfm.net.

International Veterinary Acupuncture Society (IVAS), P.O. Box 271395, Ft. Collins, CO, 80527-1395; www.ivas.org; phone: 970-266-0666; fax: 970-266-0777.

International Veterinary Information service, www.ivis.org.

International Veterinary Student Association (IVSA), www.ivsa.org.

IVSA international exchange opportunities, www.avma.org > Student AVMA > International exchange opportunities.

International Wildlife Rehabilitation Council, www.iwrc-online.org; phone: 408-271-2685.

Internal Revenue Service (IRS) Publications, Superintendent of Documents, Government Printing Office, Washington, DC 20402, www.irs.ustreas.gov; phone: 800-TAX-FORM (800-829-3676).

LaBoit, www.laboit.com.

Latin America Veterinary Conference,www.tlavc-peru.org.

Lesbian and Gay Veterinary Medical Association, www.lgvma.org.

LifeLearn, www.lifelearn.com.

Lifeline Mobile, http://lifelinemobile.com.

Maddie's Shelter Animal Medicine Program.

Links to programs at veterinary schools, www.maddiesfund.org > Funded Projects > Colleges of Veterinary Medicine. Externship, www.ufsheltermedicine.com > training >Student Externships.

Residency, www.maddiesfund.org > Funded Projects >Colleges of Veterinary Medicine >University of Pennsylvania; www.vet.upenn.edu >Education and Training >Training > Residencies, Internships, and Fellowships >Maddies Residency in Shelter Animal Medicine.

Manitoba careers, www.gov.mb.ca/csc.

Medical Library Association, 65 East Wacker Place, Suite 1900, Chicago, IL 60601-7246, www.mlanet.org; phone: 312-419-9094; fax: 312-419-8950; e-mail: info@mlahq.org.

Meeting Professionals International, 3030 Lyndon B. Johnson Freeway, Suite 1700, Dallas, TX 75234-2759; www.mpiweb.org; phone: 972-702-3000; fax: 972-702-3070; e-mail: feedback@mpiweb.org.

Monster.com.

Morris Animal Foundation, www.morrisanimalfoundation.org.

Mountain Gorilla Veterinary Project, www.gorilladoctors.org.

Myveterinarycareer.com.

National Aeronautics and Space Administration, www.nasa.gov >about > careers.

National Agricultural Library, USDA, www.nal.usda.gov.

National Alliance of State Animal and Agricultural Emergency Programs, www.nasaaep.org.

National Animal Control Association, PO Box 480851, Kansas City, MO 64148-0851; www.nacanet.org; phone: 800-828-6474; fax: 913-768-0607; e-mail: naca@nacanet.org.

National Animal Health Emergency Response Corps (NAHERC), www.aphis.usda.gov > emergency management > naherc; NAHERC coordinator phone: 301-734–8073; e-mail: NAHERC@aphis.usda.gov.

National Association for Biomedical Research, Animal Law Section, www.nabranimallaw.org.

National Association of Agricultural Journalists, www.naaj.net; e-mail: ka-phillips@tamu.edu.

National Association of Federal Veterinarians, 1910 Sunderland Place, NW, Washington, DC 20036-1608; www.nafv.net; phone: 202-223-4878; fax: 202-223-4877.

National Association of State Departments of Agriculture, 1156 15th Street, NW, Suite 1020, Washington, DC 20005; www.nasda.org; phone: 202-296-9680; fax: 202-296-9686; email: nsada@nasda.org.

National Association of State Meat and Food Inspector Directors, www.nasda.org.

National Association of State Public Health Veterinarians, www.nasphv.org.

National Association of Veterinary Technicians in America, www.navta.org.

National Board of Certification for Animal Acupressure & Massage, http://nbcaam.net; e-mail: info@nbcaam.net.

National Board of Veterinary Medical Examiners, www.nbvme.org.

National Cattlemen's Beef Association, www.beef.org.

National Certification Board for Therapeutic Massage and Bodywork,, www.ncbtmb.org; phone: 800-296-0664.

National Commission on Veterinary Economic Issues (NCVEI), www.ncvei.org > Resource library. (Note: The NCVEI recently announced the potential formation of a partnership with Kansas State University to create a Center for Veterinary Economics.)

National Council for Science and the Environment, www.ncseonline.org.

National Federation of Abstracting and Information Services, 1518 Walnut Street, Suite 307, Philadelphia, PA 19102; www.nfais.org; phone: 215-893-1561; fax: 215 893-1564; e-mail: nfais@hslc.org.

National Incident Management Center, www.fema.gov/emergency/nims.

National Institute of Food and Agriculture, www.nifa.usda.gov.

National Institutes of Health (NIH), www.nih.gov; www.aamc.org/research/adhocgp/aboutnih.htm.

NIH Recruitment and Employee Benefits Branch, Bldg 31, Rm B-3, C 15, Bethesda, MD 20892; www.jobs.nih.gov; phone: 301-496-2403; e-mail: odjobsweb@mail.nih.gov.

National Library of Medicine, PubMed, www.nlm.nih.gov > pubmed.

National Marine Fisheries Service, www.nmfs.noaa.gov.

National Marine Mammal Laboratory, 7600 Sand Point Way N.E., F/AKC3, Seattle, WA 98115-6349; www.afsc.noaa.gov/nmml; phone: 206-526-4045; fax: (206) 526-6615; e-mail: nmml.information@noaa.gov.

National Oceanic and Atmospheric Administration (NOAA), 1305 East West Highway, Silver Spring, MD 20910.

National Science Foundation (NSF), 4201 Wilson Blvd., Arlington, VA 22230; www.nsf.gov; phone: 703-306-1234.

NSF current vacancy listings,, www.nsf.gov >about >career > vacancies.

NSF human resources management, phone: 703 306-1182.

NSF publications, www.nsf.gov/publications/ods.

National Speakers Association, 1500 S Priest Dr, Tempe, AZ 85281; www.nsaspeaker.org; phone: 602-968-2552 fax: 602-968-0911.

National Technical Information Service (NTIS), Technology Administration, US Department of Commerce, Springfield, VA 22161; www.ntis.gov/about/form.aspx; phone: 703-487-4650.

National Veterinary Response Team (NVRT), www.hhs.gov > Assistant Secretary for Preparedness and Response > National Disaster Medical System > NDMS Team.

National Wildlife Rehabilitation Association, www.nwrawildlife.org; nwrawildlife.org/pubs; phone: 320-230-9920.

National Writers Union, www.nwu.org.

National Zoo, http://nationalzoo.si.edu.

Native American Veterinary Services, www.pavetfoundation.org; phone: 888-550-7862.

Newscientistjobs.com.

Nikki Hospice Foundation for Pets, 400 New Bedford Drive, Vallejo, CA 94591;. www.pethospice.org; phone: 707-557-8595.

North American Veterinary Conference, www.navc.org.

North American Veterinary Medical Education Consortium, www.navmec.org.

Northwestern School of Law at Lewis & Clark College, publishes the Animal Law Journal, www.lclark.edu/law > animal law.

Office international des epizooties, 12, rue de Prony, 75017 Paris, France; www.oie.int oie@oie.int; phone: 33 (0)1 44 15 18 88; fax: 33 (0)1 42 67 09 87.

Office of Personnel Management (OPM), 1900 E Street, NW, Washington, DC 20415; www.opm.gov; phone: 202-606-1800.

OPM online applications, www.usajobs.opm.gov.

Office of Public Health and Science, www.hhs.gov/ophs.

Oiled Wildlife Care Network, www.owcn.org.

One Health Initiative (One Medicine, One Health), www.onehealthinitiative.com; www.avma.org >Public health > One health

One World–One Health, www.OneWorldOneHealth.org.

Ontario Public Service Careers, www.gojobs.gov.on.ca/Jobs.aspx.

Ontario Ministry of Agriculture, www.omafra.gov.on.ca.

Organization of American States Student Intern Program, OAS/Public Information, 17th Street and Constitution Avenue, NW, Washington, DC 20006; www.oas.org; phone: 202-458-3754; fax: (202)458-6421.

Orthopedic Foundation for Animals, www.offa.org.

Pan American Health Organization, www.paho.org; e-mail: info@who.int.

Para Publishing, PO Box 8206-222, Santa Barbara CA 93118-8206; www.parapublishing.com; phone: 805-968-7277; fax: 805-968-1379.

Peace Corps, Paul D. Coverdell Peace Corps Headquarters, 1111 20th Street, NW, Washington, DC 20526; www.peacecorps.gov; phone: 800-424-8580.

People to People Ambassador Program, S. 110 Ferrall St, Dwight D. Eisenhower Building, 1956 Ambassador Way, Spokane, WA 99202-4800; www.peopletopeople.com; phone: 509-568-7000; international phone: 866-794-8309, fax: 509-534-5245; e-mail: info@peopletopeople.com.

Pork Board, www.pork.org.

Porta-Vet, www.portavet.net.

Poultry careers, www.poultrycareers.org.

Poultry industry, www.thepoultrysite.com.

Primate Info Net (PIN), University of Wisconsin, http://pin.primate.wisc.edu.

PrimateLit, www.primatelit.library.wisc.edu.

Program for Assessment of Veterinary Education Equivalence, www.aavsb.org > PAVE.

Public Health Agency of Canada, www.phac-aspc.gc.ca.

Public Health Informatics Fellowship, www.cdc.gov/PHIFP; e-mail: phifp@cdc.gov.

Public Health Service Commissioned Corps, www.usphs.gov.

Public Service Commission of Canada, http://jobs-emplois.gc.ca/index-eng.htm; www.psc-cfp.gc.ca/centres/employ-ment-emplois-eng.htm.

PubMed, National Library of Medicine, www.nlm.nih.gov > pubmed.

Purdue University, Veterinary Management Institute, Krannert School of Management wwww.krannert.purdue.edu > admissions > masters programs > nondegree programs > sponsored programs.

Purdue University, National Conference For Agribusiness, 1145 Krannert Bldg., West Lafayette, IN 47907-1145; htpps://www.agecon.purdue.edu/cab/programs; phone: 317-494-4325; fax: 317-494-4333; e-mail: wall@agecon.purdue.edu.

Rotary International, National Headquarters, One Rotary Center, 1560 Sherman Ave., Evanston, IL 60201; www.rotary.org; phone: 847-866-3000, fax: 847-328-8554.

Saskatchewan careers, www.agriculture.gov.sk.ca/careers.

Service Corp of Retired Executives, www.score.orgt.

Shelter Veterinarian, www.sheltermedicine.com.

Small Business Administration, www.sba.gov; phone: 800-827-5722; e-mail answerdesk@sba.gov.

Small Business Resource Center, 1101 E. 33rd Street, Suite C307, Baltimore, MD 21218; www.sbrcbaltimore.com; phone: 443-451-7160; fax: 443-451-7169; e-mail: info@sbrcbaltimore.com.

Small Publishers Association of North America, 1618 W. Colorado Ave, Colorado Springs, CO, 80904; www.spannet.org; phone: 719-475-1726; fax: 719-471-2182; e-mail: info1@spannet.org.

Smart Business Supersite, www.smartbiz.com.

Society for Human Resource Management (SHRM), www.shrm.org; phone: 800-283-7476.

Society for the Internet in Medicine, www.internet-in-medicine.org.

Society for Technical Communication (STC), 901 N. Stuart St., Suite 904, Arlington, VA 22203-1854; www.stc.org; phone: 703-522-4114; fax: 703-522-2075.

Society for Veterinary Medicine and Literature, www.vetmedandlit.org; e-mail: information@vetmedandlit.org.

Society of Animal Welfare Administrators www.sawanetwork.org.

Society of Greyhound Veterinarians, www.greyhoundvets.co.uk.

Software & Information Industry Association, 1090 Vermont Ave NW Sixth Floor, Washington, DC 20005-4095; www.siia.net; phone: 202-289-7442; fax: 202-289-7097.

Southern European Veterinary Conference, www.sevc.info

Southern Regional Aquaculture Center Publications, http://srac.tamu.edu.

Spirits in Transition, www.spiritsintransition.org.

Stanford University School of Medicine, Medical Informatics Short Course, www.smi.stanford.edu/shortcourse.html; phone: 650-723-6979; e-mail: short-course@smi.stanford.edu.

State Animal Response Teams, www.sartusa.org.

State Veterinary Loan Repayment Programs, www.avma.org > Advocacy > State legislative resources > Issues > Veterinary loan repayment.

The Nature Conservancy, www.tnc.org.

Thevetrecruiter.com.

Toastmasters, 23182 Arroyo Vista, Rancho Santa Margarita, CA 92688, www.toastmasters.org; phone: 949-858-8255; fax: 949-858-1207.

United Nations (UN)

UN Employment Information, http://careers.un.org.

UN Internship Program, United Nations, Division for Staff Development and Performance, Policy and Specialist Services, Office of Human Resources Management, Room S-2580, New York, NY 10017; www.un.org/en > Resources > Internships.

UN Personnel Management and Support Service, Field Administration and Logistics Division, Department of Peace-Keeping Operations, S-2280, New York, NY 10017.

UN Staffing Support Section, United Nations, Division for Planning, Recruitment and Operational Services, Office of Human Resources Management, Room S-2555, New York, NY 10017; www.unsystem.org.

UN Peacekeeping Operations, UN Personnel Management and Support Service, Field Administration and Logistics Division, Department of Peace-Keeping Operations, S-2280, New York, NY 10017. www.un.org/en/peacekeeping.

University of Florida, Institute of Food and Agricultural Sciences Extension, http://edis.ifas.ufl.edu.

University of Florida, shelter medicine and forensics CE, www.ufsheltermedicine.com/animalForensicsCrueltyAbuse.html.

University of Illinois Executive Veterinary Program, UI College of Veterinary Medicine, CEPS/Extension, 2938 VMBSB, Urbana, IL 61801; www.evpillinois.org; phone: 217-333-2907, e-mail: ope@vetmed.illinois.edu.

University of Missouri master's degree program in health informatics, www.hmi.missouri.edu; http://mudirect.missouri.edu > degrees and programs > graduate certificate programs > health informatics; http://mudirect.missouri.edu > degrees and programs > degrees > health informatics; phone: 573-882-3598; 800-877-4764; e-mail: MUdirect@missouri.edu.

University of Nebraska Great Plains Veterinary Educational Center, http://gpvec.unl.edu.

University of Pretoria, South Africa, Dept. of Veterinary Tropical Diseases, http://web.up.ac.za > Faculties > Veterinary Science > CE at UP; http://scarlacc.up.ac.za/CEatUP/VetSci.aspx; phone: +27 12 529 8000.

University of Tennessee, Canine Rehabilitation Resource, www.canineequinerehab.com; phone: 800-272-2044; email: nicolethistle@neseminars.com.

University of Tennessee, facilities offering physical therapy/rehabilitation, www.utc.edu/Faculty/David-Levine/Veterinary.HTM#Clinics; phone: 423-425-4111.

University of Wisconsin Fish Health Medicine Certificate Program, http://vetmedce.vetmed.wisc.edu/fhm.

US Agency for International Development (USAID), Office of Human Resources, Recruitment Unit; Room 671 SA-36 Washington, DC 20523-3609,; 1550 Wilson Boulevard, Room 658A SA-36, Washington, DC 20523-3607; www.usaid.gov; fax: 703-302-4095.

USAID jobs, www.usaid.gov >careers.

US Business Advisor, www.business.gov.

US Department of Agriculture (USDA), www.usda.gov.

USDA research, education, and economics, www.reeusda.gov/ree.

USDA vacancy announcements, www.usda.gov/da/employ.html.

US Department of Health and Human Resources, job vacancies, www.hhs.gov/careers.

US Department of Health and Human Services, Office of Public Health and Science, www.hhs.gov/ophs.

US Department of Veterans Affairs (VA), c/o Chief Veterinary Medical Officer, 810 Vermont Avenue, NW, Rm 15E, Washington, DC 20420; www.va.gov; phone: 202-273-8230.

US Office of Personnel Management (OPM), for federal jobs: usajobs.opm.gov.

US Preventive Services Task Force, www.ahrq.gov > Clinical Information > Prevention and Care Management > US Preventive Services Task Force.

US Public Health Service Commissioned Corps Recruitment, 1101 Wooton Parkway, Plaza Level, Rockville, MD 20852; www.usphs.gov; phone: 877-463-6327 (general inquiries); 800-279-1695 (recruitment; application questions); Job announcements, www.usphs.gov.

US State Department, www.usembassy.gov; www.state.gov/travel.

USA Jobs, www.usajobs.gov; phone: 202) 606-2525.

VETAID, Pentlands Science Park, Bush Loan, Penicuik, Midlothian, EH26 0PL, UK; www.vetaid.org; phone: +44 (0)131 445 6241; fax: +44 (0)131 445 6242; e-mail: mail@vetaid.org.

VETDispatch, www.vetdispatch.com.

Veterinarians without Borders, www.vetswithoutborders.net.

Veterinary Business Management Association, www.vbma.biz.

Veterinary Cancer Society, www.vetcancersociety.org; phone: 619-474-8929.

Veterinary Career Center, AVMA, 1931 N Meacham Rd Schaumburg IL 60173-4360; 800 248 2862; vetcareers@avma.org www.AVMA.org/vcc.

Veterinary Dermatology Association, www.wcvda.com.

Veterinary Economics, 8033 Flint, Lenexa, KS 66214; www.dvm360.com; phone: 800-255-6864; fax: 913-871-3808.

Veterinary Emergency and Critical Care Society: 6335 Camp Bullis Road, Suite 12, San Antonio, TX, 78257, 210-698-5575, Fax 210-698-7138, http://veccs.org, email info@veccs.org.

Veterinary Emergency and Specialty Practice Association, www.vespassociation.org.

Veterinary Forensics, www.veterinaryforensics.com.

Veterinary Hospital Managers Association (VHMA). www.vhma.org; phone: 877-599-2707.

Veterinary Information Network (VIN), www.vin.com; phone: (800) 700-4636.

Veterinary Internship and Residency Matching Program (VIRMP), www.virmp.org.

Veterinary Learning Systems, www.vetlearn.com.

Veterinary Medical Assistance Teams, www.vmat.org; www.avma.org/vmat.

Veterinary Medicine Loan Repayment Program, www.nifa.usda.gov/vmlrp Email: vmlrp@nifa.usda.gov. Plant and Animal Systems Unit, USDA – National Institute of Food and Agriculture, STOP 2220, 1400 Independence Avenue, SW, Washington, DC 20250-2220.

Veterinary Services Careers Program, www.aphis.usda.gov > about >programs > veterinary services.

Veterinarycareernetwork.com.

Veterinary Specialists in Private Practice annual conference, www.vsipp.com.

Vetlib-L, veterinary librarian discussion list, http://listserv.vt.edu/archives/vetlib-l.html; e-mail: listserv@listserv.vt.edu.

Vetlocums, www.vetlocums.com; e-mail: vfeedback@vetlocums.com.

VetPartners, www.vetpartners.org.

Vetrelief.com.

Vocation vacations, www.vocationvacations.com

Volunteer Abroad, www.volunteerabroad.com.

Volunteers in Overseas Cooperative Assistance, 50 F Street, NW, Suite 1075, Washington DC 20001; www.acdivoca.org; phone: 202-638-4661; fax: 202-783-7204.

Washington State Univerisity. College of Veterinary Medicine

    WSU bear research center www.natural-resources.wsu.edu/research/bear-center.

    WSU International opportunities, www.vetmed.wsu.edu/international; e-mail: c/o IVE Mushtaq A. Memon, Coordinator, memon@vetmed.wsu.edu.

    WSU School for Global Animal Health, http://globalhealth.wsu.edu.

Wellington Rehabilitation Institute, Wellington FL; www.caninerehabinstitute.com.

Western University College of Veterinary Medicine, www.westernu.edu > colleges > veterinary medicine.

Western Veterinary Conference, www.wvc.org.

Wildlife Conservation Society, 2300 Southern Boulevard, Bronx, NY 10460; www.wcs.org; phone: 718-220-5100.

Wildlife Rehabilitation Information Directory, www.tc.umn.edu/~devo0028.

Wisconsin National Primate Research Center, www.primate.wisc.edu.

World Aquatic Veterinary Medical Association, www.wavma.org.

World Health Organization (WHO) 20, Avenue Appia, CH-1211 Geneva 27, Switzerland; www.who.int/en; phone: 41-22-791-2111; fax: 41-22-791-2300; 41-22-791 0746.

WHO, job vacancy page, www.who.int >employment >vacancies.

WHO Regional Office (US), 525 Twenty-third Street, NW, Washington, DC 20037; www.who.int/en; phone: 202-974-3000; fax: 202-974-3663.

World Organisation for Animal Health (OIE), www.oie.int.

World Small Animal Veterinary Association, www.wsava.org.

World Veterinary Association, www.worldvet.org.

Zoo/Exotic Pathology Service, www.zooexotic.com.

Books, periodicals, and articles

Please see notes in the introduction about how to obtain these resources.

Albers, J., From the Executive Director: Thoughts on veterinary medicine, companion animal practice, and AAHA. *Trends magazine*, Nov/Dec 2009:13-15.

Alred, G.J., *Handbook of Technical Writing*, 8th ed., (Bedford/St. Martin's, 2005).

Altman, R., *Why Most PowerPoint Presentations Suck* (Harvest Books, 2007).

American Animal Hospital Association publications, www.aahanet.org.

AAHA Guidelines (Referral guidelines; Dental care guidelines; Mentor guidelines; and more) www.aahanet.org >resources > guidelines.

AAHA, *2005 Specialty & Referral Veterinary Practice Benchmark Study* (AAHA Press, 2006).

AAHA, *Associates Survival Guide* (AAHA Press, 2005).

AAHA, *Compensation and Benefits Review* (AAHA Press, published periodically), www.aahanet.org.

AAHA, *Compliance: Taking Quality Care to the Next Level* (AAHA Press, 2009.

AAHA, *Financial and Productivity Pulsepoints: Vital Statistics for Your Veterinary Practice* (AAHA Press, published periodically).

AAHA Leadership Addresses Major Association Projects, AAHA practice management software summit meetings, www.aahanet.org > Media > Press releases > 03/26/2009.

AAHA Releases Diagnostic Terms, Diabetes Guidelines, *AAHA NewsStat* May 12, 2010; 8(10).

AAHA, *The Path to High-Quality Care: Practical Tips for Improving Compliance*, (AAHA Press, 2003).

AAHA, *Veterinary Fee Reference: Vital Statistics for Your Veterinary Practice* (AAHA Press, published periodically).

American Association of Feline Practitioners, AAFP Feline Handling Guidelines, www.catvets.com (In press, 2010-2011).

American College of Veterinary Pathologists, ACVP, Veterinary Pathologist Survey: Final Report, www.acvp.org/career/employsurv.pdf.

Anderson, P.V., *Technical Communication: A Reader-Centered Approach*, 6th ed., (Wadsworth Publishing, 2006).

Andru, D., et al., Job Satisfaction, Changes in Occupational Area, and Commitment to a Career in Food Supply Veterinary Medicine, *JAVMA*, June 15, 2006; 228(12): 1884–1893.

Animal Law Journal, www.lclark.edu/law > animal law.

AVEPA, Asociación de Veterinarios Españoles Especialistas en pequeños animales, Instituto veterinario de estudios económicos, Hill's Pet Nutrition. *Healthy Pets Mean Healthy Business: How Increased Compliance Makes Good Sense In Building a Modern, Caring Veterinary Practice.* Barcelona, Spain, 2007.

American Veterinary Medical Association, www.avma.org.

AVMA, 2008 AVMA Biennial Economic survey of US veterinarians *JAVMA*, (236) 8, April 15, 2010.

AVMA, *2007 US Pet Ownership & Demographics Sourcebook*, www.avma.org > references > market statistics.

AVMA, Addressing the Role of Veterinary Medicine in Human Health Care Following Catastrophes Involving Mass Human Casualty. www.avma.org > issues > policy.

AVMA Center for Information Management, Demographic and Employment Trend Data (AVMA, various years); www.AVMA.org > veterinary resources.

AVMA Communications Division, Shepherd A., Employment, Starting Salaries, and Educational Indebtedness of Year 2009 Graduates of US Veterinary Medical Colleges. *JAVMA*, September 1, 2009; 235(5): 523–526.

AVMA Communications Division, Shepherd A., Employment of Female & Male Graduates of US Veterinary Medical Colleges, 2009, *JAVMA*, October 1, 2009; 235(7): 830–832 (similar report published periodically).

AVMA Communications Division, Shepherd A., Employment, starting salaries, and educational indebtedness of year-2010 graduates of US veterinary medical colleges. *JAVMA*, October 1, 2010; 237(7): 795-798

AVMA, *Food Supply Veterinary Medicine Coalition Report*, www.avma.org/fsvm.

AVMA, Guidelines for Complementary and Alternative Veterinary Medicine, www.AVMA.org >issues >policy.

AVMA, Guidelines for Veterinary Hospice Care, www.avma.org >products.

AVMA, Report on Veterinary Compensation, 2009, (published biennially), www.avma.org > Scientific resources.

AVMA Response to the Final Report of the Pew Commission on Industrial Farm Animal Production. 2009, www.avma.org.> advocacy.

AVMA, Relationship of AVMA-Recognized Veterinary Specialty Organizations with Veterinary Specialty Organizations in Other Parts of the World, www.avma.org > Issues > Policy > Veterinary specialty organizations.

AVMA, *US Pet Ownership & Demographics Sourcebook* (published every other year; www.avma.org > reference).

Axtell, R.E., *Essential Do's and Taboos: The Complete Guide to International Business and Leisure Travel* (Wiley, 2007).

Baker, R.L., *Pricing on Purpose: Creating and Capturing Value* (Wiley 2006).

Bannock, G., et al., *The Economist Dictionary of Economics*, 4th ed., (Bloomberg Press, 2003).

Barley, G.E., et al. Characteristics of and issues faced by rural female family physicians. *J Rural Health*. Summer 2001; 17(3):251-258.

Bear, M., Nixon, T., *Bear's Guide to Earning Degrees by Distance Learning*, 16th ed., (Ten Speed Press, 2006).

Beck, N., *Shifting Gears: Thriving in the New Economy* (Harper Collins, 1992).

Bellman, G., *The Consultant's Calling: Bringing Who You Are to What You Do*, revised ed., (Jossey-Bass, 2001).

Berger, L., *Savvy Part-time Professional: How to Land, Create; Negotiate the Part-time Job of Your Dreams* (Capital Books, 2006).

Bimnez, R., et al., *Technical Large Animal Emergency Rescue* (Wiley Blackwell, 2008).

Blech, E., *Business of Consulting*, 2nd ed., (John Wiley and Sons, 2007).

Block, P., *Flawless Consulting: A Guide to Getting Your Expertise Used* (Jossey-Bass/Pfeiffer, 2000).

Bockstahler, B., et al., *Essential Facts of Physiotherapy in Dogs and Cats* (Lifelearn, 2005).

Bolles, R., *What Color is Your Parachute?* (Ten Speed Press, 2009).

Brabec, B., *Homemade Money: Bringing in the Bucks: A Business Management and Marketing Bible for Home-Business Owners, Self-Employed Individuals, and Web Entrepreneurs Working from Home Base* (Betterway Books, 2003).

Brown, J.P., Silverman, J.D., Study of the Current and Future Market for Veterinarians and Veterinary Services in the United States. Executive Summary, *JAVMA*, 1999; 215(2):161–183; *Abridged version*: C. Smith, editor, National Commission on Veterinary Economic Issues, Schaumburg IL (2000).

Burns, K., Evolution of Shelter Medicine, *JAVMA News*, November 15, 2006; 229(10): 1543–1545.

Burns, K., Teaching Hospitals Short on Specialists, *JAVMA News*, August 1, 2006; 229(3): 337–346.

Burns, K., The Economic State Of Specialty Practice, *JAVMA News*, June 15, 2010:1278-1280.

Burns, K., Training Program Brings Veterinary Pathologists to NIH. *JAVMA News*, February 1, 2009; 234(3): 306–307.

Carter, C.N., *One Man, One Medicine, One Health—the James H. Steele Story* (BookSurge Publishing, 2009).

Chaddock, H.M., Veterinarians: Integral Partners in Public Health. (2007); www.aavmc.org/documents/VWEACongressionalPaperPDF.pdf.

Choca, E., Confidence, Not Cash, Motivates Interns. AAHA *Trends magazine* Nov/Dec 2010.

Chronicle of Higher Education (weekly tabloid), www.chronicle.com.

Cima, G., Economists: Livestock and Poultry Producers Cutting Flock, Herd Sizes, *JAVMA News*, April 15, 2009; 234(8): 985–987.

Cima G, NH Considering Licensing Nonveterinarian Livestock Care. *JAVMA News*, Mar 15, 2010, 236(6):612-613.

Cockerell, G. L., and D. R. Patterson, Closing the Supply versus Demand Gap for Veterinary Pathologists. A Multifaceted Problem in Need of a Multifaceted Solution, *Can Vet J*, 2005; 46: 660–661.

Commerce Business Daily, Subscription phone: 202-512-1800, Government Printing Office Stock Number 703-013-000007, List ID "COBD". http://cbdnet.gpo.gov.

Correa, M.T., Employment in International Veterinary Medicine: A Survey of Requirements and Opportunities, *JVME*, Spring 1995; 22: 26-27.

Council for Adult & Experienced Learning, *Earn College Credit for What You Know*, 4th ed., (Kendall/Hunt Publishing Company, 2006).

Coyle SL; Ethics and Human Rights Committee, American College of Physicians-American Society of Internal Medicine. Physician-industry relations. Part 1: individual physicians, *Ann Intern Med*. 2002 Mar 5;136(5):396-402

Crawford, T., *Business & Legal Forms for Authors and Self-Publishers* (Allworth Press, 2005).

Cron, W., et al., Executive Summary of the Brakke Management and Behavior Study, *JAVMA*, August 1, 2000; 217: 332–338.

Damp, D.V., *Book of US Government Jobs: Where They Are, What's Available, and How to Get One*, 10th ed., (Bookhaven Press, 2008).

DHHS, Comparison of Civil Service and Commissioned Corps, www.ihs.gov/jobscareerdevelop/navajojobs >Compare.

Dininny, S., Dearth of Rural Veterinarians Raises Food-Safety Concerns, *Associated Press*, March 16, 2008.

Dumas, C.R., Veterinarian Shortage Threatens Producers, Public Health, *Farm & Ranch Guide*, January 31, 2009; www.farmandranchguide.com/articles.

DVM Newsmagazine, www.advanstar.com >Our markets > Life Sciences > Veterinary; www.dvm360.com.

Edwards, P., and S. Edwards, *Working from Home*, 5th ed., (Tarcher/Putnam, 1999).

Ellsbury K.E., Baldwin L.M., et al. Gender-related factors in the recruitment of physicians to the rural Northwest. *J Am Board Fam Pract*. 2002 Sep-Oct;15(5):391-400.

Employment, Starting Salaries, and Educational Indebtedness of Year 2009 Graduates of US Veterinary Medical Colleges. *JAVMA*, September 1, 2009; 235(5): 523–526.

Environmental Care Organization, *Complete Guide to Environmental Careers in the 21st Century* (Island Press, 1998).

Fasulo, M., Walker, P., *Careers in the Environment,* (McGraw Hill, 2007).

Ferrazzi, K., Raz, T., *Never Eat Alone: And Other Secrets to Success One Relationship at a Time* (A Currency Book, Division of Random House, 2005).

Fine, D., *Fine Art of Small Talk: How To Start a Conversation, Keep It Going, Build Networking Skills——and Leave a Positive Impression!* (Hyperion, 2005).

Folio: The Magazine for Magazine Management, Cowles Business Media, www.foliomag.com.

Food Supply Veterinary Medicine Coalition Report, www.avma.org/fsvm.

Future Trends in Veterinary Public Health: Report of a WHO Study Group. Technical report series No. 907 (World Health Organization, 2002); http://libdoc.who.int/trs > WHO TRS 907.

GAO, Veterinarian Workforce: Actions Are Needed to Ensure Sufficient Capacity for Protecting Public and Animal Health. February 2009. GAO-09-178, a report to the Chairman, Subcommittee on Oversight of Government Management, the Federal Workforce, and the District of Columbia, Committee on Homeland Security and Governmental Affairs, US Senate. www.gao.gov.

GAO. Veterinarian Workforce: The Federal Government Lacks a Comprehensive Understanding of Its Capacity to Protect Animal and Public Health. Statement of Lisa Shames, Director Natural Resources and Environment. February 26, 2009. Testimony before the Subcommittee on Oversight of Government Management, the Federal Workforce, and the District of Columbia, Committee on Homeland Security and Governmental Affairs, US Senate, GAO-09-424T. www.gao.gov/htext/d09424t.html.

Gehrke, B. C., et al., Professional Income of Laboratory Animal Veterinarians Predicted by Multiple Regression Analysis, *JAVMA*, 2000; 216: 852–858.

Glassman, G., Tax Rules for Relief Veterinarians, *Veterinary Economics*, 2006.

Glassman, G., The New Era of Corporate Practice, presents interesting facts regarding purchasing and statistics, *Veterinary Economics*, November 2007; www.dvm360.com.

Gordon, M., et al., Comparison of long-term financial implications for five veterinary career tracks, *JAVMA* Vol 237, No. 4, August 15, 2010: 369-375.

Gwinner, K., et al., Attracting Students into Careers in Food Supply Veterinary Medicine, *JAVMA*, June 1, 2006; 228(11): 1693–1704.

Hare, D., Challenges in Clinical Education. *Can Vet J*, February 2007; 48(2): 121–123.

Harper, T., ed., *ASJA Guide to Freelance Writing: A Professional Guide to the Business, for Nonfiction Writers of All Experience Levels* (St. Martin's Griffin, 2003).

Hastings, A. Hastings Introduces the Wildlife and Zoological Veterinary Medicine Enhancement Act, January 21, 2010, http://alceehastings.house.gov > newsroom > 2010 press releases >January.

Hayes, H.B., The Rise of the Corporate Veterinarian, Growing Presence of National Chains in Virginia Reflects Shifts in Industry, Virginia Business News, August 2006; www.virginiabusiness.com.

Hazelgren, B., *Your First Business Plan*, 5th ed., (Sourcebooks, 2005).

Heinke, M L., McCarthy, J.B., *Practice Made Perfect, A Guide to Veterinary Practice Management* (AAHA Press, 2001).

Helms, T. D., and M. J. Bain, Evaluation of Owner Attachment to Dogs on the Basis of Whether Owners Are Legally Considered Guardians of Their Pets, *JAVMA*, April 1, 2009; 234(7): 896-900.

Herbold, J. R., et al., Vet Med Today: Public Veterinary Medicine, *JAVMA*, December 15, 2000, 217(12): 1812–1836.

Hoblet, K. N., et al., Special Report: Veterinarians in Population Health and Public Practice: Meeting Critical National Needs, *JVME*, 2003; 30: 287–294; www.jvmeonline.org.

Honeychurch, C, Watrous, A., *Talk to Me: Conversation Tips for the Small-Talk Challenged* (New Harbinger, 2003).

Hourdebaight, J-P, *Canine Massage: A Complete Reference Manual* (Dogwise Publishing, 2004).

Hubbell, J., et al., Workforce Needs for Clinical Specialists at Colleges and Schools of Veterinary Medicine in North America, *JAVMA*, November 15, 2006; 229(10): 1580–1583.

Huneke, R.B., Salary Survey of Laboratory Animal Veterinarians for the Year 2008 (American College of Laboratory Animal Medicine & American Society of Laboratory Animal Practitioners, April 2009).

Inc. magazine, www.inc.com.

Jacobs C, Association Jobs: AVMA-GRD Agriculture Policy Analyst. *JAVMA*, March 15, 1990; 196(6): 858–859.

Jelinski, M., et al., Factors Associated with Veterinarians' Career Path Choices in the Early Postgraduate Period, *Can Vet J*, September 2009; 50: 943–948.

Journal of Veterinary Medical Education (JVME), www.aavmc.org.

Kieves N, Roark A, Sparks T. Business Education in Veterinary Schools: The Potential Role of the Veterinary Business Management Association. *JVME* 34(5).

Kohls, L. R., et al., *Survival Kit for Overseas Living for Americans Planning on Living and Working Abroad*, 4th ed., (Intercultural Press, 2001).

Kuehn, B. M., Shelter Medicine: A Budding Field that is Helping to Raise the Standard of Care in Animal Shelters, *JAVMA* May 1, 2004; 224(9): 1412–1413.

Lane I., Gobue, E.G., Perspectives in professional education: Faculty perspectives regarding the importance and lace of nontechnical competencies in veterinary medical education at five North American colleges of veterinary medicine. *JAVMA*, July 1, 2010; 237(1): 53-64.

Larkin M, Board Weighs In On Foreign Accreditation, *JAVMA News*, July 15, 2010: 130-133.

Larkin M, Veterinarians Leave Their Mark on African Nation. *JAVMA News*, October 15, 2009; 235(8): 911–915.

Larkin M, Veterinary Education Receives A Workup: Academic leaders ponder teaching models. *JAVMA News* 236(12), June 15, 2010:1270-1275.

Larsen, M, *How to Write a Book Proposal*, 3rd ed., (Writers Digest Books, 2004).

Lauber, D, *Government Job Finder: Where the Jobs Are in Local, State, and Federal Government* (Planning Communications, 2009).

Levinson, J C, McLaughlin, M.W., *Guerrilla Marketing for Consultants: Breakthrough Tactics for Winning Profitable Clients* (John Wiley & Sons, 2004).

Lewis R, et al., Nontechnical Competencies Underlying Career Success as a Veterinarian. *JAVMA*, June 15, 2003; 222(12): 1690–1696.

Liff, S, *Managing Your Government Career: Success Strategies That Work* (AMACOM Books, 2008).

Lloyd, J. W., Current Economic Trends Affecting the Veterinary Medical Profession, *Vet Clin Small Anim*, 2006; 36: 267–279.

Macejko, C., Choice Veterinary Jobs Hard to Find in Tough Economy, *DVM Newsmagazine*, June 2009:1.

Macejko, C., Public-Health DVM Shortage Called "Critical," *DVM360*, April 1, 2009; www.dvm360.com

Maister, D, et al, *Trusted Advisor* (Touchstone, 2000).

Martin, J S., and L H. Chaney, *Global Business Etiquette: A Guide to International Communication and Customs* (Praeger, 2008).

Meeks, B. Animal Docs Fill Homeland Security Slots: From Farm to Fork, Veterinarians on the Agro-terrorism Frontlines. MSNBC. March 18, 2005; www.msnbc.msn.com/id/7200413.

Merck, M., *Veterinary Forensics: Animal Cruelty Investigations* (Blackwell Publishing, 2007).

Merriam Webster's Online Dictionary, www.merriam-webster.com.

Mills, D.L., et al., *Canine Rehabilitation & Physical Therapy* (Elsevier. 2004).

Mize, D.A., *Complete Idiot's Guide to Going Back to College* (Alpha, 2007).

Money magazine, Best Jobs in America, 2009, http://money.cnn.com/magazines/moneymag/bestjobs > job growth.

National Animal Control Association, Pros and Cons of Working in the Field of Animal Control, www.nacanet.org/careeropps.html.

National Aquatic Animal Health Task Force, *National Aquatic Animal Health Plan for the United States*, August 2008, www.aphis.usda.gov > animal health > animal diseases by species > aquaculture.

National Commission on Veterinary Economic Issues (NCVEI).

  NCVEI, A Veterinarian's Guide to Pet Health Insurance, www.ncvei.org/resources.aspx.

  NCVEI, *Current and Future Market for Veterinarians and Veterinary Medical Services in the United States. KPMG LLP Study Report, Abridged version*. C. Smith, Editor; National Commission on Veterinary Economic Issues, 2000.

  NCVEI resources, www.ncvei.org > Resource library

National Library of Medicine, www.nlm.nih.gov/services/veterinarymed.html and www.ncbi.nlm.nih.gov/PubMed; SNOMED FAQs. www.nlm.nih.gov/research/umls/Snomed/snomed_faq.html.

National Research Council, Committee on Increasing Veterinary Involvement in Biomedical Research, National Need and Priorities for Veterinarians in Biomedical Research. (National Academies Press, 2004), www.nationalacademies.org/publications.

National Wildlife Rehabilitation Association, *Principles of Wildlife Rehabilitation: Minimum Standards for Wildlife Rehabilitation.*

Nolen, R.S., Animal Care faulted for lax oversight of problem dog breeders, *JAVMA News*, July 1,2010; 237(1):8-10.

Nolen, R.S., Despite High Demand, Laboratory Animal Veterinarians in Short Supply: Economic Survey Shows Upward Trend in Specialists' Salaries. *JAVMA News*, October 1, 2003.

Nolen, R.S., Mahr calls for ,one health' initiative, *JAVMA News*, September 1, 2006:.

Nolen, R.S., One-Health Wonders, *JAVMA*, December 15, 2008; 223(12): 1828–1829.

Nolen R.S., Promoting One Medicine Among Veterinary Students, *JAVMA News*, February 1, 2007.

North American Compendiums, *Compendium of Veterinary Products*, 2008.

Ontario Veterinary Medical Association, 2010 Report on Veterinarians in Alternate Career Paths, www.ovma.org.

Osborne, D., Predicting the Future of Large Animal Practice, Focus, September/October 2007; 26(5): 14–16.

Pew Commission on Industrial Farm Production, *Putting Meat on the Table: Industrial Farm Animal Production in America,* final report www.ncifap.org/ www.pewtrusts.org; www.ncifap.org/_images/PCIFAPFin.pdf. Also see Letters to the Editor, *JAVMA*, October 15, 2008; 233(8): 1227–1228.

Pew National Veterinary Education Program, Future Directions for Veterinary Medicine: The Pew report. *Can Vet J.* 1989 June; 30(6): 472–476. (www.ncbi.nlm.nih.gov)

Poynter, D, *Self-Publishing Manual* (Para Publishing, 2007).

Prince, J. B., et al., Future Demand, Probable Shortages, and Strategies for Creating a Better Future in Food Supply Veterinary Medicine, *JAVMA*, July 1, 2006; 229(1): 57–69.

Public Health Reality Check. *DVM Newsmagazine*, Opinion/Letters, June 2009; 32.

Remsburg, D.W., et al., A Proposed Novel Food Animal Health Care Delivery System, *JAVMA*, Sept 15, 2007; 231: 6.

Rezendes A, Government Revises Veterinary Medical Officer Standards. Veterinarians in Federal Government Earn More Recognition. *JAVMA News*, July 1, 2006.

Rezendes A, More Veterinarians Offer Hospice Care for Pets. *JAVMA News*, August 15. 2006.

Rezendes, A., One World, One Health, One Medicine, *JAVMA News*, September 15, 2007.

Robbins-Roth, C., *Alternative Careers in Science: Leaving the Ivory Tower* (Academic Press 2005).

Roberts, H., *Fundamentals of Ornamental Fish Health* (Wiley Blackwell, 2009).

Rose, R, Smith, C., *Career Choices for Veterinary Technicians: Opportunities for Animal Lovers.* AAHA Press, 2009.

Schoen, A.M., *Veterinary Acupuncture: Ancient Art to Modern Medicine* (Mosby, 2001).

Schoenfeld-Tacher R., et al, Comparison of strength of the human-animal bond between Hispanic and non-Hispanic owners of pet dogs and cats, *JAVMA* 2010;236:529–534.

Schwartz, C. *Four Paws, Five Directions: A Guide to Chinese Medicine for Cats and Dogs* (Celestial Arts, 2004).

Scott, G.G., *Sell Your Book, Script; Column: How to Write a Winning Query and Make a Winning Pitch* (ASJA Press, 2007).

Sherman, D.M., *Tending Animals in the Global Village: A Guide to International Veterinary Medicine* (Blackwell Publishing, 2002).

Shojai, A., *New Choices in Natural Healing for Dogs and Cats* (St Martin's Press, 2001).

Sinclair, L., et al., *Investigation of Animal Cruelty: A Guide for Veterinary and Law Enforcement Professionals* (Humane Society Press, 2006).

Smith, C., *Client Satisfaction Pays: Quality Service for Practice Success* (AAHA Press. 2009).

Smith, C., *FlexVet: How to Be One, How to Hire One. The Comprehensive Practice Guide for Relief & Part time Veterinarians* (Smith Veterinary Publishing 2007).

Smith, C., Gender and Work: What Veterinarians Can Learn from Research about Men, Women, and Work, *JAVMA*, May 1, 2003; 220(9): 1304–1311.

Smith, C., Gender Shift in Veterinary Medicine: Cause and Effect, in *Veterinary Clinics of North America: Practice Management Issue* (Elsevier Publishing, 2006), Chapter 4.

Smith, C., *Housecall: The Housecall Veterinarian's Manual,* (Smith Veterinary Publishing 2007).

Smith, C., *The Relief Veterinarian's Manual,* out of print; see FlexVet.

Smith, C., *Team Satisfaction Pays: Organizational Development for Practice Success,* (Smith Veterinary Consulting, 2008).

Smith, C., (Editor); National Commission on Veterinary Economic Issues, *Current and Future Market for Veterinarians and Veterinary Medical Services in the United States. KPMG LLP Study Report, Abridged version.* 2000.

Smith, C., Rose, R, *Relief Veterinary Technician's Manual* (Smith Veterinary Publishing, 2002).

Smith, R., et al., Applications of Informatics in Veterinary Medicine, *Bulletin of the Medical Library Association,* January 2000; www.pubmedcentral.nih.gov.

SPCA Opens Largest Nonprofit Hospital in San Francisco.*DVM Newsmagazine* Feb 2009:14; also *Veterinary Practice News,* March 2009.

Sundlof, S.F. Need for Veterinarians in Biomedical Research. Comments by Stephen F. Sundlof, DVM, PhD. Director, CVM, FDA for the AAVMC Aug 2, 2007 Bethesda, Maryland. www.fda.gov > Science & Research > Science and Research Special Topics > Critical Path Initiative and www.fda.gov > Animal & Veterinary > News & Events > FDA Veterinarian Newsletter 2007 (XXII:IV).

Tremayne, J. Kansas Program to Increase Rural DVMs, *DVM News,* July 2006; 62.

Tyson, E. and J. Schell, *Small Business for Dummies,* 3rd ed., (Wiley Publishing, 2008).

US News online, America's Best Careers 2010: Healthcare; http://money.usnews.com > Money > Careers; Dec 28, 2009

VanBiema, D, Rural Churches Grapple with a Pastor Exodus, *Time magazine,* Thurs Jan. 29, 2009; www.time.com/time/magazine.

Van Laan, K., Julian, C., *The Complete Idiot's Guide to Technical Writing* (Alpha Books, 2001).

Verdon, D., Vet blows whistle on slaughter practices. *DVM Newsmagazine,* Apr 1, 2010. www.dvm360.com.

Veterinarian Workforce: Actions Are Needed to Ensure Sufficient Capacity for Protecting Public and Animal Health. February 2009. A Report to the Chairman, Subcommittee on Oversight of Government Management, the Federal Workforce, and the District of Columbia, Committee on Homeland Security and Governmental Affairs, US Senate, GAO-09-178.

Veterinarians (formerly Today's Veterinarian). www.avma.org > Animal Health > AVMA brochures > Veterinarians.

A Veterinarian's Guide to Pet Health Insurance, NCVEI; www.ncvei.org/resources.aspx.

Veterinary Economics magazine. www.advanstar.com; www.dvm360.com.

Veterinary Healthcare Communications, *Veterinary Pharmaceuticals & Biologicals.* 2001.

Veterinary Hospital Managers Association Salary Survey (AVMA, 2009).

Vetguide, *Veterinary Economics* supplement, www.dvm360.com; phone: 800-255-6864.

VetPartners, No-Lo Practice Valuation Worksheet, www.vetpartners.org.

Villarroel, A., McDonald, S., et al., A survey of reasons why veterinarians enter rural veterinary practice in the United States, *JAVMA,* April 15, 2010; 236(8): 849-857.

Villarroel, A., McDonald, S., et al., A survey of reasons why veterinarians leave rural veterinary practice in the United States, *JAVMA,* April 15, 2010; 236(8): 859-867.

Volk, J., et al., Executive Summary of the AVMA-Pfizer Business Practices Study, *JAVMA*; 2005; 226: 212–218.

Walker, J. B., Food Animal Medicine in Crisis, *JAVMA,* August 15, 2009; 235(4): 368–374.

Weintraub, A.,*Kaiser Health News,* New Health Law Will Require Industry To Disclose Payments To Physicians; www.kaiserhealthnews.org/Stories/2010/April/26/physician-payment-disclosures.aspx.

Weiss, A., *Value-Based Fees: How to Charge and Get What You're Worth, The Ultimate Consultant Series* (Pfeiffer, 2002).

Williams, B., *Complete Guide to Working for Yourself: Everything the Self-Employed Need to Know about Taxes, Recordkeeping & Other Laws,* with Companion CD-ROM (Atlantic Publishing Group, 2008).

Williams, J., *Unbending Gender: Why Family and Work Conflict and What to Do About It* (Oxford University Press, 2000).

Willis, N., et al., Envisioning the Future of Veterinary Medical Education: The Association of American Veterinary Medical Colleges Foresight Project, Final Report, *JVME,* 2007; 34(1): 1–41.

Wilson, J.F., Inviting the Elephant into the Room: A Dialogue to Co-create a Financially Healthy Veterinary Profession. Presented at the North American Veterinary Conference 2008, www.vetpartners.org >Resources.

Wilson, J., et al., *Contracts, Benefits, and Practice Management for the Veterinary Profession* (Priority Press, 2009).

Wisconsin Ag Connection, WFBF Awards Scholarship to Future Veterinarian. June 4, 2010. www.wisconsinagconnection.com.

Wohl, J, Nusbaum, K., Public Health Roles for Small Animal Practitioners. *JAVMA*, February 15, 2007; 230(4): 494–500.

Wolf, C., Lloyd, J., Black, J., An Examination Of US Consumer Pet-Related and Veterinary Service Expenditures, 1980–2005; *JAVMA* 233(3), August 1, 2008, 404-413.

Wood, F., Is Purchasing Power Shrinking? *Veterinary Economics*, August 2007; 36.

Wride, N., A Nose Job for a Sawfish: A Long Beach "Aquavet" Is among a New Breed of Specialists Bringing Human-Type Treatments to Ailing Marine Life. Fake Fish Eyes, Anyone? *Los Angeles Times*, November 10, 2006, p. A1.

Writer magazine, www.writermag.com.

Writer's Digest, www.writersdigest.com.

Writer's Market (Writer's Digest Books, published annually).

Wynn, S.G., *Emerging Therapies: Using Herbs and Nutraceuticals for Small Animals* (AAHA Press, 1999).

Wynn, S. G., and Steve Marsden, *Manual of Natural Veterinary Medicine: Science and Tradition* (Mosby, 2002).

Yetter, D, Halladay, J, Nurses Covering More Health Care: KY is among states looking to fill gaps by expanding roles of other caregivers. *USA today*, March 12,2010:3A.

INDEX